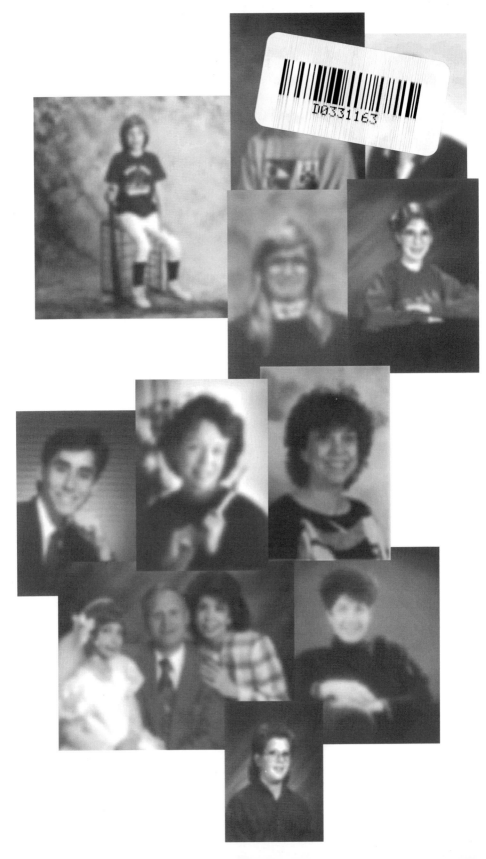

SIT down before fact as a little child, be prepared to give up every preconceived notion, follow humbly wherever and to whatever abyss nature leads, or you shall learn nothing.

—Thomas Huxley

(OPPOSITE)
VISUAL DISTORTION IN DYSLEXIA.
DESIGNED BY LISA ORANGE.

SIT DOWN BEFORE FACT AS A LITTLE CHILD, BE PREPARED TO GIVE UP EVERY PRECONCEIVED NOTION, FOLLOW HUMBLY WHEREVER AND TO WHATEVER ABYSS NATURE LEADS, OR YOU SHALL LEARN NOTHING. THOMAS HUXLEY

An Inspiring Thank-You

Elizabeth Woof

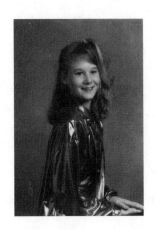

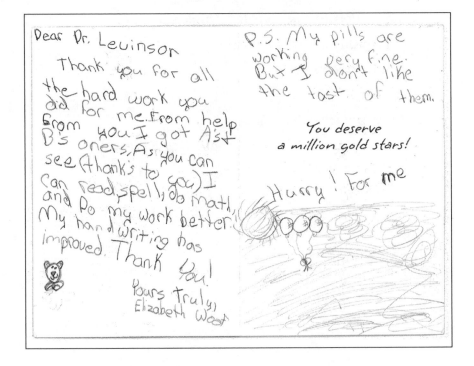

Book also available on Cassette
1 • 800 • 874-6242

Other books by Harold N. Levinson:
A Solution to the Riddle—Dyslexia
Smart But Feeling Dumb
Total Concentration
Phobia Free
The Upside-Down Kids
Turning Around—The Upside-Down Kids

A SCIENTIFIC WATERGATE

DYSLEXIA

How and Why Countless Millions Are Deprived
of Breakthrough Medical Treatment

Harold N. Levinson, M.D.

Cover and Internal Art: Lisa Orange, New York City

Design and Typesetting: Barbara & Ron, Glasco, New York

Endpapers: Hal, Barbara & Ron

Library of Congress Cataloging-in-Publication Data

Levinson, Harold N.

A scientific watergate—dyslexia: how and why countless millions are deprived of breakthrough medical treatment/ Harold N. Levinson

p.   ill.   cm.

Includes bibliographical references and index

ISBN 0-9639303-0-3

1. Dyslexia

I. Title

RC394.W6L48 1993

616.85'53—dc20   93-87064

Stonebridge Publishing, Ltd.

15 Lake Road

Lake Success, NY 11020

Manufactured in the United States of America

Poignant Questions

Were You and/or Your Loved Ones Victims of a Scientific Watergate?

Was President Bush?

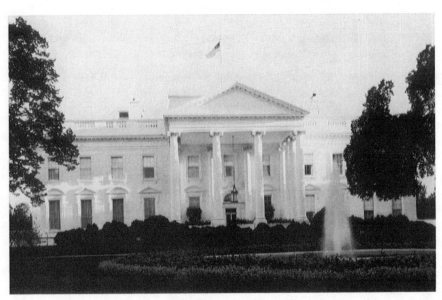

Table of Contents

[1]Appendix B (Editorial Comments and *New York Times* Articles on Dyslexia, etc.), Appendix C (Miscellaneous Correspondence), and a more complete Bibliography were deferred to Book II due to space constraints.

A Word of Explanation

Medicine and its science belong to those sincerely interested in, and dedicated to, helping mankind advance without needless pain and suffering. This book and my life's work as a physician and medical researcher—determined to heal—is dedicated solely to this end.

Over the past twenty years, I've discovered a festering medical-scientific abscess preventing—for self-serving reasons—countless millions from receiving or even knowing about a breakthrough medical treatment for a disorder otherwise untreatable and even undiagnosable. To heal these suffering millions, otherwise doomed to forever feeling dumb, lazy, stupid, brainless, crazy, I was forced to localize and lance this Watergate-like abscess.[1] But in doing so the pain was mine.

Hopefully, the medical-scientific end (solving the riddles in dyslexia) will justify this unavoidably painful means (*A Scientific Watergate—Dyslexia*). No one else would—or could—do it.

Harold N. Levinson, M.D.
Director, Medical Dyslexic Treatment Center,
    Great Neck, New York
Formerly, Clinical Associate
    Professor of Psychiatry,
    NYU Medical Center

---

[1]For those who may not know, *Watergate* represented a political cover-up and scandal leading to President Nixon's resignation. Accordingly, lancing the above-mentioned "abscess" or cover-up in dyslexia research so that millions of dyslexics might benefit from breakthrough medical treatment was called *A Scientific Watergate—Dyslexia*.

Dual Perspectives

A *Scientific Watergate—Dyslexia* is a well-achieved, unique and tantalizing attempt to integrate the emotional inner experience of a physician and scientist with the intellectual evaluation of objective evidence gathered during his (Dr. Levinson's) life span. Using real case studies of dyslexic children and adults in a novelistic style and dialogue, this work convincingly describes the discovery and implementation of a nontraditional scientific model, resulting in a dramatically successful method of medical treatment based on the inner-ear or cerebellar-vestibular origins of learning disabilities. It simultaneously exposes and explains the continued lack of any medically based diagnostic or therapeutic progress stemming from the conventional cerebral-language concepts and the traditionalists' opposition to new and successful physiologically based treatment strategies. In this context, the author confronts the astonished reader with the dramatic encounters and clashes of his scientific endeavors with superstitious criticism, opportunistic opposition, and barren conservative pseudo-science. This is an exciting text, combining touching autobiographic episodes with a systematic, scientific exposition of the controversial topic of dyslexia and its vicissitudes.

Reuven Kohen-Raz, Ph.D.

Professor Emeritus, The Hebrew University, Jerusalem

Former Chairman, Department of Special Education

A Word of Explanation

Medicine and its science belong to those sincerely interested in, and dedicated to, helping mankind advance without needless pain and suffering. This book and my life's work as a physician and medical researcher—determined to heal—is dedicated solely to this end.

Over the past twenty years, I've discovered a festering medical-scientific abscess preventing—for self-serving reasons—countless millions from receiving or even knowing about a breakthrough medical treatment for a disorder otherwise untreatable and even undiagnosable. To heal these suffering millions, otherwise doomed to forever feeling dumb, lazy, stupid, brainless, crazy, I was forced to localize and lance this Watergate-like abscess.[1] But in doing so the pain was mine.

Hopefully, the medical-scientific end (solving the riddles in dyslexia) will justify this unavoidably painful means (*A Scientific Watergate—Dyslexia*). No one else would—or could—do it.

Harold N. Levinson, M.D.
Director, Medical Dyslexic Treatment Center,
   Great Neck, New York
Formerly, Clinical Associate
   Professor of Psychiatry,
   NYU Medical Center

---

[1]For those who may not know, *Watergate* represented a political cover-up and scandal leading to President Nixon's resignation. Accordingly, lancing the above-mentioned "abscess" or cover-up in dyslexia research so that millions of dyslexics might benefit from breakthrough medical treatment was called *A Scientific Watergate—Dyslexia*.

Dual Perspectives

A *Scientific Watergate—Dyslexia* is a well-achieved, unique and tantalizing attempt to integrate the emotional inner experience of a physician and scientist with the intellectual evaluation of objective evidence gathered during his (Dr. Levinson's) life span. Using real case studies of dyslexic children and adults in a novelistic style and dialogue, this work convincingly describes the discovery and implementation of a nontraditional scientific model, resulting in a dramatically successful method of medical treatment based on the inner-ear or cerebellar-vestibular origins of learning disabilities. It simultaneously exposes and explains the continued lack of any medically based diagnostic or therapeutic progress stemming from the conventional cerebral-language concepts and the traditionalists' opposition to new and successful physiologically based treatment strategies. In this context, the author confronts the astonished reader with the dramatic encounters and clashes of his scientific endeavors with superstitious criticism, opportunistic opposition, and barren conservative pseudo-science. This is an exciting text, combining touching autobiographic episodes with a systematic, scientific exposition of the controversial topic of dyslexia and its vicissitudes.

Reuven Kohen-Raz, Ph.D.

Professor Emeritus, The Hebrew University, Jerusalem

Former Chairman, Department of Special Education

IT has been my privilege to both hear Dr. Levinson's lecture on the subject matter of dyslexia and to review his most recent and thought provoking work, *A Scientific Watergate—Dyslexia.* His research appears to be a clinically verifiable and convincing breakthrough in the diagnosis, prevention and treatment of this previously misunderstood disorder—especially since the many real patients and improvements presented within his well written and easily understood text mirrors exactly those my colleagues and I have personally observed during his recent seminar at the Chicago Medical School. Indeed, his medically based approach to this enigmatic condition—*dyslexia*—provides another entry to scientific understanding and how visual functions relate to reading symptoms specifically, and learning in general. The author is to be complimented for his courage and candor as a pioneer in discovering and implementing this new and uniquely explanatory and helpful scientific concept. The prospect of a medical treatment helping a multitude of patients is exciting and its clear presentation within this text was stimulating and refreshing.

Robert H.G. Monniger, M.D.

Professor and Director of Academic Ophthalmology,

UHS/The Chicago Medical School

Dedications

❦To my wife, Diggy.

❦To our parents and a heritage that forever tempted—but defied—extinction.

❦To our loving daughters, Laura and Joy.

❦To William Broad and Nicholas Wade for their stimulating book, *Betrayers of the Truth: Fraud and Deceit in the Halls of Science.*

❦To those dedicated healers and scientists that follow God's stars rather than their self-serving ambitions.

❦Finally, this work is dedicated to my many patients and critics. Were it not for the immeasurable inspiration provided me by the often "life-saving" favorable therapeutic responses of thousands of dyslexics such as Sue Stafford, Larry Landsberg and Joan Sparks (Chapter 10 and Book II), as well as the reactive stimulation triggered within by the determination of traditionalists to block similar improvement in millions of others, I would never have been able to easily endure, understand, and complete *A Scientific Watergate—Dyslexia.*

A Therapeutic Preview

For purposes of rapid but preliminary introduction, I thought it essential to present a few dramatically instructive medication-triggered dyslexic improvements right up front, with the dedication. No doubt a literary first. But I felt it vital to do so—hoping to highlight the crucial role played by dyslexic patients and their loved ones in solving the riddles underlying dyslexia while simultaneously portraying what dyslexics and the breakthrough medical treatment are all about. Needless to say, these therapeutic responses and the many to follow also provide a rapid contrast to the 100-year-old *therapeutic void* characterizing the traditional research efforts to date.

Larry Landsberg

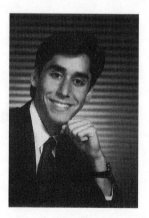

Larry, now 17 years old, spontaneously wrote me a letter of thanks.

> My name is Larry Landsberg. I do not know how well you remember me. I visited you when I was in the fifth grade; a terribly disturbed child, lacking any self-confidence at all. At that age with a problem I had yet to know, I lived with the assumption that I was (the clearest way stated) dumb. I never dreamed that the cause of my problems was due to a section of my ear called the inner-ear,

and that this portion of the ear controls the way the brain processes information.

Since visiting you my marks in school increased semester by semester. I went from an elementary school C/D student, to a straight A senior high school Honor Roll student, and a National Honor Society member who tutors students who may be suffering from dyslexia as I did.

Thanks for all your help. Without your knowledge, skill, and persistence, I would never be the person I am today.

Sue Stafford

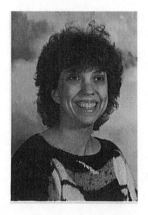

Sue is currently a learning disability teacher with the feelings and expertise that all healers vitally require to really help those in need. And so I utilized her talents within *The Upside-Down Kids* and dedicated *Turning Around—The Upside-Down Kids* to her. I first met her as a struggling 24-year-old dyslexic student seeking help. At the time, she had problems primarily with reading, spelling, balance and coordination, and concentration. *Here's her story* as initially reported—a story traditionalists never read or wanted to benefit from. Even a cursory reading *rapidly* conveys what dyslexia and its medical treatment are all about.

She writes:

The large number of children who experience school phobias and the number of academic difficulties many children experience motivated me to enter the field of special education. *Everything I read in the field convinced me the experts were missing something crucial. Accepted theories about learning disabilities and dyslexia did not sufficiently explain the scope and complexity of the disorder.*

I could not subscribe to the view that the cerebral cortex was the site of the problem. These (traditional) theories did not make any sense to me . . . . The reason I felt so strongly about this is that I am dyslexic. Although I have reading and spelling problems, I score high on differential aptitude tests for abstract and mechanical reasoning. Obviously someone with brain damage could not have a high score in abstract reasoning and math.

Since I felt the data on learning disabilities was insufficient and certainly not helping dyslexic children to deal with school-related and other problems, I decided to enter the field of research in special education and put my firsthand experience and learning to good use.

I was in the first grade when I experienced that dreaded disease "school phobia." I was unable to master the skills or the phonetics required to read. It wasn't until the sixth grade that I finally learned to read—to satisfy school requirements, not for pleasure!

Two summers ago my reading problem was very severe. I consulted an optometrist, who prescribed glasses for my problem (poor focusing) and vision therapy. The glasses did not help much; in fact, they made me feel dizzy. But the exercises did help. Unfortunately they did not get at the heart of the problem, and I found when I was tired that the exercises did not help at all.

My last year in college was easier because I had learned to organize my work better. I was also taking more education courses, which I found very interesting. When I read *A Solution to the Riddle—Dyslexia,* I thought, This really makes sense! I knew I had to see Dr. Levinson.

Testing and consultation disclosed what Sue already knew: *that she had dyslexia.* Medical treatment was initiated, and she was asked to record any therapeutic or negative reactions. Sue called two weeks later and excitedly related her favorable observations.

After only two days on medication, I was fairly sure my reading and balance were better; however, I wasn't one hundred percent sure. Within six days I was positive! Not only was my head clearer, but also letters and words were more distinct. I was reading faster with good comprehension and no fatigue and frustration. . . . My balance was better. I could close my eyes and stand on one foot. I could never do that before!

I am so excited about my reactions that I have changed the subject of my thesis; it will now deal with new theories of learning disabilities, and your hypothesis on dyslexia will head the list.

Shortly thereafter, I received a progress report from Sue:

Everything is going well. My greatly increased ability to concentrate, read, and comprehend are still with me. I finished all the required reading for all my courses this past semester—for the first time! I was even able to begin outside readings for my thesis, and I am elated. . . . For the first time I find all the reading I am doing very exciting and pleasurable.

I no longer have a focusing problem: the vision training has become beneficial, along with the medication. During my last vision training session, to my great surprise, I was able to walk the balance beam backward! The month before I saw you, I worked on balance activities quite a lot and never got very far with them. As I told you, I never could get very far with them as a child, either.

I was discussing with a friend, also in special education, my newfound ability to stand on one foot. I told him that now I feel that I have one focal point of gravity, at my heel, as opposed to many. In other words, I had the feeling that I was being pulled from all directions. He replied, "What you are saying is that you feel your vertical axis in relationship to your body, something we are aware that children with learning problems lack." I found this most interesting and thought you would too.

I have also noticed that emotionally I feel as though I am freer. I am not constantly on guard for fear that I may reveal my disabilities. I also feel more focused. My thoughts and actions are not as scattered as they once were. It is somewhat analogous to the sensation I feel with my balance, as previously mentioned—of having one focal point when I stand on one foot.

My spelling, grammar, and sentence structure are also greatly improved. My mother, who has always proofread my school papers, tells me I now make very few errors in those areas. She was particularly excited after reading some pages of my thesis.

My report would not be complete without the inclusion of my responses to an interruption of medication. Within one day after I stop taking the medication, I feel a big difference:

- The first night I have dreams of falling and of not being able to stay balanced.

- The next morning I feel "out of it" and tend to keep feeling that way until I resume the medication three days later.

- There is no desire to read, and when I try, I have trouble tracking, even when reading just a few lines. My eyes feel as though they are pulling at each other and causing me to see double.

- I feel more unsteady.

- My old habit of head shaking to clear the fog is back.

When I resume my medication, the positive results return: I feel great again; reading becomes easier and letters darker and sharper.

I am tremendously excited, not only about my improvements via your treatment, but also about the wonderful possibilities for help that now exist for the millions of children afflicted with dyslexia and related learning disabilities.

After several months on medications:

I am writing this letter by hand to illustrate to you the changes in my handwriting that have taken place in the last few months. There is a smoothness, evenness, and fluidity that I never had before. It is as though the writing literally flows out of my hand, although I am still holding the paper at a ninety-degree angle to my body, and am therefore writing away from myself.

This is my last year at Bank Street School; I will be graduating in June. My last two classes are very demanding, but I am most proud to say that I am *ahead* in all the readings. As I have written before, I used to do as little reading as possible. I can't begin to describe the enjoyment I am now experiencing by participating in the class discussions of these readings.

After a long day of teaching and being a student, I don't feel tired or overloaded. Even though my schedule is as busy as, if not busier than, it was, I seem to require less sleep—six to eight hours of sleep as opposed to ten to twelve hours I used to need. I have also noticed a change in my dream patterns and content. Previously my dreams were hectic, debilitating, and at times bizarre and fragmented. Now they are peaceful and relaxed. I think this has a lot to do with my requirement for less sleep.

I have also noticed an interesting change with regard to my spelling. I still forget and confuse the spelling of words that were learned prior to taking my medication, but new words I have read in the literature, particularly in the last two months, I am able to correctly picture in my mind. When I became aware of this interesting phenomenon, I thought it was a fascinating concept, dealing with developmental sequences in cognitive thinking.

I have been applying to colleges and universities for possible acceptance into a Ph.D. program in educational psychology/special education research! I never before entertained the possibility of such a venture, but now I realize that it is a possibility for me—and I am on an all-time high contemplating it.

My excitement and enthusiasm for your theory of dyslexia has motivated me to discuss it with many people from the local school systems in my area. In fact, I will be presenting information during a few staff meetings in several districts. I have found that I receive very little criticism because I present myself as a case in point of the success of your medication treatment. I will also be discussing your theory of the inner-ear or cerebellar-vestibular system at Bank Street College during a presentation on the use of medications in special education, along with the role of the teacher.

Additionally, I have noticed that I have developed an ability to calculate large numbers in my mind. I have always been a good math student, but I did need to work out the solution to problems on paper because I had trouble retaining the numbers and processes in my mind. However, while teaching a computer course, I became aware that I was able to calculate the solutions to problems in my mind.

There have been so many changes in the last six months that I am truly amazed. I never considered myself impulsive, but I realize now that I was. I would be upset if I did not make quick decisions about everything, from buying a dress to deciding whether or not to take a job. I would jump into a situation or volunteer my time to a project, and then find that I did not have time in my schedule to fulfill my promise. Recently, though, I have discovered that I actually enjoy thinking about arriving at a decision—I realize that I don't have to make a split-second decision. I also don't feel overwhelmed when I do decide on a course of action. Finally, I feel good about my decision and don't perseverate . . . about an impulsive choice.

Along with this loss of impulsive behavior has come the feeling of calmness, of being able to sit back and absorb what is going on without being the one always talking and monopolizing the conversation to prove that I know something. In fact, I don't think I talk as fast as I used to because I am not afraid any longer that I will forget what it is that I wish to say.

One day, for no apparent reason, it occurred to me that I read better lying on my stomach. I mentioned this one day in class, and several people have since told me that they have had some of their students try this position with interesting success. Children who display dyslexia-like symptoms tend to find this position very comfortable when reading. It seems logical that lying on one's stomach may have a harmonizing effect on the inner-ear system; it probably has something to do with the law of gravity.

My balance and posture have improved so much that I can hardly believe it! I had always had the tendency to slouch, but I now feel as if I internally stand straight. I no longer get backaches between my shoulder blades. Also, I can walk in high-heeled shoes without falling forward and looking like a klutz!

Every day I notice something else that has changed for the better in my behavior, personality, or perception about the world. All these changes together have contributed to the wonderful feeling that I have about myself, especially these last months.

Once again, I deeply thank you for everything.

Acknowledgments

Were it not for the overwhelming desire—and cry—of countless dyslexic patients for *hope* and medical help—I would never have been driven to complete the breakthrough insights characterizing my scientific text, *A Solution to the Riddle—Dyslexia*.

Were it not for the amazing reactive energies triggered within me by the self-serving criticism of the traditional "Dyslexia Monopoly" attempting to prevent breakthrough research and help from reaching countless millions of desperately suffering *dyslexic children and adults*, I would never have been catalyzed—catapulted—to complete *A Scientific Watergate—Dyslexia* in record time once started.

Were it not for the loyal and dedicated staff of the Medical Dyslexic Treatment Center, including *Larry Dopkin*—and especially the continued inspiration, encouragement and faith of *Selma Schwartz*, I might have emotionally and/or physically "retired" long before this God-inspired task was begun—let alone initiated and completed. And had *Adam R. Cohen* not been able to type, retype and edit this manuscript at the accelerating pace it was presented him, the needed momentum might have been significantly broken—and the end interminably delayed.

And finally, were it not for my father's terminal illness during this writing process and my inner need and desire to have him read *A Scientific Watergate—Dyslexia* before he died, I seriously doubt this content—flowing and racing against imminent death—could have materialized with lightning speed.

In short, this work owes its content, intent and completion to all those factors and forces mentioned here, within my dedication, and in my many scientific works.

Thanks—to all those mentioned directly and indirectly!

Section I

Introductory Content

BECAUSE readers *must* understand dyslexics and dyslexia as thoroughly as possible in order to evaluate objectively the traditionalists' resistance to, and criticism of, any and all meaningful therapeutic breakthroughs—especially the often dramatic medication-triggered responses depicted throughout this and my prior research efforts, the introductory and even pre-introductory content became crucial. As *A Scientific Watergate—Dyslexia* is a complex, multidimensional endeavor riddled with sharp contrasts, I considered it essential to present separate but overlapping and interwoven *informal* vs. *formal* overviews. And the former was subdivided into seven rather short segments (A-G) so the emotional impact of its *patient-based* vs. *critical* content could more readily be conveyed and appreciated.

CHAPTER 1

An Evolving Perspective— Informal

In a nutshell: The traditionalists maintain that all the patients and therapeutic responses presented throughout this and all prior works are fictitious. I maintain the opposite: that these patients and their responses are real! And if real, then the 100-year-old concepts of the traditionalists are as fictitious as their dyslexia expertise.

A

The Scientific Firing Line

The following material—poem, response to medication (after one week), consultation halfway around the world, cancellation letter, and a case-in-counterpoint—speaks for itself. This content highlights—indeed symbolizes—*the eye of the storm* as well as the urgent need and special design of *A Scientific Watergate— Dyslexia.*

The Ones Who Made It

Cathy A. Lanning
Jessica M. Swanson

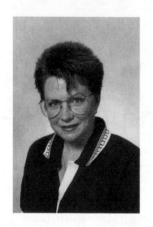 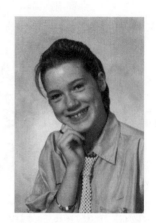

A DEDICATION TO DR. LEVINSON

Constant motion, timeless days,
  No rhyme or reason to my ways,
Eyes that read the words all blurry,
  As across the page they scurry.

Fear of height and crowds and stores,
  Only one person . . . please no more!
Senseless hurrying, frantic fits,
  No relaxing, no time to sit.

A six-year-old daughter, just like me.
  How could this happen, how could this be?
Where is the justice, where is the light?
  I've no more strength to continue the fight.

Then the book that changed our lives.
  New hope perhaps we were alright.
The decision to journey to New York . . .

From that great moment our lives would fork
To untold moments of peace and calm,
And new expectations at each day's dawn.

A treatment program which worked within days...
After 33 years of living in a haze!
How do I thank you dear Levinson
For making life easier and even fun.

So to you I dedicate this poem,
With renewed belief man walks not alone.
Though life was rough and times were down,
We're so very thankful you turned us around!

Cathy A. Lanning (age 33)
Jessica M. Swanson (age 6)

Meg Fex

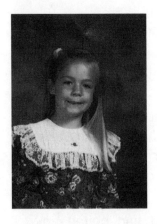

Mrs. Katy Fex described her 6-year-old daughter's improvements to me as follows (2/18/93):

As I write this letter to you, I am sitting in the children's section of the public library. Few people would appreciate the significance of this. *Megan has been taking meclizine[1] for only six days now. And her response to the medication*

[1]Meclizine is one of many inner-ear-enhancing medications found helpful in treating the many and varied symptoms of dyslexia.

has been nothing short of miraculous. So much has happened in this short time that I have had difficulty getting everything into my journal. I now face the task of condensing this into a letter to you without writing a novel. . . . Here goes.

Meg had to postpone beginning medication because she had another severe ear infection (detected by your staff). She took her first ¼ antihistamine pill Saturday morning (2/13/93) and went to ballet in the afternoon. I was very concerned that, with all the physical activity, Meg might have some kind of reaction.

Meg does not know why she is taking the medication—she believes it is for her ear. As a result I told her: "Meg, you took your ear medicine today so if you feel bad you have to let Mommy know."

Meg: "I don't feel bad Mommy, I feel great. . . . You know Mommy, I can't explain it, but I'm not so mixed up today."

David (Meg's father) and I tried to be cautiously optimistic, trying to pass it off as a good day—David being the greater skeptic. But this was the beginning of the most incredible week. *Meg has done nothing but write and read all week. We find her with books or pencil and paper in the morning.* And we have to take them out of her bed at night after she has fallen asleep.

When I asked Meg if her reading had gotten any easier, she said, "Yes." I asked her how. She explained it this way: "It's like the letters are glued down. The letters are glued on the paper. Now they don't jump around."

Sitting in your office a few weeks ago, you asked me what I wanted from all this. And I said that I wanted to eliminate her frustration. You have made that possible and so much more.

I have come to realize that her problem was much more complex than we ever imagined, affecting all parts of her life. Her ability to compensate was incredible . . . masking most of her symptoms from us.

I have throughout this, and continue to, read all the literature I can on the subject. I have read the criticism. *No placebo could accomplish this. Not all the positive thinking in the world could do this. This is real. This all makes sense.*

Meg's Graphomotor Response to Medication

And to illustrate Meg's improvements, I thought it would be helpful to provide samples of her writing prior to inner-ear-enhancing medications and *after two days* on medications.

Prior to Treatment:
Meg's letter took over 1½ hours to complete. And it was just too much for her to add Elizabeth's name.

After Treatment:
After only two days on medication [meclizine], Meg completed this very same letter in about 15-20 minutes. Meg wrote it independently and only asked how to spell words.

Despite All Odds

Jan Stevens

I came to learn about Dr. Levinson through his book, *Smart But Feeling Dumb*, which I read in Manila. I had a marker in my hand. And by the time I finished, practically the entire book was colored in. I felt this book was written about my son, Jan. So I took it to my doctor who said *it was all too simple, and if this were such a breakthrough, how come there weren't more places doing this?* When I told my husband, who is German, that I wanted to go to New York, he thought I was crazy and looking for a miracle. *It wasn't until he had "Ménière's" which caused him a lot of dizzy-related and dyslexia-like problems from his ears that he began to understand why I was so insistent to fly halfway around the world— no matter what it cost to give this a try. Somehow I just knew I had to come.*

I do believe in miracles [1]

Margie Stevens

26 April 1993

[1] Despite all odds, Mrs. Stevens sought hope and help for her frustrated and suffering 14-year-old son, Jan. What were the odds: Her instincts led her to defy the "experts" who claimed her son needed discipline and was a behavior problem. Her determination led her to "stumble" onto *Smart But Feeling Dumb*—a book derived *entirely from countless dyslexics rather than the countless test-scores and fantasies of prior "experts."* She had to fly halfway around the world to see me. And her "objectively-minded" physician and husband were both dead-set against her coming. And for very good reasons. But as "chance" would have it, Mr. Stevens suddenly acquired dyslexic-like symptoms following a vertigo attack— "Ménière's." And suddenly he understood and experienced the content within *Smart But Feeling Dumb*—without ever reading it! Suddenly he understood his son—and his wife! And suddenly they appeared—as this work was completed, just in time for all to read. And hopefully you all will come to realize—as I eventually did—that a mother's gut feelings and instincts about her children are often far superior to the scientific dogma and fantasies of biased or egoistic "experts."

As chance would have it, Mrs. Stevens communicated the following observations concerning her 14-year-old son Jan's improvements—*just* in time to be read here.

10/23/93

Jan is now riding elevators "with the greatest of ease"—his words exactly. He has also managed to sleep through 3 typhoons and thunderstorms which last year he would use ear plugs, and have 2 pillows and our king-size bedspread over his head every time it rained just to block out the sound of the rain. Jan would tell me the sound of strong rain would actually hurt—and so he would wake me up and ask me to sit with him. During the last typhoons I would lie in bed waiting for him to come in and *NOTHING*—he slept right through them. I have a gut feeling his reading has improved but unfortunately I don't think he trusts himself enough to see the change. And we still have quite a bit to work through. I am happy that I took him to see you and I already feel it has been worthwhile with what Jan has been able to overcome.

I will keep you up to date on his progress.

Caught in the Crossfire—
One who didn't make it

For those who might not know: The Orton (Dyslexia) Society is one of the oldest and best-known organizations of its type. Named after a pioneer dyslexia researcher, Dr. Samuel Orton, those in control appeared to lose sight of their initial aims—*helping dyslexics.* And as the content within this letter and work will clearly highlight, they began defending dyslexics from all insights and help that wasn't their own.

David Sakowski

February 14, 1983

Dear Carolyn Malman (Secretary to Dr. Levinson):

My husband and I regret to inform you that we have to cancel our son's appointment on March 4, 1983. *To be honest with you we have just read an article by Priscilla L. Vail and another book review by Richard L. Masland, M.D. and Celia Usprich, Ph.D. (of the Orton Dyslexia Society). They both tend to say the same thing, that Dr. Levinson fails to provide proof of his theory.*

My husband and I don't care about the money because our son is worth anything if we could help him. *The one book review points out if our son wasn't able to be helped then he would really have bad feelings about himself. He would think, boy, I'm really a freak—even magic won't work for me.*

We are going to continue to watch for any evidence that would show Dr. Levinson's theory is right.

Sincerely,

Mr. & Mrs. Robert Sakowski

The Eye of The Storm

Had the Orton Society-led *sanction* against my research not scared these and countless other parents off, might their children have benefitted from breakthrough—"controversial"—treatment, as did others? What further harm would not benefitting from medical treatment have done considering the frustration and difficulties already encountered, and if frightening promises of imaginary "magic cures" by my critics were not made? Would this similar illogic also justify withholding tutoring or special education for fear of failing—and thus making dyslexics emotionally worse? Were this true—why then should patients, parents, educators and healers try their very best, at all costs?

Thus, for example, is Ortonian Priscilla Vail correct when she compares me to the *"Wizard of Oz"* and my dyslexia research and its improvements to *"a peddler of panaceas pretending to wizardry"*? And that the failure to respond to *"an easy, instant cure . . . will lead all concerned to feel, 'This kid is a real freak—even magic won't work on him.'"*[1] Or has a book review full of verbal *dirty tricks* discouraged countless dyslexics from obtaining breakthrough insights and medical treatment while defensively covering up the ignorance and scientific void characterizing the *dyslexia monopoly* for the last 100 years.

Stated another way, at the eye of the storm, which of the following possibilities appears more credible: Are the Ortonians altruistically saving dyslexics and their loved ones from breakthrough medical treatment responses such as those presented here? Or are they saving their own self-serving status quos from these very same diagnostic/therapeutic insights?

Should not the Ortonian-led negative book reviewers have told their readers:

- that there is absolutely no scientific validation for the traditional thinking-linguistic theories of dyslexia—a view now confirmed even by Harvard researchers, who recently saw the *light*,[2]

- that Dr. Samuel Orton's 1937 theories of dyslexia are dead wrong—since the basis of his theories are dead wrong, as demonstrated by my research and confirmed by others,

---

[1] For those readers interested in fact vs. fantasy and distortion, a detailed presentation and review of this Ortonian-inspired distortion will be presented in Chapter 6, The Orton Society Sanction.

[2] The favorable visually-related dyslexia responses to colored lenses and *filtered light* clearly refuted the 100-year-old traditional language theories of dyslexia and led a group of Ortonian researchers to propose a visual concept of this disorder similar to one I described in 1973 (see Chapters 14 and 18).

- that Dr. Samuel Orton would probably turn over in his grave if he knew about the defensive and offensive distortions spewing forth from an organization using his name for their own purposes,

- that there has been absolutely *no* proven scientifically based rejection of *any* of my breakthrough diagnostic or therapeutic conceptualizations since they were first published twenty years ago, and

- that my inner-ear (cerebellar-vestibular) dyslexia research has been actively supported by many distinguished scientists such as Sir John Eccles, Nobel Laureate for his cerebellar breakthroughs, and highly regarded investigators—Alan and Henrietta Leiner and Robert Dow. Thus, within landmark research entitled "*The human cerebro-cerebellar system: its computing, cognitive, and language skills,*" the Leiners' and Dow's neurophysiological and behavioral data and conceptualizations *independently corroborated all* my inner-ear or cerebellar-vestibular findings in dyslexia, as did the favorable therapeutic results obtained when using so-called controversial therapies which enhance or compensate for impaired inner-ear or cerebellar-vestibular functioning.

Additionally, should not *all* dyslexics and their loving parents as well as caring teachers and healers also know:

- that *all* the favorable responses to the breakthrough medical treatment presented throughout this book and within all my other works are as real as the patients themselves,

- that this reality is highlighted by the countless dyslexics volunteering their real names and photos so that the impact of their improvements might help overcome the traditionalists' denial while simultaneously serving as a sharp contrast to the existing medical void reigning supreme,

- that dyslexics may benefit from multiple therapeutic insights and therapies offered them, not just Ortonian tutoring as indicated by tutor Priscilla Vail, and

- that Ortonians aside, most teachers are not "freaked out" by medication-triggered improvements in dyslexic symptoms, and many are absolutely delighted.

A Case-In-Counterpoint

Robert Charles King

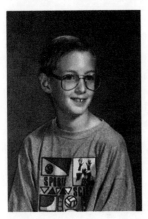

To rapidly counter the nonsensical Ortonian attack, I decided to present the readers with yet another real named and pictured dyslexic before concluding this segment. As you will note, Robert Charles King was helped not only by medication but by scientifically based insights, loving parents, and a dedicated teacher. Holistically! Most important, the explanation, interest and care given Robert in New York not only helped him overcome his prior shame and denial of academic failure even before medication therapy was initiated, it triggered within him a need to help others as he was helped.[1] Not a bad result from an alleged "peddler of panaceas pretending to wizardry."

[1]As discussed in Chapter 21, Looking Back, a similar mechanism led me to become a physician. *By the way, where is Priscilla Vail's fantasied "freak" if it isn't within my patients?*

Hopefully, Rob's stated and written appreciation, as follows, and his holistically triggered improvements will clearly and simply refute the defensive and offensive bias characterizing the Ortonian and related criticism.

Writing sample: Rob was asked to write what he spontaneously verbalized to his parents after his initial dyslexia evaluation. Obviously, he benefitted from the explanation given him for his symptoms. Additionally, his writing, spelling, and grammatical difficulties are illustrative and diagnostic of his inner-ear-determined disorder.

Rob's Improvements

Rob's mother, Mrs. Irene King, described her son's improvements as well as her appreciation (1/10/92).

> Thank you! Thank You! Thank You! When my husband Bob and I brought our son, Rob King, to your office in October 1991, little did we know how much you would help us.

> My son Rob never wanted anyone to know he had a reading problem. He always told me not to tell anyone. But when we came back from New York, his teacher, Mrs. Knispel, said she never saw such a happy little boy. He finally had an answer to why reading was so difficult for him.[1] Out of the blue, he told his cousin, Adam, he had

---

[1]The emotional benefits and relief provided patients by insight led me to write two "therapeutic novels" which simply explain the origin of the symptoms characterizing dyslexia and how the various therapies work for *children and adults*. It was anticipated that the insights within *The Upside Down Kids* and *Turning Around—The Upside Down Kids* would provide similar improvements to *all* dyslexics.

dyslexia. He also said to tell Dr. Levinson to use his full name, Robert Charles King, if needed to tell anyone about him. Something he was unwilling to do before. How far he's come. He even wanted us to tell his aunts and uncles, so that he could help his cousins with their reading problems. There have been so many reading problems in my husband's family for so many generations. When we started telling my husband Bob's brother and sisters, they were so thrilled to know that there was a name for the reading problems in their family. They are all reading your book, *Smart But Feeling Dumb*. My husband's family has searched for many, many years for an answer, but never found it until now. Thank you.

When I told Rob's psychologist at the school that Rob had dyslexia, he said to me, "I can't be bothered with you now." So, Dr. Levinson, when you win the Nobel Prize, and I'm sure you will, we'll be here, knowing you had some answers for all our dyslexic sons, daughters, sisters, brothers and parents.[1] May God Bless You.

Rob's Teacher, Cecilia M. Knispel

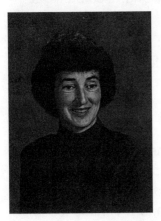

---

[1]Because I find exaggerated "positive criticism" more difficult to handle than its negative counterpart, I initially felt compelled to edit-out or modify Mrs. King's comment about the Nobel Prize.

And as is readily apparent, many professionals prefer the nonspecific term LD to dyslexia—a medical disorder they poorly understand and so attempt to deny.

Mrs. Knispel Comments

I was Rob King's fourth grade teacher. It was a very exciting year having Rob in my classroom. The accomplishments that Rob made in one school year were remarkable.

I have taught twenty-one years and I am really impressed with his growth and progress socially and mentally.

Rob came to me in September, one month prior to your New York consultation. He was shy, very unsure of himself, and lacking direction.

Prior to medical treatment, he was in the LD program and very unhappy. He joined my class for social studies, science, and math. Reading was very difficult. And he was struggling in math.

By January, after only several months of treatment, he was mainstreamed into my classroom for all subjects. He was much happier and I noticed Rob becoming a leader instead of a follower. When we worked in small groups, the other students would turn to Rob for answers. In math he was able to do his work as quickly and accurately as my best math students.

I am extremely pleased with Rob's achievements and I will be watching his progress in the future.

Mrs. King's Latest Summary

7/26/93

Thank you for all that you have done for our son, Rob. He has always been a worker in school and at home. I see, after two years of coming to you, a growth in his ability to be more independent in school and a confidence in himself. I thank God for Rob's 4th grade teacher, Mrs. Knispel, for going the extra mile for a student and for telling us about you and your work. I also thank God for you, Dr. Levinson, for helping all our dyslexic sons and daughters.

Important Questions

In summary, I think it imperative for readers to evaluate Priscilla Vail's criticism in the perspective provided and thus attempt to answer the following questions: Does my medical treatment prevent or enhance tutoring? Do my medically based dyslexia insights help or "freak out" my patients, medications aside? And is Ortonian tutoring *alone* capable of producing all the dramatic and rapid improvements characterizing the dyslexics presented and to be presented? Are the patients and their favorable responses real or merely fantasies inspired by the "Wizard of Oz"? And who is "freaked out" by my therapeutic results: patients, parents, teachers, or the traditionalists?

Finally, are there not clear and simple scientific reasons for why insight and inner-ear-enhancing medications help dyslexics and their inner-ear-determined symptoms? Indeed, are there not even psychologically based mechanisms capable of readily explaining how ignorance defensively triggers "magic," "wizards," and related primitive fantasies to account for natural and related events such as those described and analyzed within this work?

B

A First Glance

Since this book represents my attempt to ensure that *all* dyslexics needing *medical treatment* get it, I thought it essential to provide the reader with some typical clinical examples right up front. These real named and pictured dyslexics and their often dramatic responses to treatment will hopefully convey to the reader in a rapid realistic manner:

- What dyslexics and their symptoms are all about.
- The suffering they endure.
- The possible benefits from the breakthrough diagnosis and treatment to be described.
- And the lunacy of the traditionalists' attempt to conceptualize and define this disorder as merely one in which reading is severely impaired and reversals are present.

In addition, this clinical introduction to dyslexics and their disorder aims at providing the reader with the initial insight needed to better comprehend the *critical motives of the traditionalists* and their misguided attempts at preventing the results of this breakthrough research and treatment from reaching and benefitting frustrated and suffering individuals. Hopefully the improvements characterizing the varied dyslexics to be presented will ultimately extend to all in need.

Meredeth Smith Lewis

Meredeth, age 39, conveyed her improvements on medication (10/4/91).

It is so perfect that the last question in every section of your Progress Report (that patients must complete while on medication) is about anything else being easier. *My life is easier.*

Ask anyone who has ever known me and they would say I had the total package to be or do anything I wanted. Looking from their shoes it did appear to be so. So, why wasn't I? I finally summed it up to my therapist (approximately six months before I came to see you) that my life is so hard—everything is so hard for me! I realize now how there would be no way for her to *begin* to understand the complexities behind those words, and even less of a chance for her to help. I just told myself what I always had, "Just get on with it, Meredith, it's just something you'll have to live with."

I felt helpless, disheartened, misunderstood, insecure, and angry, while I continued to chip away at the process of building a life. But something would not let me give up in spite of the pain. Finally, after years of searching for the answer to that ultimate question *"What is wrong with me;"* after therapists, counsellors, groups, EST, Transactional Analysis, Yoga, and a fortune in books, *I found* Smart But Feeling Dumb. *And what I found that day was a miracle.*

I knew when I read your book that you were talking to me. Every doubt, every hurt, every symptom and emotion was as if I had written the words I was reading! I realized how my affliction was not so severe as to hold me back totally, but severe enough to keep me crippled both mentally and emotionally beneath a veneer of a "well" person. Every action and reaction of my 39 years found explanation, and I knew my healing had begun.

Upon returning from your New York office, I was ecstatic! I felt I had been given the key to my prison cell and was freed—finally! I rushed to get my medicine. Within days I could sense a difference in myself. It was so subtle, just gently washing over me. When I first started noticing that I was happy without a reason to be, I was certain I

knew what Heaven was going to be like. I was still forgetting things and running into frustrating situations, but I was
coping! I began handling more on my agenda, not becoming overwhelmed by the planning, doing, and follow-up.

My school work takes one millionth of the time it used
to. I find that I can breeze through a chapter, my notes
and handouts, and go in and get an "A" on a test. And I received an "A" in math! In fact, I was tutoring other students
in the class! I could sit for hours doing my homework, not
getting restless, bored, or frustrated, rather working
straight through from the first problem to the last. And
what's more, I liked it! Of course it helped that we had an
excellent professor. However, I am not diminishing my being able to sail through!

Dr. Levinson, I used to feel like a vulnerable little chick
who clung to the nest. All the other birds said there was no
reason why the chick shouldn't be flying with the rest of
them, that it *looked* like it was ready! But the little chick
knew he "wasn't done" and couldn't explain why it was
taking so long. I was like that little chick. Now, I'm complete and flying and soaring with the others. And people
say, "See, Meredeth, we always knew you were ready."
And I think how they never knew, but it's okay now because I'm finally "done." And not only can I fly, but I know
I'll trip and stumble, but that I can pick myself right back up
again. Now, looking from the shoes of another at the person they see, I know that I am that person on the inside
too. And everywhere I look I see a reflection of confidence,
talent, strength, and beauty.

*Dr. Levinson, you have given me the gift I have
searched for all of my life! You have given me happiness
where depression used to brood, self-esteem where doubt
and shame once prevailed, and courage where fear dominated. You have replaced my anger and frustration with
humor, while redirecting it to create purpose in my life. And*

thank you; because of you I can focus with intent on that purpose.

A Follow-Up Visit (7/29/93)

Meredeth briefly summarized her achievements, despite the trauma of a divorce and a major illness:

> This treatment made it possible to go back to college and to handle the rigorous demands of undergraduate study. For the first time in my life I was able to draw (and well!) and do math and enjoy it. I edited the school newspaper and graduated as salutatorian.

Ann Dixon

To those who consider dyslexia as *merely a reading disorder*, review 16-year-old Ann's favorable responses to medication carefully and then ask: *Are not the reading and academic-related symptoms merely the recognized tip of the dyslexic iceberg?*

Observations and Comments by Ann's Mother

> *How do I begin to thank you, Dr. Levinson—that one visit to your office last year changed our sixteen-year-old daughter's life. I came looking for help with school related problems, e.g., reading, omitted words, careless errors, concentration, etc. The medication has helped a great deal in those areas, but to my surprise and joy we now have a daughter who is much happier, feels much better about herself and is far more confident.*

> The strongest single memory I have of Ann during the last twelve months is of her about ten days after she began the medication. I looked at her as she walked toward me. She was no longer the girl who slouched, head down, but a person who walked straight, tall, looking more confident. When she reached me, I asked her if she thought the medication was helping. Her reply was: "Something is

happening to me." It was and is as if she has found a lower center of gravity. Now, whether Ann is running, playing basketball, roller blading, or biking, we no longer hold our breath fearing that she will fall.[1]

I have also noticed that during the last 12 months many of Ann's fears have faded. She's gone on several school trips and has had no fear of riding a bus, going on elevators, and even sliding on her belly in a deep, dark cave. Ann is the first to say that life is just more enjoyable. I can't tell you how happy that makes me feel!

I have also seen tremendous improvements in her school work. Ann still works as hard as she always has, but thanks to the medication her hard work now pays off.

Before starting on medication Ann always had trouble reading and understanding what she had read. No matter how much I tried to help, things seemed to get worse. It wasn't until after we were riding home from our first visit to your office that she told me that "the words change places when I read." I asked her why she hadn't told me, and she replied "because you would never have believed me." In a sense I was shocked to hear that, but also felt relief. Because now I believed we were getting some help for her. Even though our daughter has attended a private day school for the past six years where classes are small, a learning disorder was never suggested to us. Last year I was simply told that Ann had an emotional problem and needed psychiatric care. Except for you, no one understood or took the time to find out what was wrong—what a terrible burden Ann had to labor under.

Last year in her ninth grade English course Ann's teacher wrote this comment at the end of one of her

[1]When Ann was re-examined on 6/26/93, her progress continued to expand. And her report once again indicated that simple multivitamins and lecithin helped her balance. Recall this when reviewing Dr. Silver's denial of vitamins and all other "controversial" therapies in The "Magic Cure," as discussed in Chapter 8-C.

papers: "You make some excellent points, and you give good details, but you need to read this aloud so it will make sense. It sounds almost illiterate as I read it—there are omitted words, incorrect spellings, and odd choices of words. This really needs work! Conclusion is really quite good. Also—remember to avoid 'you.'" *D+*

After Ann had been on medication almost a year, the above comments may be contrasted with the comments made by Ann's tenth grade English teacher at the end of the term:

"Her writing has been consistently very good, and her *Macbeth* paper (B+) was a particularly well-written and nicely argued piece of analysis."

Again, in math class the symptoms were there for them to see—time and time again she was told that she made careless errors, had difficulty putting concepts together and lacked self-confidence.

This year these comments have ceased. Ann (who had to struggle last year to get a C-) this year in Algebra IIA received a B first semester, A- second semester, A- third semester and B+ for the fourth semester.

It has been a good year for Ann. It is as if you unlocked the door to the world for Ann. She has changed from a shy, unhappy, insecure girl to a much more self-assured sixteen-year-old.

I would like to quote once more, this time from her advisor's comments at the end of the school year. Please bear in mind, Dr. Levinson, that the school is unaware of your diagnosis or medication—that is the way Ann wants it.

"Ann finished with a very strong academic record . . . Ann seems to have had a much better year than last. She seems happy, more self confident, and carries a wonderful smile and friendly greeting wherever she goes. I look forward to having her again next year. It should be even better!"

(Ann's academic record this year was: English B, European History A-, Spanish I A-, Algebra IIA B+, Chemistry B+.)

Thank you again, Dr. Levinson, for your research, for the books you have written (because without them I wouldn't have learned about you), and for helping so many children, including Ann.

Debby Iberger

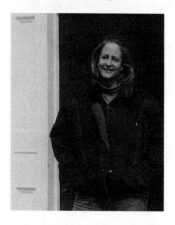

Debby, age 38, responded rapidly and dramatically to medication. Thus she reports:

2/22/92

I could never thank you enough for *giving me back my brain*. I am now in control of my life (and on top of all my husband's business paperwork)— days don't pass by *dizzyingly*; I'm out of a heavy, dense fog.

I've read much of the non-technical literature about dyslexia in the last four months. I find it amazing that you've stuck to your beliefs and research despite the verbal lashings (poundings?) you've taken from America's "esteemed" dyslexic community.

I'm waiting for the day, and I know it will come, when the *obstructionists* will be unable to refute your work. And if you need a guinea pig for any experiments on dyslexia, I'm available (and only 1 hour away).

Tom Henderson

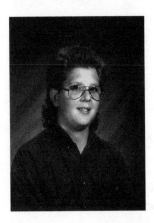

Tom is an 11-year-old dyslexic who has responded very well to 9 weeks of treatment. His parents' report on 4/30/92 follows:

General Improvements:

We have started to see a calmness in Tommy that has never been there before. His self-image has gotten so much better. He is so much more organized. His school work seems to be getting easier for him to do.

Tommy also seems to be making friends with more kids in school, and around the neighborhood.

When he gets mad, he will catch himself and say "I'm sorry," whereas before he would just stay mad.

Tommy seems to be sleeping better at night. He is not having as many bad dreams. He seems more rested.

Specific Improvements:

Reading: is easier, more spontaneous, smoother; less word and sentence skipping errors; words are clearer, less jumping around; double vision is gone; fewer reading headaches; less head tilting; greater visual span; better reading memory and concentration.

Writing: better; more spontaneous; smoother and easier to read; straighter on lined paper with better spacing; faster; more detailed.

Spelling: better orally and written, easier visualization.

Math: easier addition, subtraction, multiplication, division, fractions; less reversals; neater columns and less careless errors.

Memory: significantly improved short-term.

Time: sense is better.

Direction: sense is better; is distinguishing right/left, north/south, east/west.

Speech: increased spontaneous expression and speed in saying what he wants, improved clarity and sequencing for speech heard.

Grammar: better understood and improved memory for details, fewer errors.

Concentration/distractibility/overactivity: all improved, more alert, less impulsive.

Mood: steadier, less depressed and happier.

Frustration tolerance: better, temper controlled.

Self-image/body-image: feels smarter, more confident, more together—mentally and physically.

Socialization: better.

Psychosomatic symptoms: fewer headaches, stomachaches; dizzy spells and motion sickness gone.

Balance/coordination: better, steadier, less accident prone, better sports ability.

Organization/planning: improved for writing, drawing, thinking—even room.

Fears/Phobias: less repetitive thoughts and decreased need to check things; fear persists (i.e., needles).[1]

[1]By carefully listening to and detailing *all* the many and varied symptoms and corresponding therapeutic responses reported by dyslexic patients and/or their loved ones, I developed a dramatic multi-dimensional concept of dyslexia which is far different than that fantasized by the traditionalists.

Tom's Letter

And as a rapid introduction to Tom's dyslexic writing and spelling as well as his humor, I decided to include the following letter:

> 9364 Shawnee Cr.
> Streetsboro OH 44241
> ~~March~~ 9/1992 ?
>
> ~~Harold~~ H. Levinson, MD, P.C.
> 600 Northern Blvd.
> Great Neck, N.Y. 11021
>
> Dear Dr Levenson:
>
> Thank you for finding out what was wrong with me. I am feeling much better in what I am doing. I have only felt one side affect I think...and that is crankyness Tomorrow March 6, 1992 I have to get a blood test! (OUCH!) Dad is going to give blood first! (Good) Ha! Ha! Yo
>
> Your Patient,
> Tom Henderson.
>
> rec'd at 3/92

Antonia Baziotis

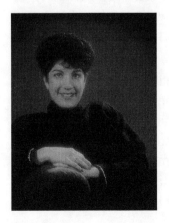

Antonia is a 28-year-old pharmacist who described both her *dyslexic* and related *agoraphobic-panic* symptoms and improvement on medical treatment.

> It has been ten weeks since the initiation of treatment. In that time I have blossomed. The fun and excitement which I have experienced in the past few weeks stands out vividly when compared to the harsh realities which I have faced for the past twelve years. The changes are too numerous to even mention. I feel a centeredness and an inner peace that I haven't experienced since I was a very young child.

> *Past*—Where do I begin? I have since spoken to several relatives who have filled me in on some enlightening aspects of my childhood. Apparently, I was unable to distinguish between my left hand and my right for many years. I remember utilizing a birthmark on my left hand as a reference point, and to recall the left-hand-birthmark relationship I made up a little jingle.

> I had a difficult time learning the alphabet and how to spell my name. I remember using a visual type of memorization in an effort to learn. I would picture what the alphabet looked like on my little desk and print my name from that picture. I had difficulty tying my shoes and until this day I still cannot spell. I developed some remarkable coping techniques. I would read with my chin on the book and I would write with my head lying sideways on my desk. In an effort to concentrate I would tilt my head severely to the right.

> I didn't learn to ride a bicycle until after my younger brother had. I now bicycle a lot and I am able to ride much faster because I don't have the sensation of falling. Sports were difficult and so I avoided most activities. I always had the feeling the ball was going to hit me in the face. And skiing was particularly frustrating because I felt as though I was always going to fall forward when I went downhill.

My piano teacher to this day commends me on my perseverance in learning how to play. I always felt as though I was going to fall off the piano bench and could never get my fingers to coordinate with the music I was reading. I had difficulty timing the music and even counting out loud would not help. As an adult I have trouble cooking and coordinating a dinner so that all the dishes are ready at the same time.

Response to Antihistamines—Needless to say, everything has improved immensely. I can read while sitting in a chair or standing. I listen intently with my head straight, my shoulders back and my spine straight. I walk properly and stand with the weight distributed evenly throughout the bottom of my feet. My writing has improved and I can keep my head a comfortable distance away from the paper and best of all I can write in a straight line. I ride my bicycle fast (even down the hills) and when the tour is finished I am able to walk without feeling motion sick. I've started to play piano again as well as tennis.

My personality has become amazingly calm. My roommate is astounded at what you have done! More than a few times a day I am taken aback by the profoundness of it all. My body and personality feel new, almost alien to me. I can tolerate stress. I can fill prescriptions and manage a crew of people, work 10 hours, go home and walk for an hour all on less sleep than I have required in ages. My restless sleep and terrorizing dreams are gone. Instead my dreams are both calm and pleasant.

I no longer work compulsively trying to run away from my anxiety. Gone is the bargaining with God, the fruitless searches, the endless reading and analyzing in an effort to still the turmoil within my body. Nor do I have to find a deep psychoanalytic reason for why the room shifts or I cannot stand in church (I am able to sit through a service!).

Gone is the feeling of helplessness. I am able to make a commitment and follow through. I can plan in advance without worrying how I will feel that day. I can command respect from my family and friends and walk away from those who I don't like without precipitating a panic attack and having to run back for help (only to have them say that I am crazy). I have my dignity now.

My impulsivity and mood swings are gone. I am able to make a decision and stick to it. I have become very organized and competent. I am no longer the victim of constant aggressive or hostile thoughts. I am able to let go of the past and live in the present. All of the events which had terrorized my childhood seem to have receded into the back of my mind and out of my present day-to-day consciousness.

Last week I went to the mall. Until recently I could not look at clothes without holding onto the rack, change in the dressing room without feeling the walls were going to close in on me, walk without the aid of a shopping cart. I walked throughout the mall calm and cool, even looking over the balcony! I can even walk quickly now. Ordinarily, I would have had to stop every 5-10 feet to recapture my balance and reorient myself.

This past weekend was remarkable. I volunteered to work at my church festival. Here was Ann in a huge gymnasium that was brightly lit with fluorescent lights and packed with 500 people, working at a steady and fast pace, calm as a cucumber! Then to top it all off I went in and danced with all of my friends. Greek dancing involves dancing in a circular motion at a fast pace with small dance steps. Last year, I remember standing in the doorway watching all the festivities and my friends. Walking inside more than a few feet terrorized me, and after a few attempts, I just went home all alone and cried.

The small wonders range anywhere from being able to ride in elevators, walk up and down stairways, go up tall buildings and enjoy the New York skyline, to tilting back in a hairdresser's chair, going shopping alone, and making some major changes in my life.

Finally the most wonderful news of all. In the past couple of months I have resumed communication with my ex-fiancé. Since I have become fully functioning I can go on with my life. We are planning a December wedding. I plan on walking up the aisle in confidence. No longer am I afraid of church and the alter. At the reception I hope to kick up my heels and dance, twirling round and round lots of times!

Summary

My hope and desire is that readers listening carefully to my many and varied dyslexic patients will begin to clearly understand:

- the diverse and interrelated symptoms (academic, concentration/activity/distractibility, balance and coordination, speech, mood and anxiety) characterizing this puzzling disorder,

- the way *inner-ear-enhancing medications* improve and thus highlight these varied symptoms and their mechanisms of origin, and

- the conscious and subconscious motives leading the traditionalists to deny all these breakthrough insights for the past twenty years.

C

Two Sides to a Coin

Under ordinary circumstances, to understand a new research effort such as the medical breakthroughs in dyslexia, all one needs is a clear and simple presentation of the diagnostic/therapeutic results. However, when this research effort is attacked on all sides by a group of traditionalists, many with very impressive titles, then more insight is needed. Then one needs to understand the criticism as well as the conflicts triggered by the research attacked. In other words, for these breakthroughs to be publicly and scientifically accepted, *the basic research has to be clearly understood and verified. And all the resistance or distortion used to deny its acceptance has to be clearly exposed and analyzed.*

In retrospect, I was forced to ask myself a number of vital questions. And the most important one was: *What was needed in order to solve the riddles characterizing dyslexia and write A Scientific Watergate—Dyslexia?* Let me summarize what I found to be the most crucial characteristics needed to tackle dyslexia and the forces preventing its understanding and acceptance:

- Being determined enabled me to stick with a scientific effort which most often drifted in elusive arcs. Repeated backtracking and false starts were commonplace, and apparent parallels often intersected.

- Being honest enabled me to see my mistakes and those of others, and attempt their correction without the slightest bit of embarrassment. Each and every corrected mistake opened up new vistas never before anticipated or dreamed of.

- Being psychiatrically trained enabled me to quickly grasp defense or bias mechanisms attempting to mask the truth for various reasons.

- Being mathematical enabled me to "feel" solutions that made sense from those that were forced together in order to maintain preconceived notions in an "unholy alliance," notions that make as much sense as $1 + 1 = 5$.

- Being Jewish enabled me to feel comfortable as a scientific outsider, a position I was forced in by the traditional majority who defensively cast aside all those with unique or challenging points of view; and which enabled me to maintain an unbiased perspective—a perspective which traditionalists *lacked*.

- Being naive, at least initially, enabled me to feel that truth and honesty would eventually prevail if only I worked hard and long enough, and if only I could prove my theories by using sufficient numbers of dyslexics and clarity of writing style—sufficient to convince a child.

- Being flexible and resilient enabled me to endure the slings and arrows of outrageous *deceit,* conscious and otherwise.

- Being independent of the requirements of many researchers such as funding, frequent publications, etc., left me free to pursue my scientific instincts without political, economic, or self-aggrandizing contaminations.

D

Some Important Questions

What would you think if suddenly you realized that a major medical discovery, potentially capable of significantly helping millions of *both children and adults*—perhaps 20% of the *world's* population—was deliberately suppressed?

How would you feel if you, your child, or a loved one could have been saved from years of needless emotional and academic deprivation, if only a proper diagnosis had been made and medical treatment administered in a timely manner? Suppose there existed no other explanation or medical treatment for the disorder in question? And what if the medications, when properly administered, were perfectly safe and could significantly help more than 75% of treated children and adults, sparing them lives otherwise plagued by repeated failures, endless frustration, impaired self-esteem, and thus feelings of stupidity, ugliness, clumsiness, and even silent doubts about retardation or Alzheimer's?

Suppose this disorder was superficially known to you by one of its varied terms, such as: *dyslexia* (impaired reading ability), *learning disability* (poor academic performance), *minimal cerebral dysfunction, minimal brain damage, static encephalopathy*? What if it was also mistakenly confused with one of its many and varied symptoms, and thus called *Attention Deficit (Hyperactivity) Disorder* (ADD or ADHD—poor concentration and distractibility, hyperactivity and impulsivity), *dysgraphia* (poor writing ability), *dyscalculia* (poor math skills), *dysnomia and disarticulation disorders or dysphasia* (word finding and speech difficulties, including stuttering, stammering, "scrambling," etc.), *dyspraxia* (poor balance, coordination, and rhythm)?

Suppose this disorder were also responsible for triggering a wide range of *psychosomatic* symptoms (headaches, vertigo, motion sickness, abdominal complaints, bed-wet-ting, excessive sweating), and even *phobias* and excessive *anxiety* and *mood* fluctuations?

What would you do if this momentous but suppressed medical discovery were yours? How would you attempt to bring *all* of the facts to light so that concerned people might meaningfully understand and evaluate circum-stances for themselves and hopefully alleviate and prevent needless suffering.

Might you also wonder how many other discoveries were and are suppressed for quite similar political, eco-nomic and egoistic reasons? And how might other *scientific Watergates* be prevented for the sake of mankind? Would you be curious who the leading culprits were and what master they served?

What if you and/or your children were deliberately de-prived of the following treatment responses?[1]

Julie Ann Compton

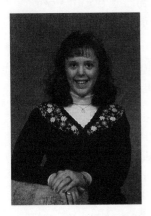

[1]For those truly interested in knowing how I came to understand what dyslexics and dyslexia are all about, read as many of their case histo-ries as possible and then clearly *highlight and outline* their described symptoms and improvements. Then compare the resulting sketch to the traditional definition of dyslexia. Hopefully this comparison will enable you to answer a vital question: Who can best define dyslexia: dyslexics or traditional experts? And no doubt the answer to this ques-tion will help answer another: Why have so many dyslexics been pre-sented throughout this work—perhaps even to the point of distraction?

Prior to treatment, 12-year-old Julie Ann's IQ mistakenly tested out below average. This is no longer true—as is apparent from repeat testing and her mother's description of improvements, dated 11/8/92.

> We could probably write a book about all of the changes we have seen in Julie. Overall, she is remarkably better! There have been dramatic changes, along with smaller ones that most people would think insignificant, but to us were remarkable.
>
> It is very encouraging and exciting to us when people who know Julie and are aware of what we have done (brought her to see you) come to us with comments like, "Julie sure is happier, isn't she?" or "Julie actually participated with the group tonight in our youth meeting!" But much, much more exciting are the ones who, unaware of her visit to you, have said, "Wow, Julie really has come out of her shell! She seems to have really overcome her fears." Some even ask what's going on with her because *she* has spoken to *them* without being spoken to first! We are then able to share with them all that we've learned about your treatment of dyslexics, and they are always amazed!
>
> Julie is more energetic, loving, pleasant, confident, outspoken, talkative, tolerant of irritations, less angry, less dismal, less confused, and less clumsy. She often says, "I'm getting smarter!"
>
> Some of the "big" changes we have seen in Julie are:
>
> 1) *Active* participation in a week-long music camp at church which culminated in a musical at the end of the week. For the first time, Julie held her head high, sang every word, and smiled and waved to us in the congregation!
>
> 2) Julie has, of her own desire, enrolled in a beginning tap dancing class! She is enjoying this immensely! She displays a newfound coordination which she is excited about. She even participated in the class on Watch Day before an audience of parents!

3) School has become easier in a lot of ways. Most of all, her reasoning processes seem to be "with it." She understands concepts better, and has for the first time in her life been able to memorize addition facts 1-10! This came only after the second week of school. She obviously had "known" them before, but been unable to "retrieve" them. How excited she was when she realized she could do this now!

As I said, we have seen many "smaller" changes in Julie that to us are just as important as the "big" ones. She has done some cross-stitch (with assistance), something that totally frustrated her before. This time, she actually finished a picture and gave it to her father for his birthday! There have also been times when she actually "plays" with her siblings—something she *rarely* ever did. One day, out of the blue, she looked at her sister and said, "Sarah, I love you!" Needless to say, she surprised Sarah as well as herself!

I could go on and on with small incidences when Julie behaved the opposite of what we used to experience. I can't tell you what a joy it has been to us to see her change so dramatically and actually begin to enjoy life.

Julie was still struggling with enough things in school that we felt she would benefit from a vision exam. We took her to Dr. David Cook. He determined that Julie has double vision and is confident that this can be corrected with a six-month vision therapy program. He was in agreement about treatment of her inner-ear problem, and felt that he could only enhance the improvement we have seen so far.

We look to the future with great hope for Julie. We are ever grateful for you and others who are willing to "go against the flow" to help others fulfill their greatest potential God has for them. Thank you from the bottom of our hearts.

Julie's Graphomotor Incoordination

Because dyslexics frequently evidence poor writing and drawing, they are often tested for this difficulty using Bender Gestalt cards and figure drawings. To highlight this difficulty, I thought it worthwhile to compare Julie Ann's drawings to the following norms and typical dyslexic figures.

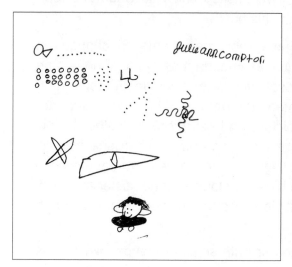

Figure 1-A Note the angulation or tilting of the drawings as well as the poor angle-formations and the approximations characterizing Julie Ann's drawings. All these errors, as well as the highly simplified figure drawings, are diagnostic of the inner-ear or *CV* dysfunctioning underlying dyslexia.

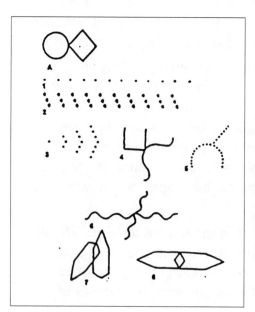

Figure 1-B The Bender Gestalt stimulus cards. Children are requested to draw nine Bender Gestalt stimuli. For children of this age, the graphomotor drawing performance should closely approximate the illustrated Bender Gestalt stimulus figures. These figures thus served as the expected norm. Taken from *A Solution to the Riddle—Dyslexia*, p. 56.

Goodenough Figure Drawings—Typical of Dyslexics

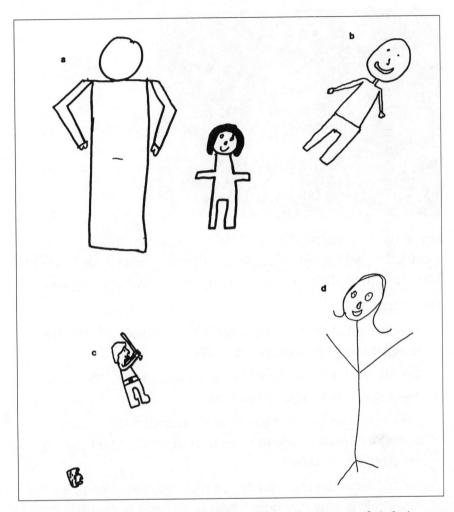

Figure 2 Typical errors provoked when dyslexics of Julie's age are requested to draw a person. As noted, the figures are frequently tilted and details such as hands, fingers, feet and facial features are omitted. A stick figure illustrates the simplification of the arms, legs, and trunk, although the facial features are detailed. These Goodenough figure drawing errors were viewed as projections indicative of underlying disturbances in CV-determined spatial, directional, graphomotor and proprioceptive integration. In addition, some of the simplification or omission errors were assumed to represent compensatory attempts at avoidance of dysmetric performance and the resulting catastrophic anxiety. Taken from *A Solution to the Riddle—Dyslexia*, p. 59.

Kimberly and Curtis Oates

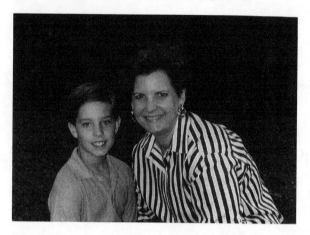

Kimberly, 34 years old, and her 6-year-old son, Curtis, responded significantly to medical treatment after only 8 weeks. She describes their respective improvements as follows:

Kimberly Oates:

> For the first time in my life, I don't have bruises all over my legs, so I must be navigating better!

> My energy level has been up and I appear to accomplish more in a shorter amount of time.

> I no longer have the nausea and dizziness I was experiencing that caused me to have to take short breaks during the day and lay down.

> My husband hasn't had to correct my sentences, as I rarely talk backwards now. I also don't think backwards either, so I am doing better at getting my points across to others.

> I can respond quicker to communication.

> My reading is better. I don't get hung up on words and therefore read faster, and without headaches from neck and eye strain.

> I am going to sleep quickly and more deeply as I don't remember my dreams as often.

> I hear numbers better though I can't always say them better.

I've worked through a mound of emotional buildup. I always thought I had a wrong perception of things. I didn't trust my own judgment. That is changing.

I am still working on body image though.

Just having an explanation for things has helped tremendously. Understanding why I do things differently.

It is great not to be a "victim" any longer, since I can trust my own judgment.

I'm not afraid to do things on my own any more.

I'm less obsessive in that my thoughts don't seem to get stuck on one thing any longer. I can get out of the rut easier.

How could one little pill do so much for [my son] Curtis and I. *Your book which led to our office visit was truly God-sent!*

Curtis Oates

After taking the antihistamine for about 2 weeks, Curtis' teacher said a light came on. Curtis could read and sit still to do so. She was so excited, and so were we!

He is beginning to speak clearer, as he appears to hear the sounds better. But he still has difficulty following a series of instructions (at least from Mom)!

Curtis is a lot calmer because he is better focused. His athletic skills requiring eye-hand coordination have greatly improved.

We haven't had but one bed-wetting incident since starting the medication. And he sleeps through the night now!

His hand coordination has also improved. Though his handwriting is sloppy, it is now within the lines on the page and more evenly spaced. He is much more interested in coloring now. The reversals are happening less and less.

I am so excited about his improvement that I share your discovery with anyone who will listen!

President George Bush

Might President Bush Have Been Helped?

In a recent article, "The Speech Thing," Jesse Furman asks, "*Is Bush brain-damaged? . . .*" Thus she states:

> The 68-year-old president's mangled speech does in fact reveal a number of characteristics associated with a brain disorder called aphasia: frequent grammatical errors, talking around subjects, groping unsuccessfully for the right word and substituting one word for another of close meaning or similar sound. Lack of substance—or "emptiness," as the specialists put it—is also a common symptom of aphasia. On "20/20" with Barbara Walters, President Bush mistakenly confused the word "divorce" with "abortion"; he often substitutes the word "thing"—as in the "vision thing" or the "law enforcement thing"—when more substantive words evade him; and his use of mixed metaphors is downright bizarre, as in his 1989 refusal to answer a reporter's persistent questions about the Oliver North trial: "Please don't ask me to do that which I've just said I'm not going to do, because you're burning up time; the meter is running through the sand on you, and I am now filibustering." In a recent statement, Bush seemed to demonstrate these aphasic symptoms all at once: "It is weird. I guess this is the normal procedure every four years—the amount of food I was eating and how did Barbara feel about it, and she said to me, what about your health. I said, well, I'm not eating too much, or something. It turned out it was the rumors."

What would or could have happened if President Bush were not either misdiagnosed or misunderstood and so inadvertently deprived of treatment by *the traditionalists*? Suppose his reported speech (and other possible inner-ear-determined) symptoms had responded to breakthrough medical therapy as did those of Kimberly and Curtis Oates and those of Meg Fex—soon to be re-presented in greater detail so as to highlight her dramatic improvements in speech as well as the favorable medication-triggered responses occurring over time, even very short periods.

Although all the neurological experts Jesse Furman consulted considered aphasia—a severe language impairment resulting from a lesion within the thinking-speaking brain—none considered inner-ear dysfunction or dyslexia. And the reasons underlying this diagnostic absurdity are simple to understand. Because the traditionalists are conceptually fixated and obsessively preoccupied with only the cerebral cortical (thinking-language) centers of the brain, they unwittingly confuse relatively mild inner-ear-determined reading and dysphasic or speech symptoms with such qualitatively and prognostically distinct "severe equivalents" as alexia and aphasia.[1] And as explained in Chapter 2, the quality and prognosis of inner-ear vs. cerebral language disorders are as different as day and night. Additionally, since the traditionalists cannot distinguish between dyslexia and alexia, they cannot conceive of dyslexics without severe reading-score impairments.

Do not Bush's reported *speech* symptoms resemble the scrambled reading, writing, spelling, math . . . and related sensory-motor processes of dyslexics? Could Bush have had "true aphasia"—and yet have gone to Yale, been a pilot and war hero, and functioned as the director of the CIA and President of the U.S.? No way!

Might he be a very bright and gifted reading-score-compensated dyslexic—similar to those you will meet in these pages? Sure thing!

According to my research, the speech dysfunctioning and all other "typical" dyslexic symptoms are due to a hidden but diagnostically detectable inner-ear or "fine tuning and sequencing" dysfunction. And as indicated, the vast majority of these inner-ear-determined dyslexic symptoms may be significantly compensated for by use of inner-ear-enhancing medications.

---

[1] *Alexia* and *aphasia* are severe reading and speech impairments of *cerebral or thinking brain origin.* By contrast, *dyslexia* and *dysphasia* are infinitely milder versions found to be of inner-ear origin. Also, politicians are known to be deliberately evasive. Thus their double talk and "rambling" away from direct answers may be of political vs. aphasic or dysphasic origin.

Thus it seemed reasonable to wonder: *Had President Bush's alleged speech and related symptoms been properly diagnosed, might he have responded favorably to inner-ear-enhancing medical treatment? Might he have won re-election?*

To rapidly illustrate the manner by which Bush-like speech and related dyslexic symptoms may dramatically change on inner-ear-enhancing medications, I decided to end this segment with the evolving improvement of Meg Fex, a dyslexic girl previously mentioned. And keep the following important considerations in mind: *The fact that speech and all other typical dyslexic symptoms respond favorably to inner-ear-enhancing medications clearly suggests that dyslexia is of inner-ear origin rather than of a cerebral-language determination as the traditionalists have mistakenly believed for almost 100 years.*

Meg Fex

In order to highlight the continued therapeutic progress of dyslexics as well as their speech and related symptoms over time—especially short three-month periods, I thought it worthwhile to update Meg's improvements as initially reported in "The Scientific Firing Line."

Her mother, Katy Fex, writes:

> *Megan is a completely different girl than the one you saw just three months ago. So much has happened in this short time span that I'm not quite sure where to begin. Academically, Meg has climbed mountains: She is reading on or above grade level with complete comprehension (nine weeks ago I would have considered her a non-reader).*
>
> She completes her school work in class most days with the occasional ditto brought home here or there. She *comprehends* all the work she does. Homework has gone from 4 to 5 hours to 30 to 45 minutes. (There is an occasional tough night, but I'm beginning to accept that this is just normal kid stuff and not reverting back. Meg usually picks up on my apprehension and will tell me, "Mom, I'm

just cranky. Don't worry, my eyes don't get mixed up any-more.")

Meg's special reading teacher has compared Meg to a blind person who has regained her sight. She does not be-lieve that Meg needs to attend the summer remedial pro-gram as long as we read at home. Further, she does not see that Meg will need to be in the program next year if she remains on her present course.

Meg's speech teacher who was unaware of the situa-tion sent home a note asking if we were doing speech therapy at home. She had never seen such dramatic im-provement. She is keeping Meg for the remainder of this year and will monitor her on occasion next year but feels Meg no longer needs the speech program.[1]

Socially, etc. . . . Meg remembers kids' names and events of the day. She no longer is "clumsy," nothing gets spilled, no hitting walls as she walks through doors. . . . No more headaches or stomachaches; she plays with large numbers of kids with lots of external confusion that no longer bothers her.

Last week Meg had a bad cold. These usually result in ear infections, but Meg has never complained about her ears until they are extremely bad. I noticed as she was do-ing her homework, her reversals increased and her letters became very disjointed again ("Ol " for "a", or "Ô " for "b" or "d"). I asked her if her ears were bothering her and she said, "Just a little." Sure enough she had ear infections in both ears. She went on antibiotics and as her ears cleared up so did her writing.[2]

[1]Keep these speech improvements in mind when reading how the tra-ditionalists repeatedly attempt to *force* similar inner-ear-determined symptoms into a "cerebral-language mold."

[2]It is crucial to note how inner-ear-enhancing antihistamines trigger improvements in dyslexic symptoms whereas ear infections may inten-sify these very same symptoms. These insights clearly and definitively substantiate further the inner-ear origins of dyslexia while simulta-neously refuting the traditionally-assumed cerebral-language theories.

So many changes have occurred and Megan has noticed each one. She said to me, "Mom, I told you my eyes
didn't see right, and Dr. Levinson fixed them." Looking
back now I interpret that as "Mom, I'm *smart but feeling
dumb* and nobody listened to me or believed me or knew
what to do, but Dr. Levinson did!"

Nine weeks ago you asked me what I wanted to happen. I asked for Meg not to be frustrated or angry and you
gave me so much more. We are forever in your debt.

Megan's Bender Gestalt and Figure Drawings

To continue to familiarize readers with the inner-ear
mechanisms responsible for impaired graphomotor coordination as well as the drawing tests commonly used for
this diagnosis, I considered it worthwhile to demonstrate
Megan's results when initially examined.

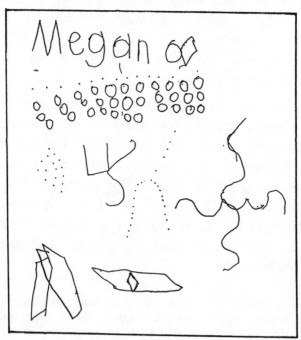

Figure 3-A A review of Megan's copy of the *Bender Gestalt
cards* shows evidence of inner-ear-determined directional and
spatial errors as well as difficulties connecting two lines when
forming angles.

Figure 3-B Megan's simplified Goodenough figure drawing emphasizes difficulties with drawing fingers, legs, etc. These difficulties as well as those responsible for her poor writing are triggered by an inner-ear-determined fine-motor or *graphomotor* incoordination.

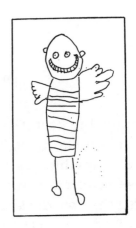

Vital Considerations

If simple *inner-ear-enhancing* medications can dramatically compensate or "cure" the speech, reading and all other typical dyslexic symptoms in those with medical evidence of *only inner-ear impairments*, how can the traditionalists maintain that the reading and speech symptoms as well as the dyslexic disorder are due to "brain damage" or "aphasia" of a thinking-brain origin?

In other words, how can the traditionalists deny both the inner-ear basis of dyslexia as well as the breakthrough benefits to be derived by using simple inner-ear medications and therapies—benefits such as those just described and the many to follow? This denial and its analysis represents the essence of *A Scientific Watergate—Dyslexia*.

In a nutshell: The traditionalists maintain that all the patients and therapeutic responses presented throughout this and all prior works are fictitious. I maintain the opposite: that these patients and their responses are real! And if real, then the 100-year-old concepts of the traditionalists are as fictitious as their dyslexia expertise.[1]

Judge this book and its *critical vs. dyslexic content* for yourselves, and arrive at your own conclusions.

[1]For purposes of emphasis and perhaps even symmetry, the epigraphs for Chapters 1 and 2 highlight and repeat this important theme.

E

Never Again

Despite the fact that politically and economically-based Watergate-like intrigues and deception are commonplace, little if anything is known about similar motives guiding those involved in medical research and related clinical efforts, i.e., *on dyslexia*. Accordingly, the primary aims of this work are: (1) to present the breakthrough research leading to the *inner-ear or cerebellar-vestibular* origins of dyslexia and related phobias, as well as to new and unique methods of *medical* diagnosis, treatment, and even prevention (further elaborated in Book II, forthcoming); (2) to describe detailed attempts by leading dyslexia experts and organizations to derail and block acceptance of this often lifesaving research—at all costs; and (3) to analyze the powerful but hidden underlying motives of the *traditionalists* and their followers.

Although this work might be considered a *survivor's manual* for budding researchers attempting to avoid the slings and arrows of outrageous fortune, it is much more than that. It represents a factual exploration and analysis of the bias-forces within seemingly dedicated men and women, unwittingly leading them to sacrifice millions of suffering individuals merely to safeguard their own status quos and egos. Hopefully, this fact-filled exposé will guide future medical researchers by the motto: *Never again!*

After recognizing blatant deceptions bordering on *psychopathy* and confused, illogical criticism bordering on *neurosis*, I attempted to delve into the specific drives triggering these outward symptoms within the many and varied dyslexia research efforts and their researchers. Obviously, power, money, status and a host of other self-serving motives appeared to be superficially fueling a small minority of these "*betrayers of the truth*" and "anti-*Hippocrates*" or "*hypocrites.*" But there seemed to be still deeper drives of unknown origin strongly motivating the traditionalist majority to shed and sidestep the scientific reality before their very eyes. And no doubt some were mere victims of unconscious drives forcing them to unwittingly worship the basest motives of a lesser god.

Eventually I wondered: Might there exist a powerful and universally acting subconscious force leading dedicated scientists and neurophysiological clinicians to believe: (1) that the *thinking-speaking brain* of man is *completely* responsible for *all* cognitive and language functioning, and thus (2) that an impairment within the thinking-speaking brain is the *unquestionable and unchallengeable cause of dyslexia—despite all evidence to the contrary?* And for reasons to be explored and elucidated, might this subconscious force be defending itself from discovery, leading us all by the nose and forcing us to dance to its various tunes, whether they be called psychopathic, neurotic, dyslexic, etc. (see Chapter 22).

F

Too Hot to Handle

- Twenty years have now passed since I first solved the diagnostic and therapeutic riddles characterizing dyslexia.

- Twenty years have passed since my analysis of Watergate-like cover-ups began in dyslexia!

No doubt you are wondering: If all this is true, why did you wait so long to publish it? The unexpected answer is: I didn't wait that long. In fact, the *first big denial(s)* and my angry dismay initially motivated me to complete a medical text: *A Solution to the Riddle—Dyslexia*. And in Chapter 13, entitled *Criticism and Its Analysis*, I presented and analyzed these scientific denials and unwitting deceptions.

But I learned something very interesting from this work. *No* scientist or clinician reading this text ever spontaneously referred to this deception. They had to be prodded by me. And only then did I hear: "It happens all the time." Kaput, finished—end of discussion. No one wanted to deal with or tackle this subject. Even dyslexics who read this rather difficult medical text with dictionaries and glossaries in hand avoided mention of this topic. *It was obviously too hot to handle.* And I was too hot to deal with it *dispassionately.* Besides, a premature and angry response would have been counterproductive. As a result, I decided to tackle this work *last* rather than *first*. And hopefully last will be best.

Most of my intended research has been completed. I had published documented evidence of *the first big denial* approximately fifteen years ago—with no denials, law suits, etc. And I let the topic *rest* until I instinctively felt the time was right to tackle this hot potato. And make no mistake about it, this is a real hot potato—really hitting home for many people. Otherwise, the topic wouldn't have been so denied, avoided—treated like a leper. *Even the many and varied Ortonian-sponsored and related critics of* A Solution to the Riddle—Dyslexia *never once referred to the content within Chapter 13. And some of these critics were "star performers" in this Watergate process. Obviously it was too hot for them to handle as well!*

In any event, I've patiently waited and analyzed the need for such a work, instinctively feeling all along that it was as crucial to science as science itself. Science and scientists should not be betrayed and diverted from their destined and intended goals. And so it is imperative that an analysis of the factors and forces underlying this betrayal be exposed before it contaminates and corrupts the whole, rendering meaningful solutions even more impossible than before.

I must add that I was also inspired by *Betrayers of the Truth* (1982), a magnificent work by two *New York Times* reporters, William Broad and Nicholas Wade. Unfortunately, they were too busy to tackle this project. Or perhaps one such work is enough for a lifetime?

I do not know the depth and scope of this corruption in science. But I can only guess that authors Broad and Wade have only scratched the surface of this phenomena in their book. Since *Betrayers of the Truth* has attempted to generalize this phenomena both historically—dating back to Claudius Ptolemy—and across all sections of science, I felt it important to add to its depth with a single case study (*A Scientific Watergate—Dyslexia*) of *currently active* ignorance and defensive bias within my own personal sphere of experience dating back some 20-30 years. Not only would this unique study *add* to *Betrayers of the Truth* but it would help enlighten those with a dyslexic disorder. It would help them understand what and why they are being told whatever they are. And better yet, what to do about it.

Thus, in their second chapter entitled, *"Deceit in History,"* Broad and Wade state: *"The great scientists of the past were not all so honest and they did not always obtain the experimental results they reported."* And they continue:

- Claudius Ptolemy, known as "the greatest astronomer of antiquity," did most of his observing not at night on the coast of Egypt but during the day, in the great library at Alexandria, where he appropriated the work of a Greek astronomer and proceeded to call it his own.

- Galileo Galilei is often hailed as the founder of modern scientific method because of his insistence that experiment, not the works of Aristotle, should be the arbiter of truth. But colleagues of the seventeenth-century Italian physicist had difficulty reproducing his results and doubted he did certain experiments.

- Isaac Newton, a boy genius who formulated the laws of gravitation, relied in his magnum opus on an unseemly fudge factor in order to make the predictive power of his work seem much greater than it was.

- John Dalton, the great nineteenth-century chemist who discovered the laws of chemical combination and proved the existence of different types of atoms, published elegant results that no present-day chemist has been able to repeat.

- Gregor Mendel, the Austrian monk who founded the science of genetics, published papers on his work with peas in which the statistics are too good to be true.

- The American physicist Robert Millikan won the Nobel prize for being the first to measure the electric charge of an electron. But Millikan extensively misrepresented his work in order to make his experimental results seem more convincing than was in fact the case.

If indeed *"the great scientists of the past were not all so honest and they did not always obtain the experimental results they reported,"* what might we find upon analyzing the content and intent of ordinary researchers—some merely aspiring to be great and others with illusions and perhaps even "delusions of grandeur"?

Considering this introductory warning, it should be no surprise to find at least similar, if not greater, degrees of *distortion* amongst scientific experts in other fields. Accordingly, my research in dyslexia clearly suggests: (1) that most experts never really talk to dyslexics nor carefully listen to their complaints but merely test them to death using a wide range of psychological, educational, and neurophysiological measures; (2) that these resulting test scores are squeezed into pre-existing theories, regardless of whether they fit or not; (3) that the vast majority of contradictory data are sidestepped, denied, or otherwise omitted from view; (4) that the traditionalist experts merely found what prior traditionalists expected them to find and rewrote or "parroted" prior versions of what they read; (5) that anything new, especially of consequence, threatens their ignorance and ingrained beliefs, and defensively results in deception—and even worse; and (6) that the *medical improvements* offered patients by *A Solution to the Riddle—Dyslexia* and presented throughout this work threatens my critics the most. Were this not so, why else would these critics continue to voice their nonsensical fantasy-fear that I "cure 100% of dyslexics" when in fact my claims—really those of dyslexics and their loved ones—are significantly more modest and realistic.

G

Concerns and Doubts

New patients or family members repeatedly ask me suspiciously or in frank bewilderment: "If what you say about dyslexia is true, how come there aren't clinics like yours all over?"

After their initial diagnosis and evaluation, when they feel more comfortable and reassured, these same individuals ask: "How come so many professionals have tried to talk us out of coming here—even without them ever having read any of your books or papers we've given them?" "Some have even claimed to have read your works—but obviously didn't." "Why did my doctor call your theories 'bunk'—even though you're the only one who describes my symptoms perfectly? And especially since he knows nothing at all about this disorder?" "How come your work hasn't been recognized by all professionals—and how come you haven't gotten some sort of prize for it?"

Following a successful diagnosis and treatment outcome, others will invariably say—once they become even more comfortable and confident: "If what you say makes perfect sense, even to my child, and though everyone has noticed Johnny's remarkable improvement, why won't these very same professionals accept your theories and methods as valid?"

"Why do they take full credit for my son's sudden and dramatic improvement or attribute it to a developmental spurt—when he never significantly benefitted from tutoring for years nor spurted before?" And why do they remain silent when I ask them: "If tutoring and spurting helped him, how do you explain all his prior symptoms immediately returning in full force once medications are stopped? And why do these very same dyslexic symptoms rapidly disappear again with medication? And how can academic tutor-ing result in balance/coordination/rhythmic improve-ments as well as disappearance of his nausea, dizziness, motion-sickness as well as his fears of heights and carnival rides—and even closed spaces and crowds?"

"Why do they say you haven't published your research in scientific journals when in fact I have your papers; but they never seem to read or reference them?"

"Why do they say that you 'cure everyone' when in fact you claim only to help?"

"Why do they say *you're* controversial when all other theories have gotten us nowhere and no proof exists to substantiate them? Shouldn't non-working and nonsensi-cal theories and theorists be considered 'controversial'—rather than the other way around?"

"Why do they get so angry when your name is men-tioned or when we say we're going to your office for hope and answers?"

"Why are some parents afraid to really know what's wrong with their children and so avoid a clear-cut medical diagnosis and possible help?" "Why do they accept a diag-nosis of LD (learning disability) from experts when in fact they know this before they went to them for more under-standing and help? Are they afraid to face the truth?"

"Why wasn't there a line outside your office to Kansas City (or wherever they come from)?"

"Why did one of my friends who clearly noted academic improvements in her son following use of antihistamines for asthma question your work—after her physician told her that antihistamines couldn't possibly help dyslexic symptoms?"

Needless to say, almost all past and current patients feel, think, or actively voice many of these concerns. And they all deserve answers. Although I have tried in my other works to present the reader and patients with the background and history highlighting the way I came to discover what I did, many of their questions remain unanswered. Accordingly, I will once again attempt to review and analyze the critics and criticism I have met along the twisting and turning road leading me to my previous books: *A Solution to the Riddle—Dyslexia, Smart But Feeling Dumb, Total Concentration,* and *Phobia Free.* And I will present as much detailed and quoted critical content as possible—similar to the detail described in the dyslexic and related case histories—so that independent conclusions may be drawn.

As a psychiatrist, I have often been accused by neurotic and especially psychotic patients of everything under the sun—both good and bad. And regardless of their unrealistic quality, all their statements invariably have an inner psychological meaning. To understand this content, analysts must serve as a "neutral screen" to facilitate a patient projecting highly charged and important emotional content—biased and otherwise—so that this content might be analyzed in the context of the person's past and present.

Thus, for example, a patient longing for a beloved but dead parent may begin to worship the treating analyst. Abused patients may rant and rave at therapists, indicating angry background content to be explored. Those lied to and/or betrayed as children may not trust others, and might even lie to and betray others, themselves, etc. Those competing with parents and siblings will attempt similar tactics with their analysts. In this way, psychoanalysts can expose important unconscious conflicts and behavioral attitudes within patients, attitudes significantly influencing their interpersonal relationships and even their professional lives and scientific beliefs—perhaps even explaining some highly distorted and unrealistic attitudes towards my research bordering on neurotic and even psychopathic.

As most readers familiar with my research must know, my neurological concepts about dyslexia have triggered similar projections from critics—good and bad. And the analyses of this projected criticism—good and especially bad—have led to important insights. Indeed, the positive criticism has clearly highlighted and thus catalyzed research points needing additional clarification or modification. And the negative criticism has indicated important resistance or bias factors within critics requiring scientific exposure and resolution. In retrospect, were it not for my attempts to understand and resolve all the criticism to date, the true depth and scope of dyslexia would never have materialized. And the nature and meaning of the bias factors maintaining the dyslexic riddles in force for almost one hundred years would have remained hidden.

Since conscious and unconscious deception and denials were found to be significant defense mechanisms utilized by many involved in the dyslexia movement for both political gain and self-aggrandizement, it seemed appropriate to call this work *A Scientific Watergate—Dyslexia.*

For simplicity's sake, the negative critics and criticisms inspiring me to complete my dyslexia, Attention Deficit Disorder (ADD) and phobia research as well as this work can be separated into *three primary phases or waves*: 1) the beginning criticism or the Orton (Dyslexia) Society Meeting in 1975, 2) criticism from 1975-1992, and 3) *Acceptance Without Reference*—the Rodin Dyslexia Conference, September 1992.

Doubt and Gossip

Before concluding this final segment, I'd like to present correspondence (12/4/84) from the dean of a college to Mrs. Carter, the mother of one of my successfully treated patients. By reading the content, you will quickly grasp the *doubt and damage* done by special interest groups such as the Orton Society as well as the distortion by those running and profiting by organizations for the learning disabled. Hopefully, *A Scientific Watergate—Dyslexia* will help clarify many of the doubts raised and answer questions to follow:

Dear Mrs. Carter:

". . . I benefitted by knowing about your referral to Dr. Levinson. I had never heard of a drug treatment program for any kind of learning disability (except those also tied in with hyperactivity) and was interested in learning more.

I had occasion to talk with Mr. Richard Pierce of the Foreman School. That high school is for learning disabled students. He visited campus recently and when I asked if he had heard of any such treatment programs, he said "Oh you mean Levinson" and shared his perspective. He was quite critical of that treatment and mentioned numerous students they had who became chemically dependent on the treatment programs.

He told me of the Orton Society and commented they had issued a publication reviewing Levinson's research. I didn't know if you had seen this, so I wrote for a copy and wanted to pass it along. Certainly any new therapy will have its critics and supporters. I believe in learning from all sides and I know you do, so I thought I would pass a copy of this along to you. . . ."

To my knowledge, *no* patient of mine ever became chemically dependent on the medications I use. Instead, *is not Pierce's LD school economically dependent on dyslexics?* Although I had initially decided to present you with my responding letter to Mrs. Carter, I decided to skip it, as *A Scientific Watergate—Dyslexia* provides a more complete answer.

CHAPTER 2

An Overview—Formal

A Simple Choice: Either my many and varied dyslexic patients are deliberately malingering (misrepresenting) their inner-ear-determined improvements and corresponding symptoms *or* my many and varied dyslexic critics are malingering expertise.[1] The choice is yours. My patients and their loved ones have already made theirs.

Ever since dyslexic children were first recognized by two English physicians, Morgan and Kerr (1896-97), there developed the natural assumption and conviction that this disorder was due to an impairment within the dominant thinking-speaking center (angular gyrus) of the brain—the cerebral cortex. They reasoned that if an autopsy-proven lesion within this angular gyrus led adults to completely lose their ability to recognize the meaning of written symbols (alexia), then children failing to normally acquire reading skills must have a defect within this very same area of the thinking brain. In other words, *dyslexia = alexia.* And since alexia is a severe reading comprehension disorder with a very poor prognosis, the same was thought to be

---

[1]Within this text, the terms *inner-ear, cerebellum, cerebellar or cerebellar-vestibular (CV)* are used synonymously. And for purposes of simplicity, they have been defined as fine tuners to the brain.

true of dyslexia. Variations of this traditionally sanctioned view of dyslexia have dominated research efforts over the last century despite a vast array of refuting data, defensively called "controversial."

Unfortunately, all these 100-year-old efforts have led to *a complete and thorough medical dead-end* despite escalating scientific investigations by brilliant minds and billions of dollars. To date, the traditionalists have absolutely no way of medically diagnosing and treating the dyslexic disorder, nor can they neurophysiologically explain the vast array of symptoms characterizing this syndrome. Something was very, very wrong. And upon analysis, it appeared clear that the cerebral-language theorists were as incapable of solving their medical void and resulting riddles as they were of accepting any breakthrough research outside their scientific domain. Indeed, leading dyslexia experts were found defending their century-old theoretical positions from external insights despite the crying need of millions and millions for hope and help. And for ego-related reasons, these experts attempted, via collusion, to maintain control of their "scientific monopoly" at all costs. And the cost was ours—not theirs.

Over the last 20-30 years, my patient-based clinical research on over 25,000 personally examined dyslexics has clearly and repeatedly demonstrated *that the quality and prognosis of the reading disorder in dyslexia is as different from alexia as day and night*. Thus, for example, in sharp contrast to the *non-reading alexics* with *primary comprehension impairments*, the vast majority of dyslexics experience *only memory, directional, tracking, concentration and delayed processing* difficulties with read content. And the latter resulted in letter and word forgetting, omissions, insertions, blurring and movement as well as spatially related reversals. With maturation, tutoring, and related therapies—especially the use of inner-ear-enhancing medications—the reading prognosis among dyslexics was found to be very favorable provided secondary emotional scarring does not occur. Accordingly, most dyslexics eventually compensate and so learn to read well and even very well, thus explaining the presence of dyslexic doctors, lawyers, politicians, scientists, etc.

And since the quality, severity, and prognosis of the reading disorder in dyslexia and alexia were found to be completely different, it seemed reasonable to assume that the respective origins of these disorders might also be different. Indeed, this assumption as well as that suggesting the traditionalists were searching for the origins of dyslexia in the wrong theoretical haystack clearly and simply explained their *lack of any diagnostic/therapeutic medical progress over the last 100 years.*

The above-mentioned observations and reasoning also readily explained the traditionalists' need to *deny* such refuting data as: (1) the presence of potent compensatory mechanisms in dyslexia and thus the existence of millions and millions of dyslexics with less than severe reading-score impairments despite the obvious presence of "typical" dyslexic symptoms (in reading, writing, spelling, math, memory, speech, sense of direction and time, grammar, concentration/distraction/activity, balance and coordination . . .); (2) the complete absence of any definitive corroborating evidence of cerebral dysfunction in dyslexics; (3) the presence of only balance, coordination and rhythmic impairments of inner-ear origin among the dyslexia majority; (4) the triggering of temporary inner-ear-determined dyslexic symptoms in normal subjects by excessive spinning and "space dyslexia" in the astronauts at zero gravity; (5) the development of permanent dyslexic symptoms following inner-ear infections, trauma (whiplash and concussion states), etc.; and (6) the successful inner-ear-enhancing therapies (eye exercises, occupational or vestibular training, tinted lenses, etc.)—especially the use of antimotion-sickness medications such as that demonstrated in countless dyslexics.

Having recognized that *dyslexia is completely different from alexia* and that *only* inner-ear-determined balance, coordination and rhythmic neurophysiological signs characterize dyslexia, it seemed reasonable to postulate that this disorder was of inner-ear rather than of cerebral origin. And to explain all the many and varied sensory-motor signs and symptoms characterizing dyslexics, the inner-ear system was assumed to process and sequence the total sensory input as it does the motor output. In other words, the inner-ear was analogized as similar to the vertical and horizontal TV stabilizers—fine-tuning each and every sensory-motor channel of information entering and leaving the brain.

Accordingly, any dysfunction of the inner-ear stabilizers results in corresponding sensory-motor "channel drifting," blurring or sequential distortion similar to what happens on TV screens. And the thinking-speaking brain "watching" and "listening" to these drifting signals has difficulty processing this temporal and spatially distorted information unless it learns to compensate via descrambling mechanisms. So the thinking brain *is* significantly involved in dyslexia but only *secondarily* so. By contrast, the signals reaching the thinking brain in alexics are clear, but they cannot be recognized and understood—resulting in severe *primary* comprehension disturbances and a corresponding poor prognosis, no matter what is done to help.[1]

Eventually, all these inner-ear conceptualizations of dyslexia were proven and found consistent with both past and recent independently formulated neurophysiological

[1]As discussed in my prior works, both the psychoanalytic and neurological views of dyslexia were characterized by one and the same error: The symptomatic outcome of the dyslexic disorder was mistakenly confused with its cause. Thus, for example, the secondary emotional symptoms were used to postulate a primary psychological dyslexia origin. And the secondary difficulties in seeing, remembering, processing and thus "understanding" read content were used to postulate an alexic or aphasic cerebral origin. In other words, psychological and neurological experts used only those observations needed to prove their preconceived notions while denying all refuting data.

theories. And new and unique diagnostic instruments were designed (3D Optical, Auditory and Tactile Scanners) to rapidly and effectively measure the respective sensory and motor processing impairments underlying the diverse symptoms characterizing the inner-ear-determined dyslexic disorder. *As a result, these and related physiologically based methods can now be used to screen very young children for those predisposed towards developing reading and related symptoms.*[1] *And thus prediction and early medical treatment can now minimize or prevent both the severity of their dyslexic outcome as well as the resulting emotional scarring.* Moreover, these diagnostic screening tests are completely independent of all the secondary compensatory vs. decompensatory variables biasing the diagnostic reliability of the traditionally used pencil-and-paper psychological-educational tests.[2]

By contrast, the traditionalists continue to erroneously define dyslexia as a severe reading-score impairment in which individuals must be at least two years below peers and/or potential. As a result, these experts must wait for dyslexics to fall into an alexia-like reading "coma" before a definitive diagnosis is made. And all "non-comatose" or reading-score-compensated dyslexics are mistakenly considered non-dyslexics and called by other names, including inattentive, lazy, spoiled, stupid, rebellious, etc. Unless of

---

[1] In addition to the *3D Scanners*, a series of other CV-based neurophysiological signs and tests, such as *ataxiometry* and *electronystagmography* (ENG), useful for diagnosing and treating the inner-ear disorder underlying dyslexia will be described in Book II. The symbol *3D* denotes my redefinition of dyslexia by the term *Dysmetric Dyslexia and Dyspraxia*. To date, my investigations of auditory and tactile sequencing have been minimal vs. visual sequencing.

Investigators Kohen-Raz and Fawcett and Roderick have independently correlated imbalance with reading impairment, further verifying the common inner-ear origin of both syndromes.

[2] There are many external variables interfering with these pencil-and-paper results, e.g., IQ, anxiety, concentration/distractibility, frustration tolerance (tester and "testee"), prior tutoring, socio-economic and parental influences, etc.

course their reading scores drop beyond the "magical" two-year mark. And suddenly they become "dyslexic," until compensation may once again deprive them of a traditionally sanctioned diagnosis. Nonsensical? It sure seemed that way to me—even 20 years ago. But then again my judgment is based on experience with dyslexics, whereas that of the traditionalists is entirely theoretical. And as you will clearly see, their theory was dead wrong.

Although *dyslexia* is clearly a complex syndrome of many symptoms occurring in varied combinations and differing intensities, the erroneous analogy of dyslexia with alexia led the traditionalists to yet another mistaken equation. Indeed, an analysis of the traditional dyslexia definition highlights the striking fallacy by which experts also unwittingly equate the total syndrome of many and varied symptoms called *dyslexia* with *only severe* degrees of *only one* of its highly variable and overdetermined reading-score parameters—also referred to by them as *"dyslexia."* In other words they nonsensically conceptualized that *dyslexia = "dyslexia."*[1]

Perhaps an analogy would be helpful. Everyone now knows that diabetes is a syndrome of many and varied symptoms and that the blood-sugars in diabetics may vary from one extreme to another. Yet many years ago, diabetics were recognized only by their comatose states and so it seemed reasonable to assume that *diabetes = coma*. However, no one would consider this antiquated equation valid today. In other words, how can the complex syndrome called *diabetes* be equated with *only* severe degrees of *only*

---

[1]As is readily apparent by the dyslexic case histories presented throughout this work, dyslexia is a syndrome characterized by a diverse array of both reading and non-reading symptoms in writing, spelling, math, memory, speech, spatial orientation and timing, grammar, concentration/distractibility/hyperactivity (ADHD), balance/coordination/rhythm, mood and anxiety as well as psychosomatic difficulties (vertigo, headaches, nausea, motion sickness, bed-wetting). To date, many of these symptoms coexisting with "dyslexia" have artificially and erroneously been fragmented into differently named syndromes and are considered to be due to separate and distinct origins. Nonsensical—but true!

one of its highly variable and overdetermined blood-sugar parameters and resulting comatose symptoms? It can't—any more than dyslexia can be equated with "dyslexia" or only severely impaired "comatose-like" reading scores. And as the dyslexics within this text will clearly and concisely tell and show you, their reading scores may be normal or even superior and yet they will still exhibit typical dyslexic reading and related symptoms with writing, spelling, math, etc. Thus contrary to the definition of the traditionalists, *dyslexia* ≠ *"dyslexia."*

Perhaps some of you are amazed by the experts' confusion over *dyslexia* = *"dyslexia."* No doubt you are wondering: How could so many bright and even gifted dyslexia experts reason in such a simplistic, tunnel view? What motivated them to do so? Obviously these very same questions occurred to me as well. And the answers were tragically clear: To maintain their dominant status quo the experts were forced to cling to their century-old conviction that dyslexia and alexia were equivalent disorders. And since the proven cerebral defect in alexia invariably results in a severe and *non-compensating* reading comprehension impairment, the traditionalists assumed, really concluded, that the same held for dyslexia—despite all the refuting evidence coming from dyslexics. But obviously the traditionalists were listening only to themselves and prior experts rather than their patients.

After publishing these "revolutionary" conceptualizations over 20 years ago and having demonstrated that inner-ear-enhancing medications similar to those used by the astronauts can rapidly and dramatically help more than 75% of treated dyslexics—further verifying the inner-ear origins of this disorder—something very strange and unexpected happened. The dyslexia traditionalists refused to acknowledge the presence of clear-cut and stated cerebellar or inner-ear dysfunctioning in dyslexia—even when objectively corroborated by independent neurological and ENT (ear, nose, and throat) inner-ear experts called neurotologists.

Brazenly, the traditionally-minded neurological dyslexia experts privately and publicly refuted—denied—their very own clearly-worded inner-ear or cerebellar findings in dyslexic case reports, whereas the ENT experts solidly backed their own inner-ear data.

Moreover, at an Orton Dyslexia Society meeting allegedly designed to scientifically and objectively review the cerebellar signs found and reported by a colleague, Jan Frank, and myself in the *Journal of the American Academy of Child Psychiatry* (1973), the Columbia Presbyterian neurologists performing the "blind" neurological studies *declined invitations to appear.* Instead, they had a colleague nonsensically claim that: (1) *The "blindly" examined dyslexics with typical symptoms who were not demonstrated to be at least two years below peers and/or potential in reading-scores were not dyslexic;*[1] and (2) *the specifically reported and documented mild and moderate cerebellar neurological signs in the "blindly" examined dyslexic sample didn't count diagnostically.* By contrast, the diagnosis of minimal *cerebral* dysfunction was maintained despite the complete absence of cerebral neurological signs. In other words, both the stated presence of clear-cut and definite cerebellar signs and the absence of any and all localizing cerebral neurological signs in the "blindly" examined dyslexics were denied and so not factored into the final diagnostic equation. Amazing? Sure seemed that way to me!

By contrast, the ENT experts, readily acknowledging their reported inner-ear abnormalities in dyslexics, were never invited to present and discuss their own data by the Ortonians despite their desire to do so. In other words, the organizers of the conference or "set-up" attempted by hook or by crook to refute the reliability and validity of the breakthrough inner-ear research as well as a clinically-based and derived redefinition of dyslexia independent of

[1]The term "blind" refers to an objective examination of data without prior knowledge of the experimental aims or objectives.

reading-score severity.[1] Additionally, the traditionalists attacked the inner-ear medication treatment of dyslexics by use of such derogatory and frightening terms as "100% cures," "magical cures," "dangerous," "subjective," and "anecdotal." And they refused all attempts at replication of these published results and corroborating verbatim patient reports of improvement, such as those presented here, despite the use of real names and locations.

No doubt you are all wondering about the word "brazen" I chose to describe the "chutzpa" motivating leading and well-respected experts to publicly and privately *deny* their findings without the slightest regret or fear of being criticized by others fully cognizant of their blatant "error." Well I was too until I listened to their colleague publicly claim, by analogy, *that women who are "mildly" and "moderately" pregnant are not really pregnant.* And no one listening to this nonsense dared challenge this traditionalist expert and card-carrying Orton member—aside from me. And no one else asked why the "blind" neurologists refused to attend any and all scientific meetings specifically designed to discuss *their* "blind" cerebellar findings in dyslexic cases sent them—findings they continued to deny both privately and publicly, e.g., the *New York Times* (1974) and *Infectious Diseases* (1974) (see Chapter 3).

Well, you don't have to be a Freudian analyst to figure out what was and still is going on, although it helps. All these dyslexia experts herd together in "scientific clubs" to protect their turf and important body parts—processes I half-jokingly call "herding," "clubbing" and "turfing." And so armed, they attempt to dominate and reign supreme while "clubbing" all outsiders with challenging views. Con-

---

[1] I redefined dyslexia as an inner-ear-determined spatial-temporal and sensory-motor dysfunction in dynamic equilibrium with compensatory vs. decompensatory vectors. By contrast, since the traditionalists viewed the reading-score impairment in dyslexia as equivalent to alexia, they had no need to build compensatory and decompensatory vectors into a "hopeless" or "comatose" condition.

sidering their "ennobled" status quos, why should they investigate the validity of so-called "controversial" diagnostic/therapeutic breakthroughs if these breakthroughs threaten to shrink their egos, finances, power, etc.? And obviously they appear unconcerned with millions and millions of dyslexics desperate for medical treatment, despite protestations to the contrary. Were they truly concerned, would they have reacted so abusively to therapeutic breakthroughs similar to those reported and documented within this text? Would they have failed to attempt replication of results or at least speaking to treated patients such as those presented and to be presented?

As described, this scientific Watergate process in dyslexia was officially recognized 20 years ago. And it was carefully documented in Chapter 13 of my medical text *A Solution to the Riddle—Dyslexia* (1980). As expected, this process continued unabated despite a wide array of supporting research until a recent Rodin Society dyslexia meeting in 1992, co-sponsored by The New York Academy of Sciences, finally presented *cerebellar-dyslexia research*—but without due reference to the content presented in my prior works and now here (see Chapter 18).

Instead of inspiring and catalyzing traditionalist dyslexia experts and their organizations to update their 100-year-old nonfunctional conceptualizations and zero diagnostic/therapeutic medical progress curves, the breakthrough inner-ear research triggered a deadly series of highly biased scientific meetings and vicious pseudoscientific attacks. And the intended outcome was clear: *The traditionalists were determined to continue their comfortable and profitable status quos.* And to do so, countless dyslexics were unwittingly sacrificed, needlessly deprived of hope and help for the past twenty years.

No doubt many readers will find all this difficult to believe. And I can't blame you—for I certainly did. But the facts presented here more than speak for themselves. Indeed, their analysis has led to an exposé of *A Scientific Watergate* process in dyslexia no less devastating than that corresponding to the political exposé during Richard M. Nixon's presidency. Indeed, the fall-out from this Watergate appeared far more reaching and the denial and resulting moral confusion within dyslexia research and researchers seemed deeper, deadlier, and potentially more catastrophic: *It directly deprived 20% of the population of meaningful medical diagnosis and treatment. And it indirectly deprived their loved ones of hope. And it did so—unchecked—for the last 20 years, despite all my efforts. No one else appeared to care or dare enough!*

No doubt you must by now be wondering about the socio-economic consequences of this Watergate process: *In short, the socio-economic ripple effect by which undiagnosed and untreated dyslexics drop-out of school and drift into crime, violence, abuse, drugs, alcohol, depression, anxiety states, homelessness, repeated accidents, joblessness, divorce—forever feeling dumb, ugly, clumsy and brainless—is staggering, perhaps even equivalent in dollars and cents alone to that characterizing the national deficit. Might eliminating this and related scientific Watergate processes not only relieve the resulting suffering of millions but also eliminate the "National Deficit Disorder"?*

To date, the Orton Society sanction and their symbiotic motivated "experts" appear driven to block out all new therapeutic attempts from reaching the homes and hearts of dyslexics and their loved ones. And unless this defensive scientific "abscess" is exposed, analyzed and lanced, the traditionalist century-old status quo and dead end may continue endlessly. Accordingly, the aims of *A Scientific Watergate—Dyslexia* are simple: (1) to end the ignorance, denial, and bias characterizing the traditional dyslexia research efforts over the last 100 years, and thus (2) to bring hope and help to all dyslexics and their loved ones.

And to attempt these aims, I have deliberately chosen to present the stories of real dyslexics and loved ones who have donated their personal experiences as well as their names and photographs so that others might benefit as they did. In other words, I anticipated that reading the case histories of picture-real patients will teach the reader what dyslexics and dyslexia are all about and what benefits might be expected from medical treatment: *For most dyslexics know much more about their disorder than do their esteemed traditionalist experts. And in retrospect, I was taught reality by patients, and fantasy and bias by the experts.* Indeed, the attempt to sharpen and thus highlight the amazing differences between traditional fantasy and dyslexic reality led me to repeatedly alternate critical vs. patient-based content, and eventually resulted in the unique content and styling characterizing *A Scientific Watergate—Dyslexia.* Additionally, I have chosen to reference my critics as well as my patients so that all readers can judge the reality and honesty of this work as well as its urgent need.

In retrospect, it appears that the traditionalists neither spoke nor listened to their dyslexic patients. They just tested them to death at arms length—often from ivory towers—using a seemingly infinite variety of psychological and neurophysiological tests. And sad to say, they unwittingly forced results into preconceived theoretical molds, regardless of the fit, for publication as well as related defensive purposes. In retrospect, I was forced to consider: Had these dyslexia experts not been overwhelmed and obsessed by the "magical" powers of the thinking-speaking brain, might they have considered it far simpler and more objective to first attempt a rough sketch of the dyslexic disorder—as subjectively described by dyslexics themselves—before blindly but "objectively" investigating and statistically analyzing complex neurophysiological and psychological unknowns in complete scientific and biased darkness.

In contrast, I listened carefully to my many patients as I encourage the reader to do. And I changed and modified the hundred-year-old preexisting thinking-linguistic brain conceptualizations to fit the evolving inner-ear-determined dyslexic reality. This led to my books *A Solution to the Riddle—Dyslexia, Smart But Feeling Dumb, Phobia Free, Total Concentration,* and a series of research papers—and ultimately to this work. In other words, for dyslexics to be helped, the traditional fiction had to be replaced by scientific reality, regardless of controversy triggered and personal gain.

And since the traditional thinking-language-brain cerebral theories were *only* able to explain the existence of severe reading-score impairments (what they called "dyslexia") in dyslexia and nothing else, I thought it essential to simplify my conceptualizations so that all of the many and varied symptoms characterizing my database of more than 25,000 dyslexics could readily be explained and understood, even by dyslexic children. Accordingly, I wrote two additional "therapeutic novels" to help dyslexic children understand their condition: *The Upside-Down Kids* and *Turning Around—The Upside-Down Kids.* My endeavor was twofold: I truly believe that if something is *really* understood, it can be simply explained to children. And when bright but dumb-feeling dyslexics—children and adults— truly understand the scientific origins of their diverse symptoms, they no longer feel compelled to blame themselves. They no longer feel as dumb, ugly, stupid, clumsy, brainless. Indeed, many feel infinitely better. Not so alone. Not so defensive and overwhelmed. They suddenly and clearly recognize that they have only one disorder with hundreds of related symptoms instead of hundreds of confusing, hopeless, and overpowering *separate* problems. They suddenly realize that they are neither freaks nor brain damaged. They merely have a simple "fine-tuning" disorder within their inner-ear systems—like millions of others—which can easily be explained and successfully treated.[1]

By contrast, the traditionalists and their theories explain and offer *nothing*—except to those with analytic minds who know what lies behind double-talk and such meaningless but frightening-sounding diagnostic phrases as *minimal brain damage, minimal cerebral dysfunction* and *static encephalopathy. Nothing*—except the unwitting and mistaken fragmentation of the dyslexic syndrome into scores of separately named and considered disorders, e.g., *dysgraphia* (poor writing), *dyscalculia* (poor arithmetic ability), *Attention Deficit-Hyperactivity Disorder* (poor concentration and activity levels), etc. *Nothing*—except the confusion of simple inner-ear-determined and treatable *dysphasic* or speech symptoms, such as those attributed to President Bush, with that of a severe language disorder of thinking-brain origin called *aphasia. Nothing*—except the ability to defend their turf by scaring away questioning parents and dyslexics with threatening diagnostic terms, pomposity, and arms-length testing procedures.

Hopefully, the message within this book will resound clearly and loudly despite my inexperienced organizational abilities and writing style. After all, this work is clinically based and aimed. And I have no illusions as to my literary abilities or, rather, disabilities. Moreover, if my style were summarized, it would have to be termed "Freudian-analytic," free-associative, and *emotional* rather than *dry, compulsively sequenced, and quantitative.* Or how about "subjectively-objective?"

And so with the above apology clearly in mind, I'd like to conclude this overview with a mother and son's new beginning. The following content highlights the traditionally sanctioned delusion whereby breakthrough treatment is denied and considered "controversial" and the current therapeutic void is found perfectly acceptable and goes un-

[1]Recall the initial insight-triggered improvement leading Robert Charles King (Chapter 1-A) to want to help others as he was helped.

challenged. Additionally, this clinical data symbolizes my instinctive desire: (1) to teach you about dyslexia and its medical treatment as I was taught—via direct patient and parent contact; and (2) to maximize and catalyze your interest with first-hand clinical experience so that ultimately you might more easily endure and independently judge the presented critical content and intent constituting this work.

Eric Cole

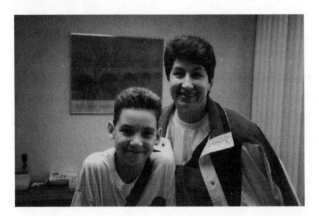

According to Eric's mother, Mrs. Susan Cole:

> By the time we brought our son, Eric, to see you in May of 1990, we were absolutely desperate in our search for answers to his problems. They included dyslexia, dysgraphia, violent out-of-control behavior episodes, impulsivity, low frustration tolerance, etc. He was then just seven years old. Life at home was unbearably stressful under these circumstances. School was a terrible experience for Eric, and I dreaded the almost daily telephone calls reporting his latest behavioral outburst.[1]

[1]Because Eric's dyscontrol syndrome, in addition to his dyslexic and related severe ADHD symptoms, was severe and had an epileptic quality, I advised Mrs. Cole to seek independent neurological consultations, and alternative forms of overlapping therapies. As a result, Dr. Hart Peterson, one of my critics, eventually examined Eric. However, he refused to treat Eric's dyscontrol symptoms until a simple antihistamine, dramatically helpful for his inner-ear-related dyslexic symptoms, was discontinued (see Chapter 5). This case and its traditional management provides the content for a chapter within Book II.

We had been making the rounds from one doctor to another from the time Eric was about 1 year old. At first we were told we were neurotic and that there was nothing wrong with him. Then he was sent for his first psychiatric evaluation at age 2½, and again at age 5 with yet another doctor. It seems that no one had a clue as to what was wrong, and worse yet, how to treat it.

Not only were you able to diagnose his problem at our first visit but you prescribed a regimen of medications that returned our life to a semblance of normalcy—because Eric's behavior was finally brought under control and his learning disabilities improved. We never realized how many aspects of Eric's being were subtly affected by all of his problems until we slowly put him on each prescribed medication and witnessed the changes.

It has not mattered what other doctors we have spoken with since meeting you, but at the mention of your name we get a lot of negative comments about your theories and medicine therapy but we are offered no alternative solutions.

We have recently had our son re-evaluated by a child psychiatrist and a neurologist specializing in neuro-developmental disabilities. We have also begun to work with a Behavior Management Therapist. They of course had the typical reaction upon hearing your name. They all advocated we take Eric off most, if not all, of the medications prescribed by you.

It was our family's decision to give this a try to see how Eric would actually do without medication after all these years. To chart any behavior changes during this time the Behavior Therapist had asked Eric's teacher and ourselves to fill out a daily checklist of ten different behavior characteristics. These checklists were begun: 1) prior to the slow removal of medication, 2) during the no medication period, and 3) after resumption of medication. Needless to say, as Eric was taken off of medication, the behavior changes were dramatic with many of the symptoms coming back with a vengeance. As we added the medication back there was a marked improvement in the ratings. By the way, the teacher was never informed about any changes to Eric's medication. She was only asked to help us by filling in the daily checklist. This proved to us yet again that while many in the medical profession consider your theories and treatment methods to be very controversial, they offer us a lot of rhetoric but have no alternative treatments.[1]

Thank you Dr. Levinson for being the pioneering spirit that you are.

A Follow-Up Evaluation

The following content was voiced by Mrs. Susan Cole immediately prior to the printing of this book.

Eric is now in the 5th grade. He is mainstreaming this year for the first time—science and social studies. He is doing A+ work and we are thrilled at his progress . . . Eric is very proud of his achievements and realizes that in spite of his dyslexia and dysgraphia he can be a success. His pride in himself makes all the difference.

We had Eric try going without medication at the recommendation of another neurologist and his pediatrician who did not feel Eric should be medicated. The results were a disaster. All the progress made disappeared. Eric's behavior deteriorated and he could not attend to his work at school. Had we listened to all the other doctors along the way who have criticized Dr. Levinson's approach, what kind of life could be expected for Eric? He would be faced with failure and frustration. Instead he now sees himself as capable of success.

---

[1]Despite the traditionalists' denials, many such formal, informal, and even blindly controlled observations have clearly and objectively demonstrated the value of inner-ear medications in dyslexia as well as the inner-ear (CV) basis of this very same syndrome.

By the way, there is even more good news in all of this. Eric was tested for and accepted into a program for the "academically talented." This could never have been realized before Dr. Levinson's help.

I say bravo—to a very brave little boy named Eric and also to a dedicated man like Dr. Levinson who has been willing to stand up against the tide of criticism to help those who would otherwise not be helped. Dr. Levinson, thank you for this very special gift.

Summary: A Simple Choice

In the final analysis, *everything* I learned about dyslexia came from listening to and examining countless dyslexic patients. By contrast, the traditionalists learned *all* they needed to know from prior experts who learned from prior experts, etc., etc., etc.—a "parroting process" going back to 1896. And sad to say, *all* their progress over the last 100 years can be summarized by two erroneous equations: *dyslexia = alexia,* and *dyslexia = "dyslexia."*

To defensively preserve their self-serving status quos while covering a hard-to-believe clinical-theoretical void, some critical traditionalists have attempted to discredit breakthrough cerebellar-vestibular or inner-ear diagnostic/therapeutic formulations using denial and related biased or distorted criticism. And since this inner-ear content was derived from more than 25,000 dyslexics, a simple choice must be made: *Either my many and varied dyslexic patients are deliberately malingering (misrepresenting) their inner-ear-determined improvements and corresponding symptoms or my many and varied dyslexic critics are malingering expertise. The choice is yours. My patients and their loved ones have already made theirs.*

Section II

Criticism
and Its
Analysis

F̲OR inner-ear-based dyslexia insights to gain acceptance, it was imperative to analyze the traditionalist critics and their criticism so that all might clearly understand both their biased symptomatic quality and underlying determinants. And since my critics were many and varied, tied together by common *self-serving bonds*, the collective content to be presented comprised the vast bulk of this work and so was symbolically responsible for the *Watergate* title.

For ease of description, the criticism was subdivided into three phases: *The First Critical Wave and Responses, The Second Critical Wave and Responses, and The Third and Last Critical Wave.* And to best appreciate these critics and their criticism, contrasting inner-ear-based insights and dramatic therapeutic improvements were interspersed at every twist and turn. Since the *second tidal wave* was far bigger than the others, it was further divided in three parts (A, B, C), to avoid drowning.

Hopefully, this rather unique and perhaps dyslexic-inspired organizational technique will achieve its basic aim— to bring hope and help to countless millions.

The First Critical Wave
And
Responses

CHAPTER 3

The First Big Denial

My first breakthrough 1973 research concepts were published with Jan Frank in a leading peer-reviewed scientific periodical, *Journal of the American Academy of Child Psychiatry*. The title, "Dysmetric dyslexia and dyspraxia—hypothesis and study," highlights significant anti-traditional concepts.

- The term *dyspraxia* was added to the dyslexia concept so as to reflect the various motor disturbances affecting balance and coordination in writing and speech, as well as a variety of fine, gross and rhythmic motor activities.[1]

[1]The cerebellum—the brain of animals—is a highly complex computer for our inner-ear system. Although traditionally thought to regulate only balance and coordination functions as well as motion and proprioception (muscle and tendon sensors throughout our body), my research and that of prior and recent distinguished neurophysiologists have recognized that it modulates all sensory-motor and related cognitive and even language functions. Traditionally, cerebellar dysfunction is detected by the "typical" balance, coordination, and rhythmic symptoms as well as slurred and disarticulated—even scrambled—speech. Specifically, there are difficulties in: (1) balancing on one foot—eyes open and closed, (2) walking a straight line in tandem—heel-to-toe, (3) touching finger-to-nose—eyes open and closed, (4) rhythmically rotating outstretched arms in opposing to-and-fro directions, (5) touching and sequencing finger-to-finger while distracted, etc. (For greater detail, refer to my prior works and references as well as Book II.)

The *dyspraxic* or *motor* symptoms I defined as characterizing dyslexics are also discussed in Chapters 17 and 18. Within these chapters you will find how these motor symptoms were presented in 1992 as if new—and even attributed to a cerebellar origin *without* proper reference.

- The term *dysmetria* reflects an inner-ear or cerebellar-vestibular (CV)-determined spatial-temporal defect underlying the many and varied symptoms characterizing dyslexia; and

- An attempt was made to distinguish this inner-ear or cerebellar-vestibular (CV)-determined *dyslexic* disorder from possible alexic-like thinking-speaking (cerebral) impairments that might exist—although I personally did not come across any during my examinations of thousands of cases.[1]

In other words, the tongue-twisting term *Dysmetric Dyslexia and Dyspraxia* (DDD or 3D) was used to emphasize: 1) that dyslexia was a complex inner-ear-determined sensory-motor syndrome rather than merely a severe reading disorder of cerebral origin, and thus 2) that this disorder could not be equated with either alexia or "dyslexia" (severely impaired reading ability). And so a new synonym was reluctantly added to the thirty-six others counted by McDonald Critchley, one of the leading pioneers in this area. *But as might be readily apparent, DDD symbolized a unique and radical departure from all prior conceptualizations of this disorder.* DDD thus clearly and simply explained this study's results:

- 97% of 115 dyslexic children were found to have definitive localizing neurological signs of a CV dysfunction—suggesting a CV origin.

- Only 3 CV dysfunctioning dyslexics within a subsample of 40 evidenced possible (not definite) signs of a cerebral impairment when using the widest traditional assumptions—suggesting the latter possible cerebral dysfunctioning, if indeed present, was a coincidental rather than a primary determinant.

---

[1]Alexia is a complete loss of the ability to recognize the meaning of letters and words. This *severe* reading impairment results from specific lesions within the thinking-speech centers of the brain—the dominant cerebral cortex.

The "Blind" Cerebellar-Dyslexia Data

In order to verify the inner-ear or cerebellar-vestibular findings independently and objectively, a sub-sample of typical dyslexic patients were sent "blindly," without any identifying data or scientific aims, to:

1) two outstanding pediatric neurologists, Drs. Arnold Gold and Sidney Carter, for independent examination so as to validate the presence of the same inner-ear or cerebellar neurological signs that I had found; and

2) inner-ear experts (neurotologists) for specialized tests to determine what percentage of the dyslexic patients examined had inner-ear dysfunctioning.

To ensure objectivity, none of the examining physicians were told anything concerning the nature of my research. And the results of their examinations were indeed rewarding. Specifically, an analysis of the "blindly" reported neurological findings confirmed that:

- 96% or 20 out of 22 dyslexics had signs and symptoms diagnostic of, or consistent with, a cerebellar-vestibular (inner-ear) dysfunction or deficit.[1]

- *None* had hard and fast neurological signs of a cerebral or thinking-linguistic brain deficit considered to be present (but never found) by traditionalists.

- *100% of Dr. Gold's dyslexic patients had abnormal cerebellar neurological signs.*

- 90% (14 out of 16) of the above cerebellar-impaired dyslexics examined by Dr. Gold were specifically stated by him to have *cerebellar deficits*. And although the cerebellar neurological signs and dys-

---

[1]Although Drs. Carter and Gold eventually examined 22 dyslexic cases by the time *A Solution to the Riddle—Dyslexia* was published (1980), only 17 cases were available for referral and discussion in "Dysmetric dyslexia and dyspraxia—hypothesis and study."

functioning in the remaining 2 out of 16 dyslexics were identical to the others, Dr. Gold merely omitted using *cerebellar deficit* to summarize the signs' cerebellar significance. Indeed, the latter should be obvious to *all* physicians—even without the *cerebellar deficit* clarification.

In addition, 90% of the dyslexics examined by the neurotologists were found to have inner-ear dysfunction as "blindly" tested via electronystagmography, known as ENG (see Chapter 5, Figures 1 and 2). Accordingly, these "blindly" reported neurological and ENG data definitively and independently confirmed that dyslexia was related to, and most probably due to, a cerebellar deficit. (For an explanation of the ENG technique and data, see my text, *A Solution to the Riddle—Dyslexia, Appendix D.*)

Following the publication of this study, I sent letters of thanks to all "blindly" involved physicians as well as copies of the research paper. All participating inner-ear experts or neurotologists were delighted by the results reported in this scientific work and the credit given them. By contrast, I never again heard directly from the pediatric neurologists, Drs. Gold and Carter. They refused to answer my letters and never came to the phone though I called them repeatedly.

The Public Denial of Cerebellar Findings

Eventually, I learned the reasons motivating Drs. Carter and Gold's rather strange behavior. Not only did they deny their neurological findings to interested colleagues, but they also denied them publicly in 1974 when contacted by the medical publication, *Infectious Diseases*, and by Jane Brody of *The New York Times*.

In *Infectious Diseases*, Dr. Carter was quoted as follows:

"Both Dr. Gold and I doubt that we interpret our findings as being consistent with cerebellar deficit. Many children with mini-

mal brain dysfunction are clumsy. This hardly justifies a cerebellar localization." Further, he went on to say, "the concept of cerebellar-vestibular dysfunction in dyslexic children is foreign to
us, and we do not understand the Frank-Levinson hypothesis."
(Infectious Diseases, 4, No. 7, July 1974, p. 15.)

In *The New York Times*, Jane Brody wrote:

Others, however, including Dr. Arnold Gold at Columbia-Presbyterian Medical Center, believe that the balance disturbance is
merely indicative of brain damage and that dyslexia is really a
cortical problem (*New York Times*, April 29, 1974, p. 20).

Although the reporter for *Infectious Diseases* did state,
upon independent review, that there were clear and direct
references to *cerebellar deficits* in Dr. Gold's dyslexic case
reports, the pediatric neurologists adamantly denied their
very own cerebellar content (see Chapters 4, 16 and Appendix A).

Needless to say, the cerebellar denials by Drs. Carter
and Gold were shocking to me. Their refusal to communicate in order to rectify all errors was even more distress-
ing. When I personally challenged Drs. Carter and Gold's
statements by speaking to the editor-in-chief of *Infectious
Diseases*, I was shown a letter written by Dr. Carter which
completely refuted any and all cerebellar findings in the
dyslexic cases I sent them. And Jane Brody of *The New
York Times* reassured me that her news article clearly
and accurately reflected Drs. Gold and Carter's stated
views.

Might someone have been mistaken? Certainly! However, this discrepancy was obviously more than just a
mistake—theirs or mine. In fact, when my research was
reviewed before the New York Council of Child Psychiatry
in 1974, the two negative reviewers—Dr. Archie Silver of
New York University Medical Center and Dr. Hart Peterson
of New York Hospital, Cornell—both claimed that Dr. Gold
personally denied finding any cerebellar deficits in the

dyslexic cases I referred to him for "blind" neurological examinations.

Although a mistake might have been made, it appeared obvious that someone was in denial. The questions remaining were: *Who* was denying? And *why?*

CHAPTER 4

Circular Logic

A closed system is a cognitive structure . . . where parallels intersect and straight lines form loops. Its canon is based on a central axiom, postulate or dogma, to which the subject is emotionally committed, and from which the rules of processing is a matter of degrees, and an important criterion of the value of the system. It ranges from the scientist's involuntary inclination to juggle with data as a mild form of self-deception, motivated by his commitment to a theory, to the delusional belief-systems of clinical paranoia. [Arthur Koestler, *The Ghost in the Machine* (New York: Macmillan, 1968), p. 264.]

So that readers might independently and objectively judge the validity of the "cerebellar denials" in dyslexia, a clear qualitative and quantitative presentation of the disputed cerebellar data became crucial. Hopefully the following abstracted verbatim case report, as taken from *A Solution to the Riddle—Dyslexia*, will provide readers with the vital initial insight needed to assess both Dr. Gold's "blind" cerebellar-dyslexia findings as well as his corresponding denial of them.[1]

[1] Initials or new names were used to preserve confidentiality. In addition, the cerebellar findings repeatedly used by Dr. Gold to diagnose "cerebellar deficits" were italicized by me. *All* cases examined by Drs. Carter and Gold were either completely or partially presented in the appendix of *A Solution to the Riddle—Dyslexia* and now here in Appendix A so the reader might better understand their cerebellar findings and my interpretation of them.

A Qualitative Analysis

Michael Rizzo

Because of severe reading and related academic difficulties, Michael, 9½ years old, is repeating the third grade. Here is a verbatim and typical excerpt from Dr. Gold's 11/1/69 neurological report:

- His [Michael's] copies of the Bender Gestalt were of poor quality. These reproductions were mildly distorted with irregular lines and poor angulation. *Graphomotor coordination was deficient with poor formation of both letters and numbers.* The child showed defective academic function in all spheres. Number concepts were primarily limited to finger counting. He was unable to tell time or perform coin conversation. Spelling was at the first grade level and he showed a prominent tendency towards reversals. . . . Reading was at a second grade level with substitutions and omissions.

- Motor examination showed normal bulk, tone, and strength of all muscle groups. The deep tendon reflexes were physiologic and the Babinski responses normal. Sensory examination was normal for all modalities including touch, position, vibration, and cortical sensation. *There was a cerebellar deficit that was manifested by a mild finger-nose-finger dysmetria and a moderate impairment of rapid alternating movement. Catching, throwing, and kicking were poorly performed.* Cranial nerve examination revealed a prominent alternating convergent strabismus which was most apparent in the right eye. *There was a prominent difficulty in the youngster fixing for any prolonged period of time. The eyeglasses tended to correct this problem.* The funduscopic examination . . . was benign. The visual acuity was 20/20 in both eyes and the visual fields were normal to confrontation.

It is my impression that this youngster. . . show[ed] unequivocal evidence of organic dysfunction of the central nervous system that is often referred to as *minimal cerebral dysfunction or minimal brain damage*.[1] The evidence to support this impression of neurologic dysfunction is the perceptual problems with visuospatial difficulties, *the deficient cerebellar deficit which primarily involved small muscle function, above all in the hands, as well as an extraocular muscle imbalance.* In addition there is a significant learning disability which involves all spheres of academic function as well as a prominent hyperkinetic behavioral syndrome which has improved with Ritalin.

Arnold P. Gold, M.D.

Professor of Clinical Neurology

Professor of Clinical Pediatrics

The Traditionalists' Circular Logic

As is readily apparent, Dr. Gold found *only* abnormal localizing cerebellar neurological signs and thus a corresponding "deficient cerebellar deficit" in this dyslexic or learning disabled youngster with hyperactivity. And contrary to simple logic, Dr. Gold used the cerebellar deficit to diagnose "minimal *cerebral* dysfunction" despite the complete absence of localizing cerebral neurological signs.

Upon analysis, Dr. Gold appeared to reason in the same way as did all the traditionalists. And their circular logic sounded something like this:

- Dyslexia or LD and related symptoms are of *unknown* origin—but are *assumed* to be due to a cerebral-language defect.

[1]These diagnostic terms were italicized by me for emphasis. In addition, the CV neurological signs reported by Dr. Gold here are similar to *all* his other "blindly" examined cases (see Appendix A).

- Definitive localizing signs of a cerebellar deficit are found in neurological tests whereas the expected cerebral signs are not.[1]

- Therefore: 1) the cerebellar signs prove the existence of a brain dysfunction, and 2) the *assumed* cerebral origins of "dyslexic" and related symptoms prove the existence of a cerebral brain dysfunction, e.g., "minimal cerebral dysfunction."

In other words, the initial cerebral assumption is used to prove this very same assumption. By contrast, I reasoned in a completely different manner: *Since dyslexia or LD and related symptoms are correlated with normal or absent cerebral neurological signs and abnormal cerebellar functioning, then dyslexia might well be of cerebellar rather than cerebral origin,* especially since independently and "blindly" performed ENG studies by neurotologists further confirmed the presence of inner-ear dysfunctioning within this very same dyslexic sample.[2]

Accordingly, I ask the reader: Is this reasoning too difficult for such eminent neurologists as Drs. Gold and Carter to understand—even if they disagree with it? Did not Dr. Gold find and report cerebellar deficits in dyslexia? And did these neurologists not *deny* the significance of their

---

[1]Specifically, the cerebellar signs reported by Dr. Gold are finger-nose-finger dysmetria (recall my 3D definition of dyslexia as *dysmetric dyslexia and dyspraxia* [DDD], impairment of rapidly alternating movements, poor sports ability and related fine and gross motor dyscoordination as well as ocular fixation and muscle balance difficulties—similar to that tested when using my 3D Optical Scanner (refer to Chapter 7 for details). By contrast, had there been a cerebral deficit, then Dr. Gold would have reported abnormal deep tendon reflexes, a Babinski response, impairments in his motor examination as well as that involving cortical sensation, etc.

[2]In addition, the presence of an inner-ear-determined visual fixation and tracking deficit was proven by me in dyslexics when using a newly developed and patented 3D Optical Scanner—a method termed "fascinating" by Nobel Laureate in cerebellar neurophysiology, Sir John Eccles. Since this method proved the inner-ear theory of dyslexia while refuting the cerebral-language concepts, it was *denied* by all traditionalists reviewing my published books and research papers.

very own data: the presence of cerebellar signs and deficits and the complete absence of cerebral signs—minimal, maximal or otherwise?

A Quantitative Analysis

In order to quantitatively analyze and clearly present the "blindly" reported—but denied—*cerebellar deficits* and the many and varied cerebellar signs used by Drs. Carter and Gold to denote this diagnosis within their sample of 22 dyslexics, graphics and tables were needed. This data appears in Figures 1 and 2 and Table 1.

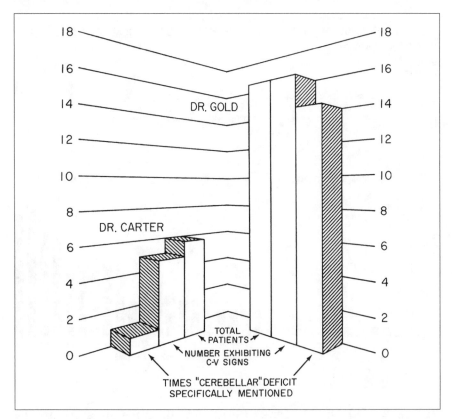

Figure 1 The total number of dyslexic patients sent to Drs. Carter and Gold for "blind" neurologic examinations, and the number of patients found to have CV signs and stated to have a "cerebellar" deficit. From *A Solution to the Riddle—Dyslexia*, p. 82.

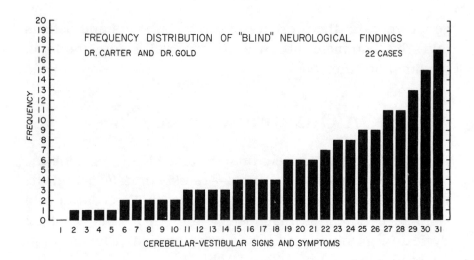

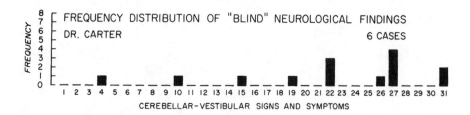

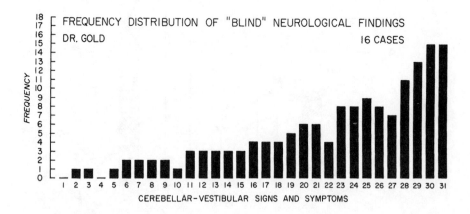

Figure 2 **(A)** Dr. Carter's "blind" CV findings in a frequency distribution form. **(B)** Dr. Gold's "blind" CV findings. **(C)** Distribution of their combined CV neurologic findings. From *A Solution to the Riddle—Dyslexia*, p. 84.

"BLIND" CEREBELLAR-VESTIBULAR SIGNS AND SYMPTOMS	NUMBER OF PATIENTS
1. Nystagmus (General)	0
2. Ocular Fixation Difficulty	1
3. Ocular Sensitivity	1
4. Difficulty Riding a Two Wheel Bicycle	1
5. Visual Motor Difficulty	1
6. Articulation Difficulty	2
7. Decreased Muscle Tone	2
8. Tandem Ataxia	2
9. Mirror Movements	2
10. Electronystagmography Abnormality	2
11. Small Muscle Extraocular Incoordination	3
12. Dysdiadochokinesis	3
13. Salivary Accumulation	3
14. Hyperextension of Muscle and Joints	3
15. Speech Difficulty (General or Non-Specific	4
16. Orolaryngeal Incoordination	4
17. Toeing Inwards or Outwards	4
18. Tandem Walking Dysmetria	4
19. Difficulty Tying Shoe Laces and/or Buttoning Clothes	6
20. Slurring of Speech	6
21. Pes-Planus	6
22. Difficulty Hopping	7
23. Difficulty Catching, Throwing and Kicking	8
24. Visual Spatial or Perceptual Difficulty	8
25. Rigid and/or Awkward Holding of Pencil	9
26. Finger-Nose Dysmetria	9
27. Clumsy and/or Awkward Coordination	11
28. Difficulty with Fine or Small Muscle Coordination	11
29. Immaturity and/or Distortion of Bender-Gestalt Drawings	13
30. Graphomotor Incoordination, i.e., Poor Letter Formation and Spacing	15
31. Impaired Succession Movements of Fingers	17

Table 1: Cerebellar-Vestibular Signs Reported in "Blind" Neurologic Examinations (n=22). From *A Solution to the Riddle—Dyslexia*, p. 83.

Summary

As the tabular and graphic display of their findings shows, Drs. Carter and Gold reported abundant and varied cerebellar neurological signs among the 22 dyslexic cases eventually sent them. Even nonprofessional adults capable of reading the above-mentioned reports and their presentation in *A Solution to the Riddle—Dyslexia* were confused by the "cerebellar denial" of the traditionalists, as were the reporters of *Infectious Diseases* and the *New York Times*. To date, *all critics have completely denied mention of those "blind" neurological and ENG findings which independently corroborated the CV-dyslexia concepts while refuting the prior cerebral-language views.*

Hopefully this presentation will lead to much-needed answers and a new boost to meaningful research efforts. In retrospect, had Drs. Carter and Gold accepted the credit given them by this author in 1973 for their cerebellar findings, *they could have accelerated the CV-based diagnosis and treatment of millions of suffering dyslexics—instead of preventing it.*[1]

---

[1]Paradoxically, while some traditionalists such as Carter and Gold refused to accept the well-deserved credit given them, others refused to reference the cerebellar-vestibular concepts they present as their very own (see Chapter 18, Acceptance Without Reference).

CHAPTER 5

Loaded Dice

The New York Council
of Child Psychiatry (1974)

Because the inner-ear theory, diagnosis, and treatment of dyslexia as initially proposed in 1973 were considered revolutionary breakthroughs, it was imperative that these data and conclusions be scientifically reviewed. Since Drs. Carter and Gold couldn't—or wouldn't—come to The New York Council of Child Psychiatry (1974), I presented my findings *alone*. Drs. Archie Silver and Hart Peterson were chosen as the independent and supposedly "unbiased" discussants. Because Dr. Gold denied his cerebellar findings when contacted by the two discussants and as they publicly stated as much to the interested audience, the reliability and credibility of the "blind" cerebellar and all my other data was questioned.

However, Drs. Silver and Peterson refused to review or read Drs. Carter and (especially) Gold's original neurological reports such as the ones included here. Could this refusal have had anything to do with their refusal to acknowledge their own cerebellar neurological findings in dyslexic patients? Could they have also been significantly "biased" toward the traditional cerebral theories of dyslexia—to the point of denial?[1] Also, the neurotologists performing the "blind" electronystagmography (ENG) inner-ear tests who solidly agreed with my findings and theories were never contacted nor invited to speak (see Figures 1 and 2).

The "Blind" ENG Data

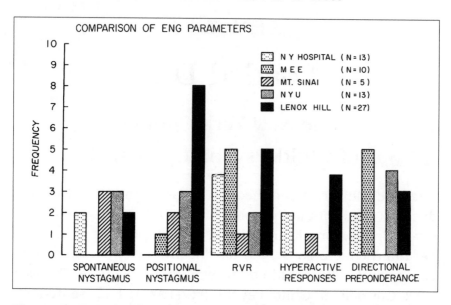

Figure 1 Positive frequency distribution of "blind" ENG's as a function of medical centers where the testing was done, and total percent positive. (Mt. Carmel Hospital, Staten Island Hospital, Mt. Sinai Hospital, M.E.E.=Manhattan Eye and Ear Hospital; N.Y.U.=New York University Medical Center; N.Y. Hospital=New York Hospital/Cornell Medical Center.) Taken from *A Solution to the Riddle—Dyslexia*, p. 85.

[1]For example, a dyslexic case examined by Dr. Archie Silver was reviewed in *A Solution to the Riddle—Dyslexia* (pp. 69-71). Silver's unrecognized or denied cerebellar signs and biased "cerebral deficit" assumptions were clearly highlighted.

Additionally, a patient referred to Dr. Hart Peterson in 1991 clearly illustrated that Peterson hasn't changed or even modified his cerebral views of dyslexia after 20 years: (1) despite the presence of neurological signs indicative of cerebellar dysfunction within his very own report, and (2) despite the child, Eric Cole, responding very well to my treatment. Considering Dr. Peterson's complete denial of both Eric's cerebellar signs and improvements on cerebellar or inner-ear-enhancing medications—as described by his mother in Chapter 2, might Peterson have been even more biased as a discussant in 1974?

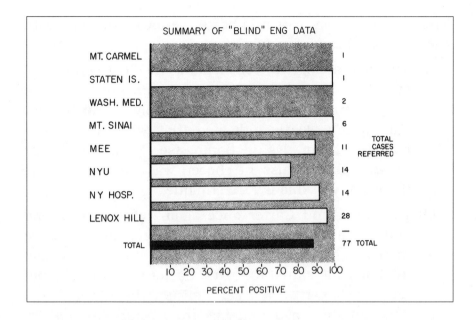

Figure 2 Frequency distribution of spontaneous and positional nystagmus and other ENG pathologic parameters (i.e., vestibular hyper- and hypo-reactivity [RVR] and asymmetric vestibular-ocular responses to caloric stimulation [DP]) as a function of hospital centers. From *A Solution to the Riddle—Dyslexia*, p. 86.

An Orton (Dyslexia) Society-Sponsored Meeting (1975)

To review "objectively" all my data used to postulate that dyslexia was of cerebellar-vestibular (inner-ear) origin and to resolve any possible confusion created by the prior meeting, another review was scheduled by the Orton (Dyslexia) Society—a society founded on, and emotionally bound by, the premise and conviction that dyslexia was of a *cerebral* or thinking-linguistic origin—after *Orton's Dominance Theory* lost favor in many scientific circles.[1]

[1]Dr. Samuel Orton originally reported (1937) a higher incidence amongst dyslexics of: left and mixed handedness, and speech symptoms (stuttering, slurring, articulation errors, etc). Since the left cerebral cortex or thinking brain was known to be dominant in regulating language functions in right-handed individuals, Orton reasoned that a *failure in this dominance* among dyslexics could explain the above-mentioned handed-

There were, however, a number of serious problems with the set-up.[1] Thus, for example:

(1) The neurotologists from leading medical centers all over New York City were once again *not* invited to present and discuss their own "blindly" obtained ENG data which clearly indicated that 90% of dyslexics had "inner-ear" dysfunctioning (see Figures 1 and 2)! Instead, the discussant chosen was *known to refute* the validity of this ENG technique.

(2) Drs. Gold and Carter once again refused to attend and discuss their own reported cerebellar findings! Instead, they sent a colleague, Dr. Martha Denckla. In short, she stated that Drs. Carter and Gold did not mean to report *cerebellar deficits* when they found and reported *mild and moderate cerebellar deficits.* That statement makes as much medical sense as saying that mild and moderate asthmatics or diabetics have nothing wrong with them. In addition, dyslexia experts Dr. Denckla and Jeanette Jansky claimed that all patients not more than two years below peers and / or potential in reading scores were not dyslexic—even if they had typical dyslexic symptoms such as those presented here and in other texts. In other words, the intent of these experts was clear. They were going to refute the *reality* of the "blind" cerebellar-dyslexia and related data by any and all means possible. And as might be readily apparent,

ness and speech correlations. There were only *three* major problems with this theory: (1) Orton himself later recognized (1942) that handedness and dyslexia were unrelated—a finding I've repeatedly noted since 1973. (2) Speech symptoms in dyslexics are of inner-ear rather than of a cerebral language or aphasic origin. (3) His cerebral theory could not explain the vast majority of dyslexia-related signs, symptoms, and improvements.

Despite these and other drawbacks, the Orton Society has attempted to maintain this erroneous theory, regardless of scientific realities. They harshly criticize all challengers.

[1]The biased set-up by The Orton Dyslexia Society was discussed in Chapter 13, *A Solution to the Riddle—Dyslexia.*

their rationalizations appeared to defy and deny common sense logic.[1] Amazing?

And against all odds, Dr. Gold is still diagnosing children with dyslexia or learning disabilities as having *cerebellar deficits* despite his prior denials. Indeed those denied cerebellar findings permeate thousands of his reports and have been read by many parents, educators, and psychologists—"Ortonians" and others—as well as referring physicians (see Chapter 16). In other words, most dyslexia professionals and experts at and after this Orton meeting were and are familiar with Dr. Gold's excellent but repetitive reports emphasizing *cerebellar deficits*. Yet none said anything!

Questions Requiring Answers

Doesn't anyone want to know the truth? And why not? These were the questions that first occurred to me. Most important, no one at the meeting *or thereafter* attempted to ask:

- Why didn't Drs. Carter and Gold show up at the meetings to personally refute "cerebellar" allegations they thought were either made in error or worse? I certainly would have—and did!

- Why didn't anyone question this rather suspicious behavior? I would have—and did!

---

[1]As of her Rodin Society lecture (9/92), I was told Dr. Denckla still believes dyslexia is a pure and severe reading disorder of cerebral-linguistic origin. Having recently examined a dyslexic boy seen by Dr. Denckla in 1990, it became crystal clear that Dr. Denckla still appears to view: (1) all reported test scores as due to an "assumed or imaginary" cerebral-linguistic impairment in the *complete absence* of any localizing evidence of a cerebral defect, and (2) a mild sequencing speech symptom similar, if not identical, to that of Meg Fex as a severe cerebral language disorder—surprising and confusing the child's parents. And she appears to deny *all* obvious and stated balance, coordination and rhythmic disturbances of cerebellar origin, including a severely impaired ocular fixation and tracking reflex during reading—resulting in *very low blurring-speeds* when measured by my diagnostic 3D Optical Scanner. In other words, scientific bias still reigns supreme in the 1990s as it did in the 1970s.

- Why didn't anyone want to see Drs. Carter and Gold's *hard and fast cerebellar evidence* in dyslexia such as that presented to the reader, so as to judge and evaluate the basic data for themselves? I certainly would have sought it out—even if it weren't handed to me on a silver platter!

- Why hadn't anyone questioned Dr. Denckla's reasoning about the *mild*, *moderate* and *severe* cerebellar signs? I certainly would have—and did!

- Why didn't anyone at the meeting or thereafter question Drs. Denckla and Jansky's traditionally accepted but misguided diagnostic view of *dyslexia* = "*dyslexia*"? Any clinical beginner had to know that many dyslexics—gifted and otherwise—often compensate for their reading scores and yet remain dyslexic, invariably manifesting many and varied "typical" dyslexic symptoms. Were they afraid? Or worse: *might they not know*?

- Hadn't any of these Ortonian experts carefully read McDonald Critchley's dyslexia research? Despite his traditional views, does he not refer to "cured" dyslexics whose reading scores are normal for their age, but who still have spelling and other typical dyslexic symptoms? In other words, even Critchley must have realized that dyslexia cannot be equated with "dyslexia."

- Hadn't anyone thought to speak up and ask Dr. Denckla and Jeanette Jansky why they could not review and discuss the cerebellar data—neurological, ENG, blurring speed—calmly, scientifically, and objectively?

- Why hadn't anyone asked: Isn't it strange that the neurologists (Drs. Carter and Gold) refuting their own cerebellar evidence in dyslexia *were invited to attend but didn't*, whereas the neurotologists who agreed with their own inner-ear dysfunctioning data

in "blindly" examined dyslexics *were not invited to
attend and speak, although they wanted to?*[1]

Two Descriptions of the Orton Society Meeting

Only those attending the Orton Society meeting could really grasp the charged climate of the discussion as well as
the defensive quality of the attacking traditionalists. As a
result, I considered it essential to present two independently written descriptions of the meeting so the readers
might clearly understand what really went on, and why.

Audrey McMahon

Audrey McMahon is well known and respected by many in
the learning disability field and is presently the head of the
Scientific Studies Committee of the Learning Disabilities
Association of America. She was invited by the author to
act as a "clinical model" in order to demonstrate to the audience her dyslexic history, cerebellar or inner-ear signs
and symptoms, decreased blurring speeds, abnormal
ENGs, and her compensatory reading spurt late in her
school life.[2] However, three of the four discussants were so
antagonistic and defensive that Audrey was spared the embarrassment of participating. Instead, she was asked to describe the meeting.

> I thought the research session at the N.Y. Orton Society (1975)
> was an unfortunate and confusing event. When new research ap-
> pears it seems to polarize the public. The traditionalists are
> threatened, and the public "grasps at anything," rushing in over-
> board with the result that thoughtful assimilation and consider-

[1]Thus, for example, Dr. Kenneth Brookler at Lenox Hill Hospital performed and read the vast majority of ENG's on the "blindly" referred
dyslexics. To date he has remained supportive of the inner-ear or CV
role in dyslexia. Currently, Dr. Brookler is clinical professor of
otolaryngology, New York Hospital.

[2]Have no fear. All these diagnostic terms will be clearly explained
throughout this work—especially in Book II. Some of these terms have
already been reviewed.

ation of a new concept with mutual respect and intellectual honesty becomes impossible—and the climate antagonistic. The meeting on April 11 turned out to be a premature presentation of "Dysmetric Dyslexia" in which the rationale, hypothesis, procedures, raw data and implications had not been sequentially codified and "translated" into audience-oriented lingo and visual aids which weakened the intrinsic impact. *In turn the three traditionalists on the panel, some of whom were visibly over-emotional (Drs. Denckla and Jansky), tore into every aspect of the reported study with such ruthless vehemence that the meeting became not a discussion but a confrontation. Few of us in an audience can respect minds which are too closed to concede any possible validity in another point of view.*

Those people in the audience with whom I spoke who were sincerely interested in getting at the basis of the phenomena evidenced in the study, including the consistency of the tracking scores in different groupings, and in learning more about the validity of the hypothesis, were tongue-tied in the face of the bombardment from the erudite big guns with whom no one wished to tangle publicly. So there were few questions at the close of the session. However, many constructive questions remained valid in my mind.

"Blurring" is a subjective response. Can it be quantified/qualified? How come *all* the special class children have tracking problems so consistently? Maybe there is something much more fundamental evidenced than only "dyslexia" malfunctions? How come the chronological age cutoff is so consistent at 10? How does this compare with known physiological developmental periods including neuronal and neurohumoral changes? Like myelination as proposed by Dr. Critchley . . . Where do adults (over 10) fit into the picture? What brain mechanisms do the motion-sickness medications mediate? If some but not all patients respond, can you find differentiations? Are the public school studies able to include medication?

Dr. Thomas Rooney

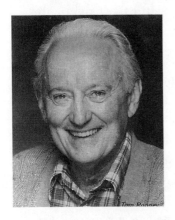

Dr. Thomas Rooney, district principal of the New Hyde Park (N.Y.) School District, attended the April 11, 1975, Friday evening session by invitation of the author, and attended Dr. Gold's presentation on Saturday morning April 12 by chance. Dr. Rooney's comments capture the essence of the Orton meetings manifest and latent content and intent, and thus independently confirm Audrey McMahon's description.

> Because the district is embarking on a special training program for teachers about learning disabilities, and since we had become acquainted and I had heard about your invention for the testing of dyslexia, I attended the Orton Society meeting in New York City for the purpose of obtaining background information which would assist me in administering district programs. I was, of course, particularly interested in hearing your presentation on Friday evening. *To the best of my knowledge, it was the one new idea, invention or suggestion scheduled for presentation at the conference.*
>
> For this reason, if for no other, I was more than amazed at the reception you were given at the conference. I mention "you" purposely because the critics who had so much to say about you did not once mention the invention, testing procedures or analysis of results. Instead, there seemed to me to be a petulant self-

righteous revelation by people representing themselves as members of the medical profession about the validity of the qualifications of the cases tested, chiefly by physicians (Drs. Carter and Gold) not present at the meeting.

As an administrator of many years' experience, I should have been prepared for hearing people slam down a person with a new idea and not discuss the merits of the idea itself. I guess I hoped that in this case human nature would not prevail and the scientific evaluation of the procedure by disinterested physicians would be presented, which was not done, as you know. *Incidentally, the next day I heard the physician (Dr. Gold) who was quoted (or misquoted) the most, say that he was not present Friday evening because it was a holy day, but he mentioned that he was not a religious person.*[1]

As I review the conference, I find confusion in my thoughts because I went to learn about a malady which has escaped real diagnosis and solution for so many generations and instead heard people who seemed to me, as a disinterested outsider, intent in promoting their previously defined positions.

Since I first heard about your investigation and approach to this problem, I have been interested because it seemed to me, as an administrator, to be logical. My colleagues in this county, with whom I have discussed this procedure, feel the same way. We intend to assist, in every way possible, to bring to fruition the testing of children through the process you suggest. We do this not with preconceived ideas of success, but with the determination that we intend to assist any or all responsible scientists in their quest for a solution to this strange problem which has beset so many children and adults for so long.

---

[1] For those unaware, Sabbath observers do not work or travel from sundown Friday to sundown Saturday. Dr. Gold lectured on Saturday at noon—hence his "joke" about not being able to attend *his* Friday night lecture.

Summary

Now that the reader is aware of both the "blindly" reported *cerebellar neurological signs* in dyslexics as well as their denial by the examining neurologists, Drs. Carter and Gold, and their associate, Dr. Martha Denckla, I will now pose a few additional questions:

- Why did Dr. Gold, Dr. Carter—and especially Dr. Denckla—*deny* the existence of clear-cut and obvious cerebellar signs and deficits in dyslexics? Could they have merely *misread* or *misunderstood* these clearly reported findings?

- Why hadn't any critic of my work ever referred to the above-reported data that was also published in *A Solution to the Riddle—Dyslexia* and *Smart But Feeling Dumb* and that has been in my possession for approximately 25 years?

- Were the traditionalists deliberately trying to mislead all those interested in dyslexia—scientifically and/or personally—for self-serving reasons?

- Why am I accused of not researching my CV-dyslexia hypotheses when, in fact, I had, and still do, although factual references to my work are frequently sidestepped?

- As highlighted in the next chapter, why am I accused of "curing" 100% of treated dyslexics when, in fact, I've never claimed to cure anyone?

- And why am I accused of not recommending a holistic therapeutic approach to my patients when, in fact, I invariably do—while only my critics appear interested in scaring dyslexics away from all new approaches—mine included?

By the time you have answered these questions for yourselves, you will also have answered another question I asked in the beginning: Why haven't traditional thinking-linguistic brain or cerebral theories and theorists solved *any* of the many riddles characterizing dyslexia over the last 100 years?

My answer is perhaps too simple: Because they've been too busy creating these riddles and resisting their solution for the past century.

CHAPTER 6

The Orton Society Sanction

In retrospect, I do not know whether my medical text, *A Solution to the Riddle—Dyslexia* (1980), or the exposure it received on the "Today Show" and "Donahue" in 1981 (and again in 1984) triggered the greatest reaction among my critics.

Certainly my description of The Orton (Dyslexia) Society Meeting (1975) in Chapter 13 of *A Solution to the Riddle—Dyslexia* did not endear me to its board members, nor the crew of clinicians and tutors that benefitted from their referrals. The Ortonian-led propaganda in newsletters and negative book reviews influenced thousands of parents sincerely interested in learning the truth about this disorder from experts in whom they believed—experts who, in my opinion, merely led parents and patients to accepting only their own views. And the experts who most often received referrals from the Orton Society had to pay homage to the "Ortonians." It was a "love affair"—albeit a symbiotic one. And suffering dyslexics and their parents not only paid for this love affair, but the affair depended upon the dyslexic status quo continuing. Thus, in retrospect, I was forced to wonder: Were the Ortonians and their symbiotic cadre of experts fearful that dyslexics might be cured?

Clearly, my discovery that simple medications could help relieve the symptoms of dyslexics must have severely threatened the Ortonians and others. Why else would they continue to state that I "cured 100%" of my patients when, in fact, my claims were far more modest. I claimed merely to have helped, never cured, seventy-five percent of treated subjects: twenty-five percent significantly, twenty-five percent moderately, twenty-five percent mildly. And unfortunately, twenty-five percent of treated patients did not respond to existing medications. No doubt the Ortonians projected their worst fears onto me: that I could cure all dyslexics. And if this is their worst fear, why are they all pretending to be interested in helping dyslexics? The answer appears tragically simple: *Might their pseudo-interest in helping dyslexics masks their underlying interest in helping themselves?*

But *cure* they repeatedly said. Cure! Cure! Cure! Might this deliberate and neurotic-sounding distortion of scientific reality have had other determinants, too? Obviously! The best way to discredit researchers is to exaggerate and/ or deny their claims. And both types of criticism were commonplace: *How can medications help a learning disability? His theories are too simple to be true! His theories are too complex to be understood!*

Some critics have even said, in the very same breath, that my concepts were too simple and too complex—attempting to discredit my clinical research from all possible angles. Others claimed that there was no scientific basis to my concepts, ignoring a vast array of data in my medical text, *A Solution to the Riddle—Dyslexia,* as well as in many scientific papers. Well-known and respected individuals behaved in difficult-to-believe ways. It appeared as if their very existence were attacked, and they were fighting off my research for dear life.

Although I will present some quoted critical attacks here for illustration and analysis, the detailed portrayal of this response is too much to handle, even within a book whose title the reader might now better appreciate.

The Value of Criticism

Since my psychiatric training has taught me that criticism (quality and intensity) and its analysis is vital for enhancing and even triggering scientific insights as well as dissolving resistance or bias forces, I thought it essential to present the reader with detailed critical data which speaks for itself. These critical data as well as their violent intensity were found derived from the "closed" or biased theoretical views characterizing the traditionalists—views best described by Arthur Koestler and used to introduce the preceding chapter.

Typical Examples

Following my appearance on "Donahue" in 1981, with Olympic decathlon gold-medal winner and dyslexic Bruce Jenner, a tremendous interest in dyslexia as well as my research was triggered. Unfortunately, some of the critical interest was of a "sour grape" nature. Once again, I encourage you to analyze how and why I have been continually attacked by defensive and offensive critics for "curing" patients—often allegedly 100% of them. (I challenge anyone to find any statement of mine claiming to cure anyone!) Since many of these critics must know the distinction between "cure" (magical and otherwise) and mere improvement, I was again forced to wonder: Do these dyslexia experts fear that my medical treatment will eventually put them out of "business"—financially, scientifically or egoistically?

Criticism—Expert Style

Gerald Ente, M.D., wrote in the Nassau-ACLD Newsletter (December '82 - January '83) following a "Donahue" rerun:

> . . . Some of you have asked me about a doctor from Fresh
> Meadows, Queens, who claims almost 100% cure for dyslexia.
> He has gotten some recent TV and newspaper publicity and has
> recently authored a book on the subject, relating it to inner ear

problems. I am not saying that his method doesn't work, but I question that only "he or his associate" can perform this amazing cure, that the fee is $500, that this fee is totally payable before the cure is produced, that there is a 5-6 month waiting time, and that he cures "almost 100%" of his cases. This is all too "pat" for me. With a problem so complex, with causation so diversified, and with such variable manifestations, this sort of advertising gimmickry reminds me of the "Tell you what I'm going to do," garter-sleeved, wax-mustached, early-days huxter selling Lydia Pinckum's Vegetable Compound, the elixir of youth, or those guys who had us all believing that we must make our poor readers crawl on their bellies for a few years. How many desperate people will clutch at this straw, spend big bucks, and be disappointed . . . (*Ask the Doctor*, Gerald Ente, M.D., Nassau-ACLD Newsletter, Dec. '82-Jan. '83.)

Dr. Ente's criticism no doubt came after he read—*or completely misread*—the following material sent by my office to those interested in my diagnostic/therapeutic methods:

1981

Dear Correspondent:

As a result of the influx of individuals interested and inquiring about Dr. Levinson's methods of diagnosing and treating dyslexic individuals, this form letter was expediently drafted.

The diagnostic procedure takes approximately 2.5 hours and is completed in one visit. It includes all neurological, ocular, "inner-ear" and psycho-educational testing to make an adequate diagnosis. This diagnosis can be made and explained in almost 100% of the cases seen.

In addition, a treatment plan is determined on the basis of the test findings. Thus far, 75% of individuals will have a favorable therapeutic response to various combinations of medications and 25% will not. The favorable responses will vary from mild to dramatic, and are thus far not predictable.

The total fee for this diagnostic-treatment evaluation, including follow-up telephone consultations, is $500. This fee must be paid at the time of the examination.

In light of my form letter and its interpretation by traditionalist expert Dr. Ente, I ask the reader several questions: Is there any wonder why new and innovative "controversial concepts" take so long to break through the traditional barriers? What would have happened to dyslexia research and millions and millions of heretofore misdiagnosed and untreated dyslexics had critics merely acknowledged—without bias and denial—the reality of the findings presented by me thus far in *A Solution to the Riddle—Dyslexia, Smart But Feeling Dumb,* and my many research papers? Considering Ente's significantly distorted remarks, is it any wonder that countless dyslexics find it impossible to be properly understood, diagnosed, and medically treated by others like him? And as you will see, there are far too many others.

Two Orton (Dyslexia) Society Critics

Dyslexia critics with apparent tunnel vision invariably attack my medical treatment, claiming that it prevents parents and children from obtaining other help. This criticism is nonsensical for several reasons: (1) Parents and/or patients often come to me when *all* other attempts at help fail. (2) I advise patients, when appropriate, to combine medical and related treatments with tutoring for best results. In reality, when the medications help, they help not only "tutored subjects" but a wide variety of functions not capable of being tutored—as presented throughout *Smart But Feeling Dumb* and here. (3) Many of my patients—some already presented in this work—are adults whose many and varied symptoms can't be solved by tutoring. (4) Indeed, this ridiculous criticism clearly indicates that experts like Dr. Ente erroneously view dyslexia as merely a simple *academic disorder* rather than a complex *medical syndrome* of neurophysiological origin. And obviously these tradition-alist experts mistakenly believe that tutoring the symptom-atic reading outcome cures the disorder. By analogy, does reducing the blood-sugar in diabetics *cure* diabetes?

Once again, these criticisms highlight bias and re-lated underlying motives: Might *the critics* fear that the in-ner-ear-determined breakthrough improvements or "*cures*" will expose their scientific and personal inadequacies? Per-haps they inwardly realize there currently exists a tradi-tionally sanctioned diagnostic/therapeutic medical vacuum regarding dyslexia and that tutoring alone leaves much to be desired and economically afforded.

A Typical Ortonian Attack

In a highly but typically defensive and offensive letter fol-lowing my appearance on a WOR radio program with two of my successfully treated dyslexics, Lois Rothschild, a branch president of the Orton Society, wrote to the radio show host. She claimed that my views were controversial and that allowing me to present them lent credibility to my theory and "does an extreme disservice to your listening public." (Are the Ortonians against free speech?) Thus she continues:

> Meclizine (Antivert) does not *cure* dyslexia. . . And those searching for an *easy cure* pay Dr. Levinson's consultation fee and obtain only a prescription for an *innocuous drug* . . . (Lois H. Rothschild, President, Orton Dyslexia Society, New Jersey Branch, June 12, 1985.)

A Quick Response

Do I cure dyslexia? Is Rothschild, a reading tutor, really an expert on meclizine and other similar medications used by physicians for such inner-ear-determined symptoms as vertigo, imbalance, dyscoordination, and motion sickness? Is this drug really innocuous meaning worthless? And if so, why had it been deemed effective by the FDA and NASA for preventing vertigo and "space dyslexia"? And if it is innocuous—harmless—as expert Rothschild states, then why do her medical counterparts fear using it, especially since they claim it's "dangerous" and an "easy cure"?

The analysis of this repeated criticism invariably leads to the very same conclusion: Perhaps these traditionalists fear that my treatment works, as evidenced by the countless patients who they *never* contact and the improvements they *deny* during forced confrontations, e.g., scientific seminars, consultations, radio and TV appearances, etc? After all, my yearly consultation fees are a lot cheaper than their costly psychoeducational testings and years of tutoring and/or private schools (which can run to more than $20,000 per year in tuition alone). And how do you measure the "cost" my treatment saves by preventing the resulting emotional scarring in millions of dyslexics who fail to respond significantly to tutoring and thus require years of psychotherapy or emotional "remediation"? Why was no mention made by Rothschild of *two* favorably responding patients—a child and adult—who appeared on the WOR radio show with me? Does this omission not further suggest bias? And does Rothschild's bias not betray a fear, *a fear that my treatment works and "cures" rather than the opposite*? And did not her fear trigger an attempt to prevent the media from airing alternative views of dyslexia to their interested audience? Are the Ortonians against free speech? Or just that of researchers with a point of view that is different from theirs?

Perhaps another example regarding the danger of *meclizine* to traditionalists will be helpful. Dr. Hart Peterson, one of my traditionalist critics mentioned in Chapter 5, refused to treat a successfully responding dyslexic, Eric Cole (Chapter 2), until he was taken off this helpful but "innocuous" medication. Accordingly, Dr. Peterson stated in his 1991 neurological report: *"I also do not agree with the*

*diagnosis of cerebellar-vestibular dysfunction, nor do I agree
with his (Dr. Levinson's) approach to treatment. . . . I have offered the family a trial of Tegretol (for the episodic
dyscontrol syndrome), but not so long as he is being treated
with meclizine at the same time."*

No doubt the intelligent and curious reader will wonder:
How is it possible for Peterson, a well-respected neurologist
and professor, to view a simple over-the-counter antihistamine such as meclizine to be "dangerous"? He used this
term specifically before the New York Council of Child Psychiatry in 1974, while simultaneously contemplating the
use of Tegretol for Eric's dyscontrol symptoms—a truly
dangerous drug resulting in liver toxicity, according to the
Physician's Desk Reference (PDR). And why should Eric be
deprived by Peterson of the known benefits of meclizine
while testing the unknown reactivity to Tegretol—considering there are absolutely no contraindications to using
them both together? How and why could meclizine be considered both "innocuous" and "dangerous"? Might not
these opposite but distorted criticisms highlight one and
the same underlying motive—fear? Perhaps you can now
better understand why a Freudian-trained psychiatrist was
needed to unravel the traditional riddles characterizing
dyslexia and its esteemed experts.

The Closed-Scientific Loop—A Monopoly

Finally, I would like to present data that indicate the presence of a closed scientific loop and a monopoly among traditionalists who use each other politically to validate or negate whatever they want, regardless of scientific reality.
Thus, for example, in her Ortonian-sponsored and published book review of *A Solution to the Riddle—Dyslexia*,
Priscilla Vail claims:

- *A Solution to the Riddle—Dyslexia* is a dangerous
  book.

- This book promises a simple solution to a complex problem.

- Its language and message—"the gospel"—is too technical to be understood.

- It "teases" the reader into positive expectations only to then overwhelm their understanding.

- Its "miracle cures" and simple promises and "formulas" to "complicated human questions" are "dangerous" and trigger secondary conflicts in both children and their teachers—delaying and denying "valid diagnoses" and "remedial training" as well as making kids who fail to benefit from these "miracle cures" feel like "freaks."

- There is danger in clarity—the danger of overlooking the subtleties of truth.

- And while claiming to be delighted by dyslexics "instantly cured by Dr. Levinson," she states that her skepticism is bolstered by similar critical responses from such eminent neurologists, scientists, and investigators as Sidney Carter, Arnold Gold, Martha Denckla, Jeanette Jansky, and Richard Masland.[1]

- Her "sense of familiarity with Levinson" came from a devastating parallel between his book and *The Wizard of Oz*. And thus she compared me, by analogy, of course, to "a peddler of panaceas pretending to wizardry . . . " (*Independent School*, February 19, 1982, Copyright 1982 by NAIS.)

Note how the same "eminent neurologists, scientists, and investigators as *Sidney Carter, Arnold Gold, Martha*

---

[1]Dr. Richard Masland *negatively* reviewed both *A Solution to the Riddle—Dyslexia* and *Smart But Feeling Dumb* for the Orton Society in its Bulletin. Although he was professor of neurology at Columbia Presbyterian Hospital and a colleague of Drs. Carter and Gold, he refused to acknowledge Drs. Carter and Gold's obvious cerebellar findings in dyslexia, data that were all clearly and precisely presented within the above texts he allegedly "read."

Denckla, Jeanette Jansky and Richard Masland" are "magically" invoked to negate my cerebellar or inner-ear-dyslexia concepts. In fact, these same individuals appear to misread and misconstrue their very own—and each others'— clinical scientific data. And mine as well, to the detriment of all others.

Might my "message—the gospel" be simple enough to read were Priscilla Vail less biased? By contrast, countless dyslexics have read and clearly understood this medical text—even though they needed medical dictionaries and glossaries! This contrast validates what seems almost unbelievable: Many dyslexics know more than their esteemed traditionalist experts! Or, as Nobel laureate physicist Richard Feynman stated, "Experts don't know more than the average person."

Since no dyslexic ever found this work "dangerous," might this danger be personal and thus express a threat to Ortonian officials? In retrospect: Why hadn't any of the Ortonian-led and related critics ever mentioned my analysis of the "blind" cerebellar-dyslexia neurological and ENG data as well as the biased Orton society meeting in 1975? Is it true that this "dangerous" book contains no substantiation for my cerebellar conceptualizations? *Or, via a Herculean effort, has a book full of substantiating cerebellar data been denied—as was the content within Chapter 13? Have not the traditionalists neurotically displaced the danger they personally experience from the cerebellar origins and treatment of dyslexia to my documentation (e.g., A Solution to the Riddle—Dyslexia, Smart But Feeling Dumb, etc.)? And even onto me?*

Considering the biased Orton (Dyslexia) Society responses to my research in the 1980s, is it reasonable to assume that these defensive criticisms in the 1980s were consistent with, and a continuation of, the "biased" and fixed Orton Dyslexia set-up in 1975?

Equal Time—Without Rebuttal

Following my appearance on the "Today Show" and "Donahue" in 1981, Orton Society officials repeatedly called both shows and *demanded* equal time as if what was presented were political rather than scientific. However, the Ortonians refused to appear with me for discussion (see the following letter by David Elliot). In other words, they preferred to say and do whatever they pleased—unopposed, as usual.

Since I never mentioned the Orton Dyslexia view on these shows, why did they appear so threatened? And why did they seem to fear a direct confrontation and discussion? Might they have had nothing meaningful to say or no one to say it in a face-to-face factual debate?

And why do they have the chutzpa to *demand* equal time from the media? Upon reflection, the reason appeared tragically simple to understand: *because their monopolistic view has been sanctioned by time and the lack of those daring to take them on. And so they use their tax-exempt foundation status and political connections to further their own views and personal agendas, when in fact their governing rules demand that they be open to all new and helpful methods for dyslexics.* How open have they been? Do they really appear interested in helping dyslexics and their loved ones? And are people who contribute money and time to this organization getting what they really need and want?

Media Refusals to the Ortonians

As David Elliott, editor of the "Today Show," confirms in his letter, there was no reason to give the Ortonians exclusive TV time—since they had nothing new to say. But that never stopped them from repeating the same old content— over and over again. And although Pat McMillan, producer of "Donahue," was called at her home by Ortonians at all hours of the night after my 1981 appearance, she felt the same as David Elliott.

The Today Show

March 15, 1982

Dear Dr. Levinson:

In regard to our conversation of a month or so ago, I'm afraid our plans for the "Today Show" segment we discussed fell through. Although the Orton Society had written us and requested time to present its views on dyslexia, it now appears the Society wants to appear alone or not at all.

We were in contact with a Mr. Eric Manterfield to propose that the Society designate someone to appear with you. However, he indicated they were not interested in a joint appearance. And since that is what our executive producer had wanted to set up, I'm afraid the deal is off . . . at least for the time being.

Anyway, thank you for your cooperation and perhaps we'll be in touch with you again.

Sincerely,

W. David Elliott
Editor
"Today Show"

An Independent Rebuttal to the Orton Society Attack—Never Published by Them

Educator and Orton member Harold Blau, Ph.D., clearly and independently responded to the Ortonian attack on my research. And as expected, his letter was neither published within the Orton Bulletin, nor even personally answered. It was *denied*, as were my many successful treatment responses. Accordingly, Blau's letter and the Ortonian "denial" clearly summarize the Ortonian bias and intent—to maintain their dyslexia monopoly, at all costs. And the cost is not theirs—it is ours!

Following are Blau's cover letter to me and his response to Priscilla Vail's attack.

April 12, 1982

Dear Dr. Levinson:

Presumably you have seen the attack by Ms. Vail on your approach to dyslexia. I would like you to know that a member of the Orton Society saw fit to reply. A copy of that reply is enclosed. I expect that within a reasonable period it will be printed in the bulletin of the society.

If not, I see no reason why you should not feel free to use it as you choose.

Sincerely yours,

Harold Blau

March 31, 1982

Dear Priscilla Vail:

As a member or the Orton Dyslexia Society I am writing this letter out of a sense of professional obligation, to make sure an issue, Dr. Levinson's approach to dyslexia, is presented in balanced fashion. I would have been happier to have seen, along with your comments, a contrary view. Also I know you would not want a child deprived of possibly effective help because of negative views expressed in what amounts to a semi-official publication. *Because there is another side.*

First, there are very few maladies for which, over the years, we have not made gains in identification and cure. With respect to dyslexia, your description of it as "complicated" is an understatement. Identification? A hope. See Duane (1979), *Towards a Definition of Dyslexia: A Summary of Views.* And treatment? See Masland (1979) who was surprised that "with the diversity of the underlying disabilities within a population of dyslexic children, there has not been more evidence of a need for a corresponding individualization of teaching strategies." I interpret this as a kindly way of asking why there are not more curative or at least clearer roads to improvement. Inevitably, radical alternatives must emerge, given such circumstances.

Now for the facts that seem not to have come to your attention:

1. Dr. Levinson's concept of cerebellar-vestibular dysfunction and optic nerve nystagmus happens to link up with deviant eye movements reported among dyslexics (Pavlidis, 1981 and Elterman, et al, 1980). Both investigators photographed eye movements with highly specialized equipment.

2. *Blindfolding dyslexics or visual processing as the villain*: An obscure group, some years ago, argued, a priori, that if a child, not visibly different from his peers, reported to school to learn to read and write, and couldn't do so while his peers could, it might be argued that something was wrong in the area of visual processing. And that a different modality was required for learning these skills.

Sandra Witelson (1976) provided a new perspective and for the new and revised theory and experimental data, see the *Journal of Learning Disabilities* (June-July).

Now as to Dr. Levinson's dangerousness: not so. There is little substantiating data: He is a respected practitioner and there are no malpractice suits clustering about him. He does have a highly individualistic style which suggests more "intuition" than actually turns out to be the case. But I can think of a lately departed extremely prominent educator-psychologist whose work required more than a little interpretation, much more.

(Now, you may find it convenient to print only the foregoing or part of it and please feel free to do so.)

I think the real issue is Dr. Levinson's use of medication. There is something about changing thoughts and behavior with medication that disturbs some individuals. It distorts objectivity. If there are even a few subgroups among dyslexics (Masland, 1979), it may be necessary to resort to what is called a trial of medication.

This is fairly common in medical practice and long periods of time are sometimes involved.

In addition to Dr. Levinson's recommendations, *we now have Piracetam*, as you undoubtedly know. Heavily funded private research suggests *this is also helpful to dyslexics and has no side effects* (Wilshire, 1982). *There will of course be others.*

It seems to me that we are between a rock and a hard place, as the saying goes. As the media invades the time and attention of children more and more, old methods must be revised or abandoned to fit into increasingly narrow time constraints. At best, Dr. Levinson is sounding an alarm which we will ignore to our regret. Or at worst, some youngster will be a little sleepy on Dramamine. *I would not describe Dr. Levinson as "dangerous," but certainly thought-provoking.*

Sincerely yours,

Harold Blau

References

Duane, D. D. Towards a definition of dyslexia: A summary of views. *Bulletin of the Orton Society: Current Issues in Dyslexia*: Towson, MD, 1979.

Elterman et al. Eye movement patterns in dyslexic children. *Journal of Learning Disabilities*, 1980, 13 (1).

Masland, R. L. Subgroups in dyslexia: Issues of definition. *Bulletin of the Orton Society: Current Issues in Dyslexia*: Towson, MD, 1979.

Pavlidis, G. T. *Dyslexia Research & Its Application to Education.* New York: Wiley, 1981.

Witelson, S. F. Abnormal right hemisphere specialization in developmental dyslexia. In Knights, R.M. & Baker, J.J. (eds.) *The Neuropsychology of Learning Disorders*. Baltimore: University Park Press, 1976.

Wilshire, C. R. Presentation at the Ninth Annual Conference of the N.Y. Branch of the Orton Dyslexia Society, March 1982.

A Final Thought

As you might recall, Dr. Blau mentions a drug for dyslexia called Piracetam, which has been shown to improve reading, memory, speech, etc. Do you know it is also an antivertigo drug—similar to ones I use for dyslexia? (Refer to Levinson, 1991, "Dramatic favorable responses of children with learning disabilities or dyslexia and attention deficit disorder to antimotion-sickness medications: four case reports.") Indeed, prior to my research and the above study, no one connected the dyslexia-related improvements of Piracetam with its antivertigo or inner-ear-enhancing properties! Might not this correlation independently serve to validate the inner-ear basis of dyslexia as well as the treatment responses reported throughout this and my prior works?

CHAPTER 7

Cures or Merely Improvements?

Since I have been repeatedly accused of "curing" dyslexics by my critics, using "magical" rather than scientific methods, I think it only fair to present some additional typical *improvements* obtained when using diagnostic/therapeutic techniques repeatedly called "dangerous." Surely even those readers without a Freudian or psychoanalytic background intuitively know how to interpret such seemingly nonsensical "sour grape" comments as: "magic," "cure," "dangerous." And do not these sour grape and scare mechanisms attempt to refute and deny the reality of the dyslexia improvements described in my research efforts?

Surely you all by now must understand that my improvements or alleged cures are not dangerous to the "cured" and/or their loved ones, nor are they performed by magic. Obviously, these improvements are only dangerous to those experts whose egos, finances, and power bases depend on the continued suffering of dyslexics. On the status quo remaining as it was. As it is. And as it will be, unless the interested majority take things into their own hands, for the sake of many currently doomed by the traditionalists to endure unnecessary pain, humiliation, and tortured lives. At the extremes, lives driven to joblessness, helplessness, depression, alcohol and drug abuse, violence and even crime.

Before continuing with my defensive critics and their often offensive criticism, let me take an important time-out for some very important patients with dyslexia and their "lifesaving" treatment responses. Hopefully you will listen to them all very carefully, as I did. Hopefully you will learn what dyslexia is really all about, as I did. As a result, you may better understand what I've repeatedly said: *Dyslexics—not experts—define their disorder.*

Indeed, you will better understand the differences between "cures," improvements, and the 100-year-old diagnostic/therapeutic void of the traditionalists. And you will clearly understand how and why these improvements threaten my critics![1] For I never did, until I gathered and analyzed the content of this book and until I read Broad and Wade's *Betrayers of the Truth: Fraud and Deceit in the Halls of Science*! Until I recognized that the traditionalists have absolutely no way of medically diagnosing and treating dyslexics—none! And as a contrast to the traditionalists' "blind" rejection or denial, all the "controversial" or "magical cures" and their respective methods of action have been presented—symbolically, of course—in Chapter 13.

---

[1]Somehow this rather strangely neglected fact never arises during scientific, newspaper, or TV discussions. The burden of proof is only on newcomers or "status quo breakers"—unless of course the latter are also part of the established "club." And then the word "new" or "original" rather than "controversial" is used—even if the theory is neither "new" nor "original" (see Chapter 14 and Appendix C in Book II). So the sophisticated media invariably sides with the traditionalists for reasons that are easy to figure out.

Some Typical Improvements

Eve Grande

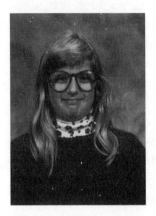

Three Sides to an Improvement

Eve is a 10-year-old dyslexic whose favorable responses to treatment were observed by all.

Eve's Self Report (3 / 93):

> Hi, my name is Eve. I'm 10 years old and life is good. But it hasn't always been. Before I met Dr. Levinson, I thought I was stupid, dumb, and ugly. I was learning slower than everyone else. And I thought I would never be able to get better. I couldn't read very well. And I couldn't concentrate. My teachers and my parents told me I was really very smart. But it didn't feel that way. I would hit myself and feel like crying inside. I was starting to think I didn't even have a brain.
>
> I met Dr. Levinson and he told me I had a fine brain but the messages were getting mixed up. Now I feel great. My school work is fine. But I still have to work hard. I am able to do things I couldn't do before, like finish a project, read a book, and even understand it. I even do math. I feel like a regular kid now. But I know I'm special. I was

even Citizen of the Year in my class last year. Some days when I don't take my medicine I am too hard on myself. And I feel down. I feel like I am out of control and can't think.

I love Dr. Levinson because he helped me a lot. I want to be an LD teacher when I grow up so I can help kids with Dyslexia. I know how they feel. Now I feel good.

Eve Grande[1]

Parental Observations

We are the parents of an Upside-Down Kid who is now Right Side Up. Before our daughter, Eve, was treated by Dr. Levinson, she was a very unhappy, frustrated child and we were a very concerned family. We come from a small town with a very wonderful and supportive school system. They gave Eve so much help and worked with her from an early age. The last day of second grade we had a PPT (Parent-Principal-Teacher Conference). No one knew what to do with poor Eve. We considered extended LD at this point. Everyone was very frustrated with the situation. Eve was a very bright child but just wasn't getting it. Her self esteem was at the lowest point ever. She was convinced she was stupid. All the love and support in the world couldn't make her believe she was really bright. We left the meeting in tears with nothing really resolved. The very next day, Eve's grandmother saw Dr. Levinson on television. He described Eve to a _T_ as he talked about dyslexics. We made an appointment to have Eve evaluated and it changed our world.

Changes in Eve were evident immediately. She was able to concentrate and sit and read a book. She was able to sit and finish a project and was much more organized. She was finally a happy child. We thought it was too good

[1]Eve was on Connecticut cable TV with me in March 1993 to discuss her symptoms and improvements. And we were seen by Andrea Lee's father (see "An Exception Highlights the Rule," Book II).

to be true. And that maybe we just wanted her to be better so badly that we thought we saw an enormous imaginary improvement. Thinking this, we stopped the medication to see what would happen. Well, she immediately reverted to the way she was before. We still do this every once in a while just to be sure.

Eve is now doing very well. She is reading and writing and she is even able to spell and do math beautifully. But the most important aspect of Eve's success story is the way she feels about herself. She is O.K. with herself and genuinely happy. We are sure she will succeed at whatever she wants to do.

David and Barbara Grande

Eve's Teacher—Barbara Chapman

Eve is an adorable ten-year-old girl who I had the pleasure of working with when she was in my nursery-school class. I have kept in close contact with Eve and her family . . . *and consider Eve's transformation from an "Upside-Down" kid to a "Right-Side-Up" kid nothing short of miraculous.*

At the nursery-school level, I noticed her very young (immature) fine motor skills, difficulty concentrating, and lack of self-esteem . . . particularly in light of the fact that Eve was a good deal older than the rest of the children in her class . . . as much as a year in some cases. Eve was *always* keenly aware that she was different . . . and she unfortunately assumed that this meant she was "stupid" and "bad" . . . when, in fact, she was very bright and very affable.

Thanks to her caring parents and an enlightened doctor, Eve's dyslexia has been properly diagnosed and treated. She is working at or above grade level in the fourth grade and displays coordination, self-control, confidence, and enthusiasm in all she does. *Her progress is truly remarkable—and has, in my opinion, saved her from a lifetime of frustration and defeat. It is great to see her enjoying her life and liking herself. She is truly a success story.*

In retrospect, although the traditionalists might consider Eve's dyslexia "cured" because her reading-scores are now normal, Eve still manifests dyslexic symptoms, despite her dramatic improvements on medication. Moreover, when taken off medication she regresses to what traditionalists would call "dyslexia." Does not Eve's improvement on medication and regression off medication highlight the basic fallacy of the traditionalists in defining this complex and highly variable disorder on the basis of only a severe reading-score impairment—the latter being also a highly variable and overdetermined parameter? Needless to say, the same considerations hold for all dyslexics—compensated and non-compensated.

Since the vast majority of bright dyslexics feel dumb, it became clear to me many years ago that reading is the *least* of a dyslexic's problem. How they feel about themselves is infinitely more important than reading scores, spelling scores, etc. All too often, "curing" the reading scores via tutoring is insufficient to improve their self-esteem since the underlying inner-ear problem remains unchanged, as do all the other non-reading symptoms found characterizing their syndrome. And to emphasize this crucial understanding as well as the need of compensating therapies, I wrote *Smart But Feeling Dumb.*

Observations such as Eve's initially led me to recognize that dyslexic symptoms occur and remain despite the best parental and educational care, clearly highlighting:

- that dyslexia was not of a primary emotional or educational origin, and

- that love and tutoring alone—although crucial—cannot reverse or "cure" the underlying origin and multiple effects of this devastating disorder.

Until the breakthrough insights and "magical cures" discussed within this book were uncovered, confusion, helplessness, and frustration frequently prevailed. Clearly, new hope and help currently exists. And as noted, this help is deeply appreciated and holistically reinforced by all professionals sincerely interested in dyslexics instead of their pet theories.

Mat Kautz

Mat is a 12-year-old dyslexic. His improvements are reported by his mother.

> Mat noticed in just a few days after starting on the Atarax (an antihistamine) that he could read easier. *He was very excited and pleased. We are too.* His written compositions have also improved greatly. There are still words that are misspelled but they are legible. Mat continues to have good and bad days in regard to concentration level, mood swings, and self esteem. But the good days by far outnumber the bad days. He is a much happier person. Mat is also gaining control of his fears for the very first time. Now he actually prefers to have his bedroom door closed at night. A year ago, prior to treatment, Mat had a night light in his room, the hall light on, and his door open. Within the last six months, Mat has been able to control his fear to accomplish a desire. His desire was to be able to ride a horse. He is doing beautifully. He is even considering riding in a show this summer.

Note how Atarax—an antihistamine—improved not only reading, writing, spelling, and concentration, but *mood* and *fears* as well, not to mention self-esteem. Do not the above repeatedly observed improvements in academics, concentration (ADD), mood and anxiety (fears/phobias) on inner-ear-enhancing medications suggest a common inner-ear origin? In other words, this clinical evidence, albeit "subjective," as well as that objectively determined in scientifically convincing studies have clearly led to new insights into the origin and treatment of physiologically determined academic, emotional, behavioral, and concentration/distractibility disorders.

Candee Lee

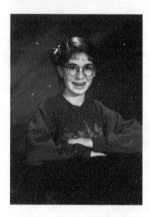

Candee (11 years old) showed remarkable improvements which were reported by her mother, Elizabeth (3/10/93).

> My husband and I brought our eleven-year-old daughter Candee Lee to see you on October 2, 1992. You asked us to write in story form how we determined Candee had dyslexia and what we have done to help her compensate for it. After the information you requested, I have asked several questions of you. You are more knowledgeable about dyslexia than anyone I know of in the world today. *You may not have all the answers to dyslexia, but you are willing to listen to your patients and learn from them. Because you listen, you are more likely than your contemporaries to find further answers to dyslexia in the future. Thank you for what you have done for my daughter and for the positive message of hope you bring to all dyslexics.*
>
> "Why am I different?"
>
> "If I am smart, why do I have to work so hard?"
>
> "Why do I feel so dumb?"

"Why is everything so much harder for me than for everyone else?"

These were the questions Candee asked me and asked of herself as she sobbed in my arms. We spent years tutoring Candee and years building a positive self-esteem in her. In spite of the right things we had done, Candee was now asking herself the same questions I had grown up asking myself all my life. Here we were with Candee about to enter the tumultuous teenage years, and she was not as well equipped to meet them as I had hoped. I had believed if I taught her to compensate academically and built her up emotionally, then she would not have to struggle as hard as I had. What were we to do? What could I do that I had not already done to help her?[1]

Response to treatment

Although the Lees logically presented Candee's many and varied dyslexic and frustration-related symptoms before her therapeutic responses, I thought it helpful to report her improvements first and relate her parents' thorough and informative description of symptoms and attempts to help compensation in Book II. For those interested in learning how a determined and struggling girl with A's and B's can have dyslexia, the following account is crucial.

Were experts as informed and intuitive as Candee's dyslexic mother, *A Scientific Watergate—Dyslexia* would never have needed writing and millions of other "upside-down kids" might have had similar therapeutic responses during the last twenty years.

Dr. Levinson, we cannot thank you enough for the help you have given Candee. I hope this letter will somehow be

---

[1]Despite the best parenting and tutoring, Candee wasn't "cured." She was still in need of a medically-based treatment which would strike at the core of her dyslexic disorder and thus minimize or eliminate the frustrating symptomatic fallout. For obvious reasons, the traditionalists believe otherwise, despite all the clinical evidence to the contrary. Their denial of this reality is difficult to believe.

useful to you as you help others with dyslexia. We enjoy our privacy and felt reluctant for you to use a picture of Candee or of us. My husband has agreed to allow it now, if it will help others who are facing a similar problem. May God bless you for the good you are doing.

Our local doctor agreed to a six-month trial of the medicines as they were all positive medicines with only minimal potential side effects. We saw no change the first week on the antihistamine. The second week, Candee's allergies were slightly better. The third week Candee could concentrate better and was less easily distracted. She finished her usual six to seven hours of homework in one hour! *The dramatic difference impressed my husband who had been even more skeptical than our doctor.* Candee's teachers noticed improvement in school, stating, "She is much more outgoing and confident." Candee's ballet teacher noticed "marked improvement" in her balance and coordination after starting the Sudafed.

At first I misunderstood the directions about her medicines over week-ends. I had been taking her off them instead of reducing the doses by half. Every time I took Candee off the medicines her dyslexic symptoms would return in full force. She would cry and whine more easily, was more easily frustrated, and was more forgetful. Also, she would have an increase in spelling errors and reversals, would have more difficulty remembering her multiplication tables, and have a longer homework study time. Over the holidays when she was off the medicine for an even longer time, the high-pitched buzzing (like crickets singing in her ears) would return.

The enormous difference in Candee on and off the medicines convinced me that Dr. Levinson's theories have merit. Not only are his theories more logical to me than preexisting ones, but the results of his treatment of our daughter are significant.

We feel delighted with Candee's progress. Our doctor has encouraged us to continue the medicines just as prescribed by you. Candee maintains her high grades with less effort and frustration. Most importantly, Candee feels pleased with herself.

Joey Rincione

Joey is a 10-year-old diagnosed with Attention Deficit-Hyperactivity Disorder and fears, phobias, and anxiety attacks of inner-ear origin. Shortly after treatment with only antihistamines, his mother wrote:

Joey had little or no tolerance with peers or younger children, particularly if there was a lot of noise or activity. He now joins in the activities. Joey couldn't enter a new area (mall, hotel, etc.) this past spring without having a panic attack. In July he was able to fly to California and enjoy all the activities without a problem. He finally showed interest in sports this past summer (baseball, football, swimming).

Joey was a frustrated child. Only days after starting the antihistamine, we saw a remarkable improvement in his moods and personality. He is much happier than he's ever been and has a positive attitude about himself. Joey has had a few spells but was able to get himself under control immediately. He became only slightly panicky, but talked himself or was talked out of the attacks before they became serious. He no longer hesitates to go out.

When Joey takes the Meclizine and Atarax on a regular basis, he no longer has panic attacks. He spent a week with a friend in N.J. last summer and got off his regular schedule of pills. Shortly after returning home, one week prior to entering the middle school (under more stress or worry), Joey had a mild attack, causing him to drop to the ground, heart pounding, pulse racing, and feeling fearful.

Once on a regular schedule of medication, he was under control. At the end of school last year, his teacher recommended testing for Attention Deficit Disorder. Joey was put on Ritalin (by your office). He became even more attentive and organized with his school work. However, he is still uncomfortable and rigid with his peers and puts himself under stress.

P.S. Handwriting is straighter, too.

Once again, observe the relationship between ADHD, fears/ phobias/anxiety attacks and favorable responses to inner-ear-enhancing medications. The fact that these allegedly different symptoms or syndromes are frequently associated with one another and all respond favorably to inner-ear-enhancing medications strongly suggests that they are all derived from a common inner-ear source. By contrast, the traditionalists view these mixed-appearing symptoms as due to separate or diffuse cerebral and related brain origins—hence their use of such diagnostic terms as diffuse brain dysfunction, minimal cerebral dysfunction, static encephalopathy, etc. In addition, the traditionalists failed to recognize that the stimulants for ADHD as well as the antipanic and antianxiety medications are all inner-ear-enhancing drugs—as are the antimotion-sickness antihistamines.

The reason Joey wasn't initially put on Ritalin or other stimulants typically used for ADHD was because of his *panic attacks*. Since the antihistamines controlled these panic symptoms (and improved his ADHD symptoms, as well), there was less need to risk using the stimulants—which not infrequently intensify and /or trigger panic attacks. In this case the combined use of medications resulted in the greatest improvement.

Elizabeth Winter

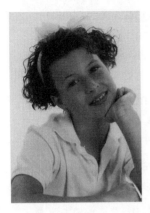

Elizabeth is an exceptionally bright and verbally gifted 10-year-old dyslexic who was initially diagnosed and successfully treated in 1992. Her case study is important for several reasons:

- Her verbal IQ was reported by a very competent psychologist to be superior, highlighting the traditional paradox whereby dyslexia is considered to be of a cerebral-language origin despite above average language functioning.

- Her balance, coordination, and rhythmic motor functioning were severely impaired and diagnostically seen to be of obvious inner-ear or cerebellar-vestibular origin.

- She was easily able to evaluate her own responses to therapy, including improvements in academics, concentration/distractibility, fears/phobias, balance/coordination, and self-image.

- Her mother, a nurse (Ph.D.), and her dyslexic father are both fully capable of supplying detailed and "objective" evidence of observed changes as well as prior symptoms (Book II).

Elizabeth's Self-Report

I feel more together on the medication. When I'm not on them, my mind wanders off when people are talking to me. And I don't hear clearly or easily what they are saying.

I now understand things more. If someone asks me, what color is the sky today, I'd usually say "what" or guess. Now I know and understand what's going on.

I used to be very restless and active when sitting in class or your waiting room. Now I'm calmer.

I'm less afraid of being alone and that there's someone else hiding in the house. When I'm off the medication, I'm scared all the time.

I've started to enjoy reading more. It's smoother, faster, and I understand more—easily. My eyes don't glue on to the words like they used to. No more headaches when I read—I can sound out new words and even old ones for the first time.

There's a big difference in my writing. For instance, it's not so all over the page and going down and up. On the medication, my writing is straighter—even on blank paper. It's smoother and faster—just like my reading.

In spelling, I can sound out the phonics more. Before it was hard—and I'd get very frustrated.

When I'm on the medication and reading, I won't hear anything else around me, even my mother asking me a question or telling me to do something. Off the medication, I can't even concentrate on reading at all. My mind is all over the place—like my handwriting used to be.

My balance is much better on the medication. I don't wobble when I close my eyes. When my medication wears off, I can't catch a ball—just like before.

When dancing, I can do much better on the medication. I won't turn the wrong way. I'll automatically know which way to correctly turn. And my dancing is smoother—very natural.

When off the medications, sometimes I stutter. *No stuttering when on the medications.* I understand what people are saying to me—more and easier and faster. I'm not sure why.

I now feel good about myself—while on the medication. Before I felt bad—stupid. Because I couldn't do very many things that other kids could do.

Although all reported data obtained from patients, parents, and teachers are vital and eventually led me to my current diagnostic/therapeutic insights, for "economy" sake I will merely call your attention to a few important details needed to overcome the denial characterizing the traditionalists. Recall Elizabeth's stuttering and other related improvements in auditory processing and speech when reading the critical misinterpretations of *Dr. Anne Huston.* Nonsensically, she claims that I *cure* the deaf and stutterers (Chapter 8-C).

Brian Conrad

Brian's father describes his 7-year-old son's dyslexic symptoms and improvements as follows:

What convinced us as parents to come: Brian's physician, Dr. Mark Piacentini, is working with Candee Lee, a patient of Dr. Levinson's. Candee Lee is doing wonderfully . . . a different kid (see pp. 134-137).

Brian has never been able to play soccer and score a goal. He had a cold—and suddenly played like an animal, scoring like crazy. We read *Smart But Feeling Dumb*—and immediately understood! We stopped his cold medication and his athletic performance ability disappeared. Restarted medications—great performance again!!! Before this "explosion," Brian was confined to sit out all prior games. Were he not determined, I doubt he would have been able to stick out his sitting and the hazing he got.

I was skeptical before coming. Suddenly I became a convert. Brian's mother read up on dyslexia to help him. And she handed in a paper on Dr. Levinson's research— which her professors felt "converted them" to Dr. L.'s theories vs. those currently in existence (traditionalists).

Observe how Brian's soccer-coordination suddenly and dramatically improved and then disappeared, for reasons understood only years later. Was it chance alone that a "cold" and related use of antihistamines led to this improvement and that the very same improvement disappeared with cessation of antihistamines?

Countless "blind" observations such as these led me years ago to the conviction that if inner-ear-enhancing antihistamines could significantly improve inner-ear-determined balance, coordination and rhythmic symptoms as well as academic, concentration, mood, and anxiety disorders, then *all* these interconnected and overlapping problems must be inner-ear-related, especially since only inner-ear neurological signs were found characterizing large samples with similar disorders. Perhaps now readers will better understand why I redefined and thus renamed dyslexia *Dysmetric Dyslexia and Dyspraxia* (DDD).

Indeed, a large series of clinically based reports such as Brian's, contained within Book II, provide a clear and definite refutation of expert Ente's misguided contention that my colleagues and I are the only ones who can obtain "magical cures."

Gary R. Chapman

Gary is a 34-year-old successful dyslexic who describes the following improvement on medication (4/9/93):

As I started taking the medications Dr. Levinson prescribed I was hopeful for improvement, but also fearful that it wouldn't help. Within a few days of my taking the antihistamine I felt better, more "with it." I heard another person (Sue Stafford) describe it as fog lifting—and that is how I felt. The change was gradual and at the time hard to perceive. But whenever I would compare current feelings to those before the medication, I knew there was a difference.

I have felt gradual improvement with all the medications except the second which has made me feel tired. I think even the vitamins and DMAE (dimethylamino-ethanol) have contributed a lot—but the strongest improvement came with the first antihistamine.

On two occasions I was in such a hurry to get to work that I forgot to take my medication. On both days I could feel the "fog" returning. By the end of each day I was tired, had headaches and was grumpy. My wife could tell I had not taken my medicine.

There has been a great improvement at work. For the past two years I've been responsible for compiling an annual statistical review of my division's activities. Last year it was very difficult for me to accomplish the task. It required a lot of "number crunching" and I could not concentrate. I made a lot of "careless" errors that required much re-work. This year the task went smoother and was accomplished faster with fewer errors. This alone has convinced me that the medications have helped.

The days seem less long! While working with my computer, I'm not as distracted as before. Concentration is much easier. And it was really bad. I don't fall asleep in front of the computer like I used to, with my hands still on the keyboard. And I'd wake up when it started to "beep." Before, this could happen several times a day despite constant breaks. Now it's twice a week.

It's scary—but now I see so much more when I drive. My peripheral vision is immeasurably greater. I can follow the traffic patterns. I can only wonder how I got by safely before.

Before, I'd just focus on the car in front of me. And
once when I forgot to take the medications, it was rain-
ing. And I was forced to fixate on the windshield wipers. I
must have always done that—but it was so normal I didn't
think twice about it. It's only now that I really know what
normal is.

On the antihistaminic medications, in meetings I'd be
significantly able to concentrate more. And I stutter and
forget names much less. When listening to conversations,
I can process information faster. And I can concentrate on
it better—but they're both different. And they both help!

I bump into things less—it's like I know where the
ends of my arms and body are more.

I must also admit the problems have not disappeared
completely. I still have symptoms at times. And I know I
"see" the world differently than others. But coping is easier
now. And with the same efforts, I can do so much more.

I think I wanted the medications to be an absolute
cure, to make it all go away. Even with the medications I
have to work to overcome. But with the medications I accomplish so much more for my efforts.

Gary's wife observes:

He's better at listening to me. It used to irritate me . . .
He was in "Never-Never Land" . . . And he's not as tired
and grumpy as before . . . It's not a magical transition.
It's subtle.[1]

---

[1]Although both Gary and his wife *wanted* more improvements than
they obtained, the improvements experienced were not directed by *desire*. Indeed, the vast array of improvements I initially observed while
treating dyslexics were different than expected. At first, only reading-
score or "dyslexic" improvements were anticipated. But to my surprise,
a diverse group of non-reading changes were reported. Instead of denying the unexpected data before me, I changed my prior views to fit
the dyslexia reality. As a result of resolving the 100-year-old traditionalist denial, I stumbled upon all the breakthrough insights characterizing this work. And millions of dyslexics can now look forward to improvements similar to those presented here.

Observing the Elephants

Mrs. Chapman writes:

I was in the room with my children, Christopher and Elizabeth, when they were given the visual (elephant) test. The elephants were projected in a line on a screen. I could see them clearly, but Chris, even up close, could not. They blurred very quickly for him when the elephants just barely started moving. They did not for me. Similarly, when the elephants were projected and bars in front of them moved, nothing blurred for me and I did not feel as though I was moving. It didn't seem to take much for the blurring to occur for either Christopher or Elizabeth. The elephants had barely started to move! When Dr. Levinson made the elephants go very fast indeed, then they did blur into "blobs of paint," as Chris said, but they were still blobs having some general shape. I had a similar experience when Elizabeth was given her test. VERY little movement started the blurring for her (she thought they got bigger and hairy), but I experienced no blurring at all, even against a flowered background. It might be noted that, while my husband and children have very good vision, mine is very poor. I wear contact lenses and can see reasonably well with them in, but the corrective factor is very high—over 10.

The "Elephant" Testing Method

For those curious about the *3D Optical Scanner and the "elephant" testing method,* Figures 1 and 2 and a brief introduction here might be helpful. Chapter 8 and Book II will discuss this diagnostic procedure in much greater scientific detail.

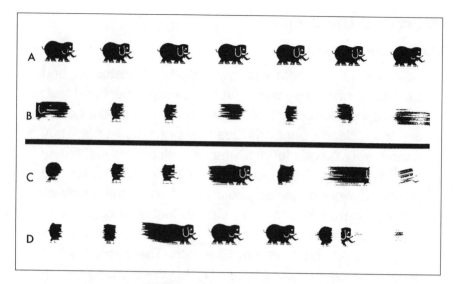

Figure 1 When a series of seven black elephants are set in motion **(A)**, a majority of dyslexics will experience the whole sequence as blurred at one half or less the speed of normal subjects **(B)** unless they consciously or deliberately begin to track one or two elephants at a time **(C and D)**.

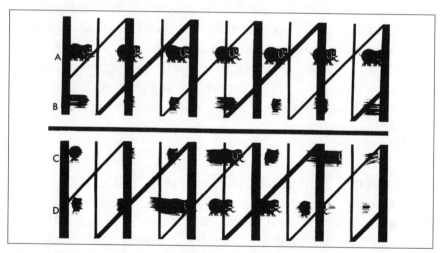

Figure 2 When a moving grid-like pattern moves across a stationary series of seven black elephants **(A)**, a majority of young dyslexics will experience either the total sequence as blurred **(B)** or all but one or two elephants as blurred **(C and D)**. Additionally, many dyslexics will also experience *movement illusions*, i.e., they see the stationary elephants or feel as if they are themselves in motion.

Dominic Barbagallo

Ann Barbagallo describes her 13-year-old son's improvements:

We have been delayed getting Dominic on all of the medication because of illnesses. He had a bad cold, went to camp (with school) just as we were ready to start another medication, and had chicken pox. However, I am seeing improvements already. As I reported to the nurse, I see a direct correlation between congestion and his stuttering.

Dominic has been stuttering since he was three years old. Sometimes it has subsided, other times it has been so bad that he could barely get through a sentence. When we started the antihistamine, I never dreamed that we would see results immediately. Despite your admonition that results would "take awhile," *the stuttering all but stopped that very day.* When I picked my son up that day after work, the first thing he said was: "Mom, I only stuttered twice today!" He was thrilled; I was on the verge of tears.

Seven years of speech therapy for my son, eight and a half years of teachers (day care and elementary) and therapists implying, suggesting and/or telling me that it was Dominic's fault and/or my fault that he stuttered, only to find that a pill relieved the problem. I even took Dominic to counseling for five months in 1989 on the advice of a speech therapist because he felt there was an "emotional component" to the stuttering. We were released from counseling without any improvement in the stuttering.

About 3 weeks after Dominic started the antihistamine, he caught a cold. As the congestion increased so did the stuttering. *When I started giving him Sudafed in addition to the other medicine, the stuttering was reduced or eliminated. I am trying to keep a tab now on how much Sudafed it takes. Dominic keeps sniffling most of the time because of his allergies. I think it takes about three regular Sudafed to stop the stuttering. I have not given him*

Sudafed continuously. I don't want to overmedicate him.[1] Also, as I said, he was away almost a week and he is still getting over a very bad case of chicken pox. We'll keep you posted.

I now have a doctor who has agreed to follow Dominic locally. When I tried to discuss our visit with you and your diagnosis with my pediatrician, he felt very threatened and would not listen to anything I said. He was upset that he did not see a problem and that I did not come to him first. Never mind that I had discussed some of these problems with him for years. We parted company.

Thanks for all of your help, prompt replies to all of my questions, and support. It is greatly appreciated!

Jennifer Simms

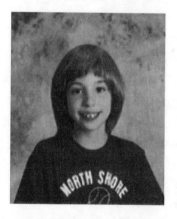

Jennifer's mother describes her daughters symptoms and improvements as follows (3/93):

Background—When our daughter Jennifer was entering kindergarten she was given the standard DIAL [Devel-

---

[1]As previously noted, the chance observation that colds and allergies intensified stuttering whereas antihistamines helped or "cured" this so-called "language" disorder clearly and independently verified that dyslexia and related symptoms are most probably of inner-ear origin, especially as only inner-ear neurological signs of dysfunction were present.

opmental Indicators for the Assessment of Learning] test. Her test results and IQ were all below average. At 5 years of age she was testing like a 3½ year old. And she was found to have very poor hand-to-eye coordination. As a result, Jennifer was placed in a Resource Room, which is where the learning disabled children get additional schooling—in her case an additional two hours a day. The school re-tested her when entering first and also second grade. And as usual, she was placed in the same program year by year. In addition, the school recommended that we involve her in piano lessons and some sort of physical exercise program. So we enrolled her in a Yamaha Music School. And for exercise, Jennifer requested karate and little league baseball.

Response to Treatment—Jennifer was in the middle of second grade when we read Dr. Levinson's book, *Total Concentration*. My husband William and I decided that he should try coming first. After all, it would be easier for him to evaluate the effectiveness of the treatment. After we saw the dramatic improvements in him, we immediately made an appointment for our daughter. As per Dr. Levinson's suggestion, we told her teacher about the treatment.

Within a week after antihistamines, the teacher sent home a note telling us of improved handwriting, and the fact that Jennifer was able to concentrate better and follow along with her regular class academically. Her grades improved. And she started getting 100s in her math tests.

Her piano teacher commented that Jennifer must be practicing a lot, because her playing had suddenly improved. The karate teacher also had commented about her improved balance and coordination abilities, and so promoted her to the next belt. And in the summer, her baseball coach noticed that she was batting a lot better. Obviously her eye-hand coordination had significantly improved as well.

Jennifer was again tested prior to entering third grade. And the school psychologist called my husband and I for a meeting to discuss the results. But when we spoke with him, it was clear that what he wanted to know was what had happened to Jennifer this past year. And what did we do with her that was different. The test results now indicated she was performing academically average or above for her age; even her IQ jumped to above average. Only her hand-to-eye coordination was deficient. But even that had actually improved considerably since last year. And because of all these changes, it was decided that Jennifer attend Resource Room only two days a week until they were convinced her improvements weren't temporary. We were notified last week that she will not be attending Resource Room next year.

There are no words to describe the other changes in her life. She used to be very shy, did not make friends easily, now she is outgoing and friendly, and a very happy child.

Thanks Dr. Levinson.

Justin Poythress

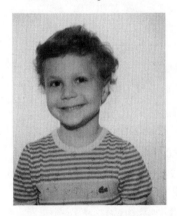

Justin was only five years old when initially examined and treated—too young to be diagnosed dyslexic by traditional measures. But as his favorable responses indicate and his detailed case (in Book II) highlight, Justin had an inner-ear dysfunction and typical dyslexic and related balance, coordination and rhythmic symptoms. Thus, for example, despite a verbal IQ higher than 160, he could not distinguish "A" and "B" after hours of practice. And as a rapid indicator of his reasoning and verbal abilities at two years of age, his parents recalled him saying, "God doesn't like worms. He put them on the ground where people can step on them." And at four years of age, "I know how we got the word 'female' for 'woman.' It comes from adding the French word 'fille' for girl to 'male'." Despite his superior IQ, his mother noted: "Justin failed his pre-kindergarten readiness exam. . . . The school wanted him to be kept out for another year. Why?"

Dr. Diane Poythress' Note

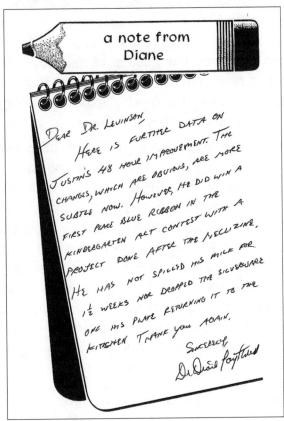

Dr. Vern Poythress, Justin's father, reports:

We could see that Justin was going to have many difficulties to overcome. Often we pleaded with God. And his mother cried before the Lord knowing something was wrong with her child. One day at a school prayer meeting we heard of a 34-year-old student who had just discovered she was dyslexic and was virtually healed by you within a week.[1] After talking with her we were excited. We could hardly sleep until our son was examined. We tried to be realistic and not get our hopes set on this one appointment, since we didn't even know for sure whether our child was dyslexic.

The appointment and associated testing proved definitively that our son was dyslexic. We actually watched him look at a horizontal row of dots and copy it into a vertical row of dots. In fact, when asked to copy a series of figures, he copied almost every figure turned 90 degrees counterclockwise (see Figure 3-A). That night we started him on the beginning low dosage of meclizine. The next day, about 21 hours later, he ate a snack in three minutes. We never saw him eat so quickly, especially without constant prodding and reminding him to eat.

The following day, about 40 hours after beginning medication, he again ate in a concentrated way. He colored two horses on his Sunday-school paper in whole units of color, not in "rainbow" fashion (Figure 4). Also, for the first time, Justin followed written lines in his Bible, moving his head from left to right. He played four-square ball for 15 minutes, only missing a few times. Before, he had normally caught balls with his hands against his chest. Now he was catching them off his fingertips above his head, to the side, and out in front of him. Even he exclaimed, "I'm good at this!" He even tried hitting the balls off his knees.

[1]This case presentation will be included in Book II.

Later that day I was showing someone a copy of the graphic patterns that Justin had been asked to copy when tested for dyslexia. Justin looked at one of the patterns and said, "Daddy, that is not what it was like before. The square was on top of the circle." We asked him how the figure looked now, and he described it correctly. Our other son got a piece of paper for Justin and asked him to re-copy the figures. They were almost exactly right. And all had the correct orientation, not turned 90° (see Figure 3-B). This change was stunning to all of us, because he had been on the medicine less than 48 hours. We were thrilled.[1]

Justin Poythress' Bender Gestalt Drawings

Before Medication:

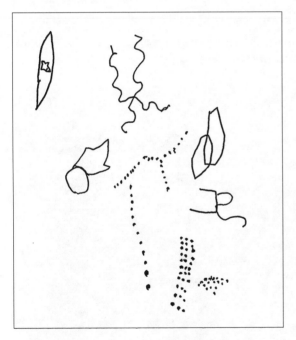

Figure 3-A Note how all of the Bender Gestalt designs were copied and perceived to be rotated 90°.

[1]The perceptual-motor improvements on a simple inner-ear-enhancing medication in a patient with only inner-ear or cerebellar dysfunction should be kept in mind when reading Chapter 16, Chutzpa. Dr. Gold appears to consider this perceptual impairment evidence of cerebral vs. cerebellar dysfunction—despite the presence of only cerebellar neurological signs and absent cerebral dysfunction. Judge the diagnostic significance of this finding for yourself!

48 Hours After Starting Medication:

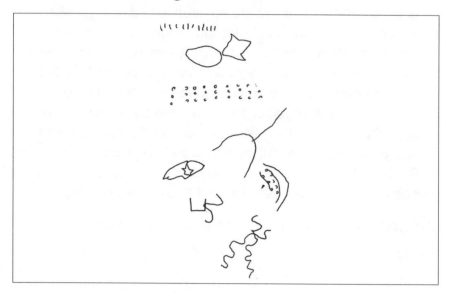

Figure 3-B Notice how all of the Bender Gestalt designs were more "normally" oriented on the page.

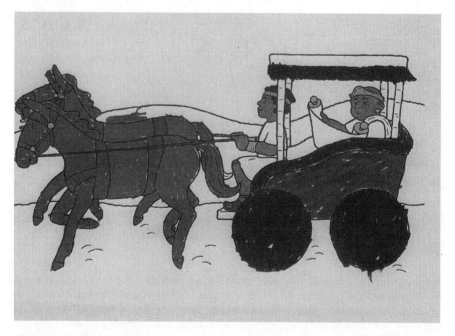

Figure 4 After 48 hours on meclizine, Justin was able, for the very first time, to color within the lines. Note how a single "color" is used instead of multiple ones prior to treatment.

After dinner Justin played a hand-held baseball game. Previously, his highest score had been 300. Suddenly he ran to us exclaiming that he had reached a score of 633. We all danced for joy that night, praising God for his mighty work and great mercy. With tears and gladness we phoned family and friends that evening with the good news.

Since then, Justin has continued to improve in many areas. He only spilled something less than once a week, whereas previously it was once a day. He won a blue ribbon first prize in the kindergarten art contest. He carried his dinner plate to the kitchen and did not drop silverware off, as was his previous habit. His responses, attention level, energy level, quickness in eating and performing other tasks have noticeably improved. *His reading ability is taking leaps.* He used to take two-hour naps every afternoon, but now sleeps only thirty minutes or not at all. His memory of recent events and instructions is vastly improved, as if a gauzy veil were suddenly lifted from his thinking. Now he tells in detail about incidents from his day at school, whereas before it was hard to get him to say more than a few words.

In terms of sequencing, he now has an interest in clocks and calendars. In fact, he could correctly say the hour and minutes although before he could usually not even say the hour. He actually played a piano piece without having to be told he was playing with the wrong hand. He began to peddle his tricycle, not walk it, and express a genuine interest in a two-wheeler. He attempted to ride one at the store. He jumped into a friend's swimming pool and picked up four rings lying on the bottom in 2½ feet of water. He began to swim under water boldly, at his own initiative. Before, he just stood, never wanting to put his head under water.

The results reported by the school at the end of his year at kindergarten were also encouraging. All the "problem" areas were now corrected. He was noticing when other children made reversal mistakes. The teacher reported that his art work had clearly improved and some work was done without any reversals now. He also showed off in front of his teacher, saying "Look at me!" as he walked backward on a balance beam. This would have been unthinkable two months ago.

The only "drawback" we have seen is a new impatience with himself if he can't do something well quickly. His personal expectations are higher. When the changes became clear he began to distance himself from what he was like previously, by deriding those children who made reversal mistakes or had athletic inability. We had to encourage him to have compassion on others as Jesus had compassion on him.

As a result of Justin's expanding improvements, his mother wrote me again, May 17, 1993.

Thank you for giving us the gifts which God has given to you. We are thrilled with our son's improvement. We will be recommending you to all our contacts both nationally and internationally. Thank you again. May the Lord God bless you with His Presence and His Holy Spirit.

Gratefully,

Dr. Diane Poythress

Summary

Although the improvements presented here were often dramatic and appeared to target many typical academic-related dyslexic symptoms—including balance, coordination, rhythm, speech, fears/phobias, mood, concentration/distractibility—these favorable results were not "cures." Symptoms and the underlying disorder remained despite the improvements.

Obviously my critics never listened to my successfully treated dyslexics any more that they did to their own patients. As a result, they failed to recognize and understand the above-mentioned insights—as well as those previously discussed. Unfortunately, the traditionalists listened only to themselves and their worst fears. And by now you all know what they were and still are: "Cures!" And a "dangerous" new inner-ear-based concept of dyslexia that finally works—a concept which will hopefully replace the 100-year-old traditionalist theories that lead only to unsolvable riddles, frustration, and continued suffering.

The Second
Critical Wave
and
Responses

Part A

The Saviors and Related Content

CHAPTER 8

The Saviors

Since *all* the experts critical of my CV research altruistically attempt to *save* countless dyslexics from the resulting diagnostic/therapeutic benefits and "dangerous cures" thus far presented, it seemed reasonable to group these critics together as *saviors* so that their common *realistic vs. defensive* and related underlying motives might be psychoanalytically explored and thus elucidated. This chapter will merely try to dissect and display the distortion and denial characterizing traditionalist critics so that the reader might more readily see through their manifest content and savior-type disguises. And a deeper exploration of the subconscious determinants underlying and apparently motivating their critical responses will be deferred to Chapters 20 and 21.

Hopefully the following content will also highlight how analysts attempt to isolate and explore biased or erroneous views so that the latter might be scientifically understood and explained. Indeed, a similar analysis led me to solve the dyslexia riddles by recognizing the fallacy, bias, and denial underlying and determining the traditionalists' equations: *dyslexia* = *alexia* and *dyslexia* = *"dyslexia."*

A

The Critic

I first stumbled across another medical-type critic at the 1975 Orton Society meeting where the Ortonian "set-up" was first rigged and the origins of *A Scientific Watergate—Dyslexia* initially began. No doubt his presence there, together with the memory of Dr. Arnold Gold and his savior, Dr. Martha Denckla, should have been a warning. But I was told by Audrey McMahon, who described the Orton Society meeting in Chapter 5, that Dr. Larry Silver[1] was open-minded when she knew him at Rutgers University. So she encouraged me to have my publisher, Warner Books, send him an advance copy of *Smart But Feeling Dumb* for review—which they did.

Dr. Silver's Responses

Following are two of Dr. Silver's written responses to Warner's request for a review of *Smart But Feeling Dumb.* Both were received by Patti Breitman, my editor at Warner Books—since Silver's letter to me, dated June 11, 1984, was sent to an address I hadn't been at for about three years. And for reasons that must by now be obvious, Dr. Silver claimed my book was "dangerous" because "Anxious

[1]As this chapter unfolds, the reader will quickly realize that Dr. Larry Silver is considered to be an eminent authority on dyslexia, LD, ADHD, etc. Currently he is clinical professor of psychiatry at Georgetown University. Additionally, he has held such distinguished positions as professor of psychiatry, Rutgers Medical School; acting director, National Institute of Mental Health; and director of the National Institute of Dyslexia. And from the traditionalists' point of view, his book, *The Misunderstood Child*, and critical papers on so-called controversial therapies and "magical cures" are thought to be excellent. As a result, he has lectured widely on the above-mentioned topics. Justifiably, his opinions on dyslexia, LD, ADHD, etc., are taken seriously, reflecting the collective understanding and perspective of the traditionalists.

families, desperately seeking a solution to their child's problem, will jump at his [my] ideas with hope." *Might they jump at my ideas because no other book or concept offered them a logical explanation for their own or their child's disorder as well as a possibility for help?* And guess what? Dr. Silver shared this book's content with none other than Dr. Martha Denckla and two others. And all, for some unknown reason, arrived at the same conclusion.

July 31, 1984

Patti Breitman

Editor

Warner Books, Inc.

Dear Ms. Breitman:

On July 10th I wrote to decline your offer to write a comment for Dr. Levinson's new book, *Smart But Feeling Dumb*. Since then I have struggled with elaborating on my reasons or not. I finally decided I should. I feel that Warner Books should know other views on a book they are about to publish.

After reading the advanced copy you sent me I shared it with a researcher in the National Institute of Neurological and Communicative Disorders and Stroke, Dr. Martha Denkla, [sic] and with two neuroscience researchers within the National Institute of Mental Health. Each of the three reached the identical conclusions. This book is not based on research, his definition of dyslexia is not necessarily that of most, the case studies are mixed clinical problems with no clarification as to what medications were used for each, and the neurological conclusions about dyslexia and about the function of the inner ear versus the brain are incorrect.

In summary, we see the book as dangerous. Anxious families, desperately seeking a solution to their child's problems, will jump at his ideas with hope.

Perhaps you could talk to the editor at Springer-Verlag about the comments and criticisms they received from professional and parent-based groups after publishing his first book on dyslexia.

Sincerely,

Larry B. Silver, M.D.
Acting Director, Alcohol, Drug Abuse, and Mental Health
Administration, National Institute of Mental Health

Dr. Silver's Letter To Me

June 11, 1984

Harold N. Levinson, M.D.
Associate Professor of Psychiatry
New York University Medical Center
61-34 188th Street
Fresh Meadows, New York 11365[1]

Dear Dr. Levinson:

Patti Breitman sent me an advance copy of your new book, *Smart But Feeling Dumb*. I read your previous book, *A Solution to the Riddle of Dyslexia* and just finished reading your new book.

I am left with two conflicting personal opinions. One view is based on the response I received upon showing your first book to the researchers who do work related to your areas of research and to the research managers who fund such research both at my institute and at the National Institute of Neurological and Communicative Disorders and Stroke. Their feedback suggested problems with your research design similar to that which you discuss in your new book. They also distinguish between primary and secondary functions of the vestibular, cerebellar, vestibular-cerebellar, and cortex in a way that differs from your views. They could cite no research to support your findings. I will now share your new book with the same professionals to seek their input.

---

[1]Because this letter was mailed to an address I hadn't been at for three years and as NYU Medical Center is not in Fresh Meadows, Queens, it must have been returned to Dr. Silver. Eventually it was sent to me by Warner Books.

My other view is based on my 15-year research and clinical career involving similar children, adolescents and adults. I agree with your clinical views; i.e., these individuals have mixed problems with learning disabilities, hyperactivity, distractibility, and secondary emotional, social and family problems. I, too, have treated the hyperactivity or distractibility with stimulant medications and the anxiety or depression with the appropriate psychotropic medications. Each works for the targeted problem. I have tried meclizine as you proposed, but with no success. My personal difficulty is that I have a problem accepting your theory, clinical models, and rationale for treatment; yet, it is difficult to ignore your clinical findings. I am also familiar with both the theory and research relating to megavitamins, trace elements, allergies, Feingold's approaches, and optometric training. None have been shown to be effective. Yet, you suggest that you get success. Your case examples do not specify what medications were used for what behaviors and what you observed to be the specific findings. For example, if you treated the distractibility with Ritalin or the depressions with Elavil I would expect improvements in performance. But, I could not sort out what was used with each case; thus, I was not able to relate treatment to outcome.

I do not want to be one of "those critics" who quote research protocol and ignore clinical findings. Would it be possible for me, or a small group of neuroscience researchers, to follow your suggestions to come over to your office to speak to your patients, observe them, and discuss your work with you? Maybe such an interaction could lead to the type of replication work you suggest.

I would appreciate your thoughts. Please write or call (301) 443-3673.

Sincerely,

Larry B. Silver, M.D.

Acting Director, Alcohol, Drug Abuse, and Mental Health

Administration, National Institute of Mental Health

Negative Criticism, Positive Insights

As repeatedly discussed throughout this work on *Dyslexia*, the intensity and quality of the negative critics and criticism forced me to recognize the bias and denial characterizing the traditional views. And the analysis of their bias and denial as well as their need to save dyslexics from the benefit of my related CV research led me to neurophysiological and psychological insights that could not have been obtained in any other way. Thus, for example, the following analysis of Silver's repeated and dedicated criticism will hopefully provide you all with these vital insights.

What's In A Letter?

In Silver's letter to me, I call your attention to a few major points:

(1) Dr. Silver claims to have tried *meclizine* (one of many inner-ear-enhancing drugs I use) without results. He then goes on to criticize me for not telling parents and patients in *Smart But Feeling Dumb* what specific drugs and doses to use. *Didn't he realize I tried to discourage patients from treating themselves—especially since this book was written primarily for nonprofessionals?* And although Silver claimed to prescribe *meclizine* while in complete scientific darkness concerning its use for dyslexia, and so mistakenly concluded it didn't work, he neglected to give me—a physician and researcher—any clues as to how many patients he treated with meclizine, what doses he used, etc. Nor did he inquire about vital therapeutic specifics beforehand any more than he did after our written and verbal communication. By analogy, would someone—even with Dr. Silver's qualifications—who was completely ignorant about computers be justified in concluding that computers didn't work, when in fact they did for knowledgeable others?

Since Dr. Silver apparently didn't know how to use *meclizine*, or the many related inner-ear-enhancing medications, and didn't believe in its efficacy, I question whether he even tried it on more than one or two patients, if any—and even long enough and with the right dosage. As can be seen by some of the successfully treated dyslexics presented thus far, this medication and others related to it have a good chance of helping—provided the doctor knows what he or she is doing.

(2) He asks me if I would permit neuroscientists to come to my offices with him so that they might observe and attempt to duplicate my work. He states, "Please write or call (301) 443-3673."

I called. I wrote. I discussed my research with him in detail and invited him to come to the Medical Dyslexic Treatment Center with as many of his colleagues as he would like—at *any* time convenient to them. And I even gave them my correct address and telephone number to make sure that they could get here—should they want to.

I never again heard from Dr. Larry Silver directly. Instead of coming and evaluating my research as befitting someone in his position, he continued to behave in a manner contrary to his letter, where he states: "I do not want to be one of 'those critics' who quote research protocol and ignore clinical findings."

In retrospect, I was forced to also wonder after rereading Silver's letter to Patti Breitman: If Dr. Silver truly reviewed my book, as he claimed, didn't he realize that *Dr. Martha Denckla* helped deny Dr. Gold's cerebellar findings in dyslexia? And if he did realize it, then why did he use her "objective" and "unbiased" opinion without first asking me about Dr. Gold's "blindly" reported cerebellar findings in dyslexia—clearly described, indexed, and graphed throughout *A Solution to the Riddle—Dyslexia*? And which now is clearly presented to readers in *A Scientific Water-*

gate—Dyslexia. Why did he send this comment to my editor, Patti Breitman—who no doubt didn't know much about Dr. Denckla? Why didn't he write this comment to me?

And the more questions I asked, the more confused I became about what Dr. Silver said he did, what he really did, and even why he did what he did. Thus, for example, if Dr. Silver really tried *meclizine* and it didn't work, why hadn't he published these negative and refuting results in a *scientific journal*—especially since he considered this treatment method "dangerous?" Surely, as an acting director of the National Institute of Mental Health, he could easily have conveyed his important findings to the scientific community. I certainly would have and did—even with my own data when they were at odds with my stated convictions.

No doubt my editor Patti Breitman and Warner Books felt the same way—hence their reply to Dr. Silver, below. And we all wondered: Did Dr. Silver believe that his letters to Warner Books would be shown to me? For the sake of countless millions, why hadn't he and his colleagues visited my medical dyslexia treatment center and evaluated my diagnostic/therapeutic results first hand—*before* calling them dangerous and attempting to use his titles and those of his colleagues to censor or bury them? Was he just too busy? Was it too unimportant? Or did he fear finding that my patients and their therapeutic responses were as real as those presented in all my works?

Patti Breitman's Response to Dr. Larry Silver

August 13, 1984

Dear Dr. Silver:

Thank you for your letter about Dr. Levinson's forthcoming book *Smart But Feeling Dumb*. I have sent a copy of your letter to Dr. Levinson.

We believe that Dr. Levinson's work deserves to be published. The methods he uses and the conclusions he draws are entitled to be read by the public. We have spoken with the people at Springer-Verlag, and they report that Dr. Levinson's first book was a tremendous success for them. We have confidence that *Smart But Feeling Dumb* will be a success for Warner Books as well.

As to offering hope to readers, we agree with Dr. Levinson that finding that hope is often the hard, first step toward finding a solution to the many problems caused by dyslexia as he defines it.

Again, I thank you for writing about the book.

Sincerely,

Patti Breitman
Editor
Warner Books

Simple Insights vs. Complex Fantasies

Upon rereading Silver's letter to me and stumbling over comments concerning 1) his treatment of dyslexia-associated ADHD or ADD with *stimulants* and related anxiety or mood disorders with *psychotropics*, and 2) his colleagues' views of *secondary* vestibular, CV, and cerebral functioning, I realized that several major issues had been overlooked. And in the absence of rapid clarification, I also realized that readers might be needlessly confused by simple concepts unnecessarily rendered complex and even frightening by the traditionalists and their denial mechanisms.

Because the traditionalists equate dyslexia with alexia, they are also driven to view dyslexia as a "pure" reading disorder—hence their need to equate dyslexia with "dyslexia."

As a result of these nonsensical equations, the traditionalists—Silver and his NIH colleagues included—tend to view the non-reading symptoms in dyslexia (i.e., ADD or ADHD, mood and anxiety disorders, etc.) as due to separate and distinct CNS (central nervous system) origins. And to justify and maintain all these complex and un- proven *diffuse* brain dysfunction theoretical fantasies and convictions, they must deny significant realities such as those to follow.

Thus, for example, my research clearly indicated that:

- The vast majority of dyslexics or learning disabled (90% or more) referred to me for diagnosis and treat- ment have co-existing or overlapping ADD-related symptoms, and the reverse (Levinson, 1988).

- Less than 0.1% of 4,000 consecutively referred and neurophysiologically examined learning disabled were found to have *only pure* reading-score impair- ments and related reading symptoms and nothing else (Levinson, 1988), clearly refuting the "purity" of dyslexia.

- The vast majority of learning disabled also have overlapping anxiety and/or mood-related symptoms, and the reverse (Levinson, 1989).

- Diverse samples with primary diagnoses of either ADD or anxiety (and mood) disorders are statistically characterized by only inner-ear (CV) dysfunction- ing—findings similar to those in dyslexia or learning disability (Levinson, 1988, 1989).

- Antimotion-sickness or inner-ear-enhancing *antihis- tamines* and related vitamins often improve *all* the many and varied symptoms characterizing dys- lexia—and not just the reading or "dyslexic" ones (Frank and Levinson, 1976-1977, 1977; Levinson, 1980, 1984, 1986, 1990, 1991).

- All the *stimulants* used for ADD or ADHD (Ritalin, Dexedrine, Cylert) and most of the *psychotropic* drugs used for mood and anxiety disorders are also *anti-*

vertigo agents, as is Valium and related anti-panic medications (Kohl, Calkins, and Mandell, 1986; Sekitani, McCabe, and Ryu, 1971; Wood, Cramer, and Graybiel, 1988; Wood and Graybiel, 1970; Levinson, 1984, 1986, 1990, 1991).

- Piracetam—a medication independently shown to improve the reading, speech, and memory symptoms in dyslexia—is also an *antivertigo drug* (Boniver, 1974; Fernandes and Samuel, 1985; Helfgott, Rudel, and Kairam, 1986; Lenzi and Milanesi, 1969; Oosterveld, 1980; Wilsher et.al., 1987).

In other words: If the vast majority of dyslexics have overlapping academic, ADHD, mood and anxiety symptoms, and since the dyslexic disorder is characterized by only inner-ear (CV) dysfunctioning and responds favorably to the above mentioned inner-ear-enhancing antihistamines and related drugs, should we not consider dyslexia and its statistically related and overlapping mixed symptoms to be only one syndrome of inner-ear or CV origin, pending contrary or refuting evidence? And since the CV circuits secondarily interconnect with all vital CNS or brain structures, should we not also assume that both a primary CV dysfunction as well as the resulting CNS structures secondarily impaired by these interconnecting feedback circuits determine and shape the ensuing dyslexic syndrome? Stated another way, what is the probability of bright and gifted dyslexics, such as those presented here, having separate brain dysfunctions for each and every symptom described? And as you recall, dyslexics often have many, many symptoms. Is it not more probable for dyslexics to have one central or core disorder with resulting multiple symptoms and syndromes?

On the other hand, Silver and his traditionalist colleagues maintain that the majority of dyslexics with overlapping or mixed ADHD, mood, anxiety, etc. . . . symptoms must have multiple and separate disorders—despite the presence of *only* inner-ear or CV dysfunctioning. And for the sake of denial, might the traditionalists also now assume that the cerebellar deficits found in dyslexia are perhaps *secondary* to an *assumed* primary or diffuse cerebral dysfunction—despite the absence of any detectable noncerebellar CNS dysfunction and despite the rapid and dramatic improvements in *all* dyslexic symptoms offered by the various and diverse groups of inner-ear-enhancing medications, each such drug group targeting some CV-CNS circuits more than others?[1]

Are the traditionalists' assumptions and convictions scientifically reasonable and probable? Or might their concepts concerning diffuse brain dysfunctioning, minimal cerebral dysfunctioning or static encephalopathy in dyslexia be significantly determined by bias and denial? Considering that all the above content and much, much more was clearly and simply reviewed in my books and scientific papers, is there any wonder why these very same books were considered "dangerous" and my supporting research and papers were denied by the traditionalist critics?

Have not the traditionalists and their denial mechanisms taken simple and independently proven inner-ear-related concepts and rendered them unnecessarily complex and even intimidating? Stated another way, are not the traditionalists attempting to maintain their erroneous cerebral concepts in dyslexia by unwittingly scrambling or distorting scientific reality to the detriment of all? Paradoxically, have they not also taken the complex depth and scope of the cerebellar-CNS-determined syndrome called dyslexia and erroneously simplified it by their equations: *dyslexia = alexia*, and *dyslexia = "dyslexia"*? Has not the Freudian-like analysis of the negative criticism and critics

---

[1]As you recall, these very same cerebellar deficits in dyslexia had been *denied* by the very same traditionalists "blindly" finding and describing them (refer to Chapters 3 and 16).

led me to vital neurophysiological and psychological insights that could not have been obtained by any other
means? Were not the traditional dyslexia concepts and
their monopoly as well as their 100-year-old void in need
of psychoanalysis?

Hopefully the following segments and chapters will enable readers to understand simply and clearly *how and
why countless dyslexics were deprived of breakthrough
medical treatment.*

Summary

Looking back, it appeared that Dr. Silver may have never
intended to come with his interested NIH colleagues to the
Medical Dyslexic Treatment Center, *since he (and they)
opted not to.* Perhaps his written and oral request to do so
was the expedient thing to say for someone in his political
position as a government employee. It sure sounded good.

And if indeed Dr. Silver is correct that "research managers who fund such (dyslexia) research both at my Institute and at the National Institute of Neurological and Communicative Disorders and Stroke . . . could cite no
research to support your [Dr. Levinson's] findings," then I
truly feel sorry for the sad state of affairs at these "Institutes" funded by our tax dollars. I venture to predict that
most readers of *A Scientific Watergate—Dyslexia* will know
more about inner-ear or cerebellar-vestibular dysfunction
and dyslexia than the experts cited by Silver in his letter—
if indeed his comments are accurate. For it sometimes appears as if he doesn't always say what he means or mean
what he says.

Hopefully readers of this book and *A Solution to the Riddle—Dyslexia* will find *all* the cited and referenced evidence needed to independently support and confirm my inner-ear or cerebellar theories and concepts, even if Dr.

Silver and his stated colleagues, for some strange reason, couldn't. But we haven't heard the last of Dr. Silver, for he appears to have the scientific zeal of a missionary on a roll.

Considering that Dr. Larry Silver found the patient-based data and insights within *Smart But Feeling Dumb* "dangerous" and *denied* a massive quantity of supporting cerebellar-vestibular and related data within my medical text, *A Solution to the Riddle—Dyslexia*, is there any wonder that traditionalist experts such as Silver were not able to find and thus solve *any* of the diagnostic/therapeutic riddles in dyslexia for the last hundred years? *It sure makes sense to me! But judge things for yourselves!*

B

More Critical Stuff

No doubt you thought this chapter and theme was over, despite my prediction. Just the opposite. But I felt the reader needed a break, even a symbolic one. I sure did. And so I broke up this seemingly endless but interesting saga into separate segments. Hopefully this break will recharge your concentration and thus prevent drifting or "ADD," at least until we're finished with Silver. And is it also symbolic that we restart with his book, *"The Misunderstood Child"* (1984)?

Considering Dr. Silver's 1984 book title, *The Misunderstood Child*, I could only wonder: Had he really read and understood my research and writings and had he come to my Medical Dyslexic Treatment Center, would dyslexic or learning disabled children still have been misunderstood, even in 1984? Had he properly read and reviewed my medical text *A Solution to the Riddle—Dyslexia*, *Smart But Feeling Dumb*, and the research and scientific papers I published—which he claims I didn't, might he have used a different book title—especially in 1991? In any event, I'm mentioned again in his book under "Controversial Therapies."

Cerebellar-Vestibular Dysfunction

In 1981, Dr. Harold Levinson published a book in which he suggested that some forms of dyslexia are caused by dysfunction in the nerve pathways and in interactions between the balance, or vestibular, system in the ear and the cerebellum, that part of the brain which coordinates balance. He proposes that this disability can be corrected by using medications such as those used for motion sickness. He reports that the dyslexia improves or disappears in patients on this medication.

I have read the book. Levinson cites his research, but most of it has not yet been published in scientific journals and other researchers have not yet been able to test out his results. At this time, then, there is no evidence on which to conclude that this approach is correct. The research to prove or disprove the theory and treatment has yet to be done.

(Larry B. Silver, M.D., *The Misunderstood Child: A Guide for Parents of Learning Disabled Children.* Tab Books, 1984, p. 165.)

Guess what? I'm also mentioned in his second edition, published in 1991.

Vestibular Dysfunction

Several investigators have suggested that the vestibular system is important in learning. The vestibular system consists of a sensory organ in each inner ear that monitors head position and the impact of gravity and relays this information to the brain, primarily the cerebellum. *These investigators claim that there is a clear relationship between vestibular disorders and poor academic performance involving children with learning disabilities.*[1]

[1]Emphasis has been added. Note here how clearly Silver recognizes a relationship between sensory integration and/or vestibular therapy while denying it later on.

The first to stress this view in the United States was Dr. Harold Levinson. In several books published since 1980 he proposes the causative role of the vestibular system and the vestibular-cerebellar systems with dyslexia. He proposes the treatment of dyslexia with antimotion-sickness medication to correct the vestibular dysfunction. *If one reads Dr. Levinson's books, one will not find research to support his theory or the effectiveness of his treatment.* His books refer to his clinical observations and case examples. In his most recent book, he proposed multiple other interventions along with the antimotion-sickness medication, including many other medications and special education. Much research has been done on the vestibular system. The consistent finding is that there is no significant difference either in the intensity of vestibular responsivity or in the prevalence of vestibular dysfunction between children who are normal and those with learning disabilities. Furthermore, these researchers point out that *the technique used by Dr. Levinson to diagnose vestibular dysfunction (i.e., a rotating cylinder with a picture on it, with the child reporting when the picture is no longer clear) is a measurement of "blurring speed" and, thus, a measurement of visual stimulation and not vestibular stimulation.*

Dr. Levinson continues to write his own books. He has not published in professional journals. Much of the publicity for his approach is through appearances on television talk shows. *Despite the evidence against his theory and treatment approach, he remains very busy with a long waiting list.*

(Larry B. Silver, M.D. *The Misunderstood Child*, Second Edition, Tab Books 1991, pp. 257-258.)

Analysis of Content

To best critique the accuracy of Silver's "objective" review of my research, I'd like to abstract part of his discussion for comment. Considering his current position as clinical professor of psychiatry at Georgetown University and his having been an acting director of the National Institute of

Mental Health, his incorrect statements become even more important. Thus, for example:

- "If one reads Dr. Levinson's books, one will not find research to support his theory or the effectiveness of his treatment." *One need only check the references in my medical text and my many research papers—and even here.*

- ". . . researchers point out that the technique used by Dr. Levinson to diagnose vestibular dysfunction (i.e., a rotating cylinder with a picture on it, with the child reporting when the picture is no longer clear) is a measurement of 'blurring speed' and, thus, a measurement of visual stimulation and not vestibular stimulation." *Had Dr. Silver come to my medical offices as he requested and was invited, it would be readily apparent to him (as it is to thousands of my patients) that his description of my 3D Optical Scanner is not only wrong but amazingly incomplete. Had he read my books and research papers, he would have come across a quote from Sir John Eccles, Nobel Laureate for his cerebellar research, claiming my blurring-speed technique was "fascinating" for diagnosing cerebellar-vestibular or inner-ear dysfunctioning. Any medical student having taken even an elementary course in neurophysiology should know that a moving visual target invariably triggers a guided-missile-like to-and-fro eye tracking reflex or nystagmus of inner-ear origin. Accordingly, the blurring of this visual target measures the maximum ability of the eye to fixate and track a moving target—the latter indicating the function or dysfunction of the inner-ear circuitry.*

- "Dr. Levinson continues to write his own books. He has not published in professional journals." *This is outright nonsense, as my books and references show. In fact, my first research paper discussed in Chapter 3 was published in the prestigious* Journal of the

American Academy of Child Psychiatry (1973). *And what is wrong with my writing my own books? Who else should write about my research and clinical experience?* Besides, are we to conclude that anything published outside of professional journals is invalid and not worth reading and investigating? And if my research is correct, then might much of the dyslexia research published in professional journals be incomplete—or in error? Have not recent scientific publications refuted data and conceptualizations in past publications? So what is Silver really trying to say—and do—with his critique? Perhaps it's best to read on before reaching hasty conclusions.

• "Despite the evidence against his theory and treatment approach, he remains very busy with a long waiting list." *As anyone reading my books and research papers will discover, no one has disproven any of my research. I'm busy because my diagnosis and treatment methods work—not because they don't. And I remain busy, despite the bias and scare techniques used by the traditionalists—Silver included. Shouldn't Silver, an eminent psychiatrist, also understand "sour grape" responses to my being busy?*

A Few More Questions And Clarifications

In retrospect, I can only ask Dr. Silver, for the sake of his patients, to reread my content! Reread my references! Reread the scientific works of Ray Snider, Lord Edgar Adrian, Guiseppe Moruzzi, Sir John Eccles—and especially the recent research of three other outstanding cerebellar neurophysiologists, Henrietta Leiner, Alan Leiner and Robert Dow! Above all, read their *many pages of scientific references* supporting their—and my—cerebellar conceptualization and its relationship to dyslexia.

And since the above-mentioned cerebellar neurophysiologists and their research clearly and independently corroborate *all* my cerebellar-dyslexia and related conceptualizations while simultaneously highlighting the corresponding traditionalists' denial, I consider it essential to present both new (1991) and old (1944, 1958) abstracts. *Hopefully this content will enable the reader to decide who is malingering (misrepresenting) cerebellar expertise: The above quoted and referenced neurophysiologists or the traditionalist critics?*

Thus, for example, in their landmark 1991 research paper entitled "*The human cerebro-cerebellar system: its computing, cognitive, and language skills,*" neuroscientists Leiner, Leiner, and Dow summarize a vast array of evidence leading them to conclude:

> "The role of the cerebellum in these (cognitive and language) human functions has tended to be obscured by the *traditional preoccupation* with the motor functions of the cerebellum which have been widely observed in other vertebrates as well. . . . Anatomical evidence and behavioral evidence combine to suggest that *this enlarged cerebellum (in the human brain) contributes not only to motor function but also to some sensory, cognitive, linguistic, and emotional aspects of behavior.*"

The Cerebellar Role in Sensory-Motor Functioning

Although my critics find *A Solution to the Riddle—Dyslexia* "dangerous" and claim it contains no supporting research, let me present the following cerebellar content abstracted from Ray Snider's 1958 *Scientific American* article (originally derived from "Receiving areas of the tactile, auditory, and visual systems in the cerebellum." Snider, R. S., and Stowell, A. (1944), *Journal of Neurophysiology*).

> "For a long time it was thought that the plotting of these (equilibrium and proprioceptive) areas had completed the map of the cerebellar cortex in line with the notion that the cerebellum was restricted to the management of the body's equilibrium and muscular activity. However, at the Johns Hopkins University in 1942

Averill Stowell and I undertook an investigation which has established that the cerebellum is equally involved in the coordination of the sensations of touch, hearing and sight. . . . It becomes increasingly evident that if 'integration' is a major function of this organ, trips into the realm of mental disease may cross its boundaries more frequently than the guards in sanitariums suspect."

—*Cited in* A Solution to the Riddle—Dyslexia, *p. 117, and denied by the various "saviors."*

To highlight and illustrate the role of the cerebellum in modulating or processing sensory-motor and related cerebral cortical functions, I felt it worthwhile to present the following three diagrams from Snider's 1958 article. Hopefully you will better understand how the cerebellar circuits interconnect and interact with all other vital brain centers, and how these secondary centers help shape the symptoms derived from a primary CV dysfunction.

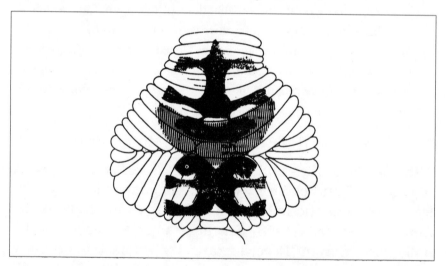

Figure 1 "Homunculi" or projection areas show localization of function in the cerebellum. They show some correspondence to similar projection areas of the cerebrum. Stimuli from the sense organs of touch and from the "proprioceptive endings" that monitor muscle behavior are projected both on the upside-down figure at the top and on the partially split figure at the bottom. Another projection area, which differs from these in not resembling the body shape, is indicated by the shaded area (center). Here auditory and visual stimuli are received. From Snider (1958).

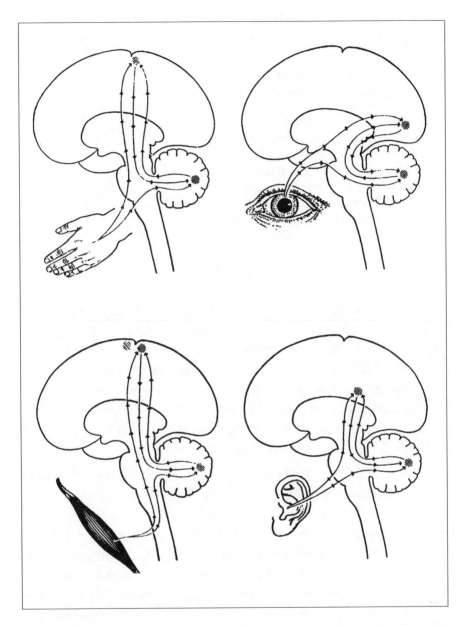

Figure 2 Reverberating Circuits link the cerebellum (the fissured organ at right-center of each picture) to the sensory nerves which connect tactile, visual, proprioceptive, and auditory sense organs to the cerebellum. While part of the message from these organs goes to the cerebrum, part detours through the cerebellum, then "reverberates" through the cerebrum to the cerebellum. It is thought that these circuits serve a feedback function. Proprioceptive impulses from muscles (lower left) may reach more than one cerebral center.

Figure 3   Nerve Circuits connecting cerebrum, cerebellum, and muscle are outlined. The main circuit (left), through which the cerebrum commands the muscle, is supplemented by feedback circuits to the cerebellum (right). Through these feedback circuits the cerebellum monitors the main circuit, comparing command impulse from cerebrum with response (sensory) impulse from muscle.

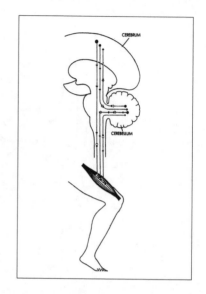

Since the above and related independently performed and corroborating cerebellar research was frequently reviewed throughout my medical text, and as this text contains fifteen years worth of my CV-based dyslexia and phobia research, I'm sure the reader by now will clearly understand why this cited and abstracted research was *denied* by the traditionalist critics, and thus why they found this work "dangerous." Are not the two related?

Clearly, the traditionalists and their scientific void were as threatened by the above cited breakthrough neurophysiological research as they were with *A Solution to the Riddle—Dyslexia, Smart But Feeling Dumb,* and all my other related cerebellar-dyslexia works. Accordingly, I reasoned: To remove this threat, they defensively resorted to denial and criticism. And so they unwittingly displaced the "danger" from themselves to my therapeutic results, the medications used, as well as to dyslexics in need of hope and help. Once again I ask: Are the traditionalists not in need of analysis?[1]

---

[1]An analysis of the subconscious forces driving traditionalist critics to deny and attack the cerebellar reality of dyslexia and its diagnostic/therapeutic insights has been provided in Chapters 20 and 21.

C

And Even More Conflict

Don't give up now. There's still more Silver-related content to come. And it's all vital. So I decided to once again subdivide Dr. Silver's data and present it to you in this final segment.

My research on Attention Deficit Disorder (ADD) indicated that *dyslexia and ADD as well as a whole group of other synonyms were syndromes derived from a common inner-ear or cerebellar-vestibular origin.* These data were clearly documented in several research papers, one containing a sample of 4,000 dyslexic or LD subjects, and a book entitled *Total Concentration* (1990). (And for an introductory validation of these inner-ear-related concepts, I refer you to the ADD and dyslexic cases presented in this book.) My letter to the editor published in the *New York Times* stated as much:

Attention Deficit is Traced to Inner-Ear

To the Editor:

As a physician specializing in diagnosing and treating patients with attention deficit disorder, dyslexia and other learning disabilities, I thank you for your June 21 Health page article on attention deficit disorders.

Dr. Paul Wender's brilliant research of attention deficits in children and adults, and the work of the other physicians you discuss, have been vital in identifying the symptoms of this traumatic ailment.

However, we must also be concerned with the cause and treatment of attention deficit. My research with thousands of patients demonstrated that in most cases there is a common source—an impairment within the inner ear (the cerebellar-vestibular system). *Balance, coordination and rhythm are controlled by the in-*

ner ear, which is a vital part of the brain's concentration and learning centers.[1]

Any disturbance within the inner ear can cause attention deficit symptoms. A three-dimensional optical scanner, a new diagnostic instrument, allows screening for inner-ear dysfunction.[2] With this and other testing techniques, we can now detect those suffering from or predisposed to attention deficit disorder.

A series of antimotion-sickness antihistamines and stimulants, similar to those used by astronauts, has been found significantly to improve inner-ear functioning. My experience is that these medications may alleviate the symptoms having to do with concentration, learning, balance and coordination in more than 90 percent of patients with attention deficits.

Readers should be aware not only of the symptoms of attention deficit disorder and other learning disabilities, but also of diagnosis and treatment available. By effectively diagnosing and treating attention deficits and related symptoms before emotional scarring occurs, we can minimize and ultimately eradicate the psychological fallout for individuals and society.

Harold N. Levinson, M.D.
The New York Times, Monday, July 9, 1990

And, as might have been expected, Dr. Larry Silver replied in another letter to the editor commenting on my letter.

Inner-Ear Origin of Attention Deficit Disorder Lacks Proof

To the Editor:

I am concerned with Dr. Harold N. Levinson's July 9 letter on the cause of attention deficit disorder, dyslexia and other learning disabilities. No other researcher or research team has found his claimed cerebellar-vestibular (inner ear) dysfunction as the probable cause of these syndromes.

---

[1] Note my attributing the control of *rhythm* to the inner-ear in 1990 here when you read Chapter 18, *Acceptance Without Reference.*

[2] I had stated 3D Optical Scanner. The editor misinterpreted this to mean "three dimensional."

There is only one known neurological measure of cerebellar-vestibular functioning, nystagmus. This is a rapid, uncontrolled movement of the eyes. There are tests to measure this behavior. The optical scanner Dr. Levinson mentions measures visual blurring, a visual perception task and not cerebellar-vestibular function.

Ten percent of school-age children and adolescents have learning disabilities (dyslexia) or attention deficit-hyperactivity disorder. Many professionals work with them and try to help them overcome or compensate for these disabilities. Be knowledgeable before using any treatment for your child.

Larry B. Silver, M.D.
Clinical Professor of Psychiatry
Georgetown University
Washington, July, 19, 1990
The New York Times, Saturday, August 4, 1990

Ignorance and/or Bias?

Once again, Dr. Sliver claims: "The optical scanner Dr. Levinson mentions measures visual blurring, a visual perception task and not a cerebellar-vestibular function." Since his misconception of my test and its CV measurements have been reviewed in segment A and will be discussed below, I will skip further comment here.

Is Dr. Silver correct when he states: "There is only one known neurological measure of cerebellar-vestibular functioning, nystagmus"? Clearly Dr. Silver is in error two ways. Not only are there *multiple* neurological signs and symptoms diagnostic of CV dysfunction, but nystagmus may not even be of inner-ear or CV origin. Nystagmus is a symptom indicating rapid to-and-fro eye movements. It may occur spontaneously or be triggered by moving visual targets such as that used by my 3D Optical Scanner. It may be of inner-ear or non-inner-ear origins. Thus, for example, any elementary text on nystagmus and my own works note that albinos with deficient retinal pigmentation develop compensatory nystagmus so that the incoming and non-filtered light doesn't injure their retinas. And there are other ocular and central nervous system origins to nystagmus as well. As a result, this multidetermined symptom cannot be used by itself to diagnose inner-ear or CV dysfunctioning.

In addition, there are multiple neurophysiological signs and symptoms, nystagmus aside, currently used to diagnose CV impairments. Since there are *medical texts* written about the many and varied inner-ear or cerebellar-vestibular neurological signs and symptoms, including those described, tabulated, graphed, and *denied* by Drs. Arnold Gold and Martha Denckla (Chapters 3 and 4) as well as those reviewed by Leiner, Leiner and Dow, might Silver's oversimplistic statement be incorrect? Should not Dr. Silver have read Dr. Robert Dow's classic text, *The Physiology and Pathology of the Cerebellum* (1958), as well as its review within *A Solution to the Riddle—Dyslexia?*

Perhaps Dr. Silver ought to observe police officers examining people suspected of driving while intoxicated. Although police are not medically trained, they clearly know how to test inner-ear-determined balance and coordination functioning (balancing on one foot with and without eyes-closed, finger-to-nose, finger-to-finger and tandem walking testing, etc.). If Dr. Silver had difficulty with these inner-ear or cerebellar tests, why didn't he read Dr. Gold's neurological reports in *A Solution to the Riddle—Dyslexia*, which he alleges to have reviewed? And finally, perhaps neurologist Dr. Denckla can be helpful.

In retrospect, since there are many, many hard and fast traditionally recognized cerebellar neurological signs, nystagmus aside, and *as there are many non-cerebellar-vestibular origins of nystagmus*, aren't Dr. Larry Silver's errors more related to bias and denial than knowledge? Had he really read *A Solution to the Riddle—Dyslexia*, as he claimed in his letters to Warner Books and to me and his readers, he would clearly have seen Tables 1 and 2 listing the neurophysiological signs in cerebellar disorders, as well as their references! Shouldn't well-respected experts like Dr. Silver be more responsible for their scientific criticism as well as the bias influencing their content and intent?

The more of Dr. Silver's content I read, the more I wondered: How could he have missed all those tables depicting

Table 1: Symptoms of Cerebellar Deficiency

Neocerebellar Lesions
Muscular hypotonia
Disturbances of posture
  Abnormal attitudes: Shoulder, body, and/or head tilt or rotation
Static tremor
Disorder of movement (ataxia)
  Dysmetria
  Tremor (movement)
  Adiodochokinesis
  The rebound phenomenon
  Associated movements
Ocular disturbances
  Weakness of conjugate ocular deviation
  Skew deviation
  Nystagmus
Disorders of articulation or phonation
Disorders of gait
Abnormalities of the reflexes
  "Pendular" knee-jerk
Barany's pointing test

Lesions of the Flocculonodular Lobe
Balance and gait disturbances
  Vertigo

Data from *Diseases of the Nervous System* by Brain, 1955, pp. 52-55. Taken from *A Solution to the Riddle—Dyslexia,* p. 60.

Table 2: The Most Common Symptoms of Cerebellar Deficiency, Classified According to the Division of the Cerebellum Thought Primarily Responsible for the Symptom When Diseased or Damaged (Dow and Moruzzi, 1958)

	Division of the Cerebellum Responsible for Symptom		
Symptoms, in Order of Frequency	Focculo-nodular Lobe	Anterior Lobe of Corpus Cerebelli or Medial Part of Corpus Cerebelli	Posterior Lobe of corpus cerebelli or Lateral parts of Corpus Cerebelli
1. Distubance in gait	x	x	x
2. Ataxia of isolated movements of upper extremity			x
3. Spontaneous nystagmus	x		x?
4. Adiodochokinesis			x
5. Ataxia of lower extremity			x
6. Abnormal head posture	x		
7. Hypotonia			x
8. Disturbance in station	x	x	x
9. Past pointing and spontaneous deviation of the limbs			x?
10. Stewart-Holmes Phenomenon			x
11. Dysmetria			x
12. Tremor			x
13. Cerebellar speech disturbance			x
14. Pendular knee jerk			x
15. Cerebellar "fits"		x?	
16. Cerebellar catalepsy		x?	
17. Positive supporting reaction		x?	

Taken from A *Solution to the Riddle -- Dyslexia,* p. 61.

cerebellar signs as well as all the other cerebellar-dyslexia "blind" data and related evidence, especially since he was focused on this specific topic? How could he have missed my scientific papers, which he stated I didn't write? Surely all these consistently and repeatedly made and directed *errors* weren't of a conscious or deliberate nature. Yet they weren't *random* either. Indeed, *all* errors were driven or biased in only one direction—to refute the CV diagnostic/therapeutic insights on dyslexia. *Not one* of Dr. Silver's or the traditionalists' critical errors to date happened to accidentally fall the other way. Considering this rather clear and blatant evidence of loaded "scientific dice," I wondered: *Might all these errors have resulted from denial and the subconscious forces motivating it?*

Perhaps readers now better understand Koestler's remarkably worded insight in the epigraph for Chapter 4:

A closed system is a cognitive structure . . . where parallels intersect and straight lines form loops . . . It ranges from the scientists' involuntary inclination to juggle with data as a mild form
of self-deception, motivated by his commitment to a theory, to
the delusional belief-systems of clinical paranoia.

And I'm equally sure readers of Broad and Wade's *Betrayers of the Truth* will clearly recognize that even gifted
traditionalist researchers, even those publishing in professional journals, are human and so might benefit from
Freud's insights.

My response to Dr. Silver, which follows, was not published. I guess the *New York Times* lost interest and its attention span on ADD.

August 9, 1990

In my July 9th letter to the editor, I simply and concisely highlighted a relationship found between attention deficit disorder
(ADD), dyslexia or learning disabilities (LD), and balance and
coordination (klutzy) signs and symptoms—the latter reflecting
inner-ear dysfunctioning. No doubt Dr. Larry Silver in his August 4th letter was confused by this relationship and unaware of
the wide range of independently published scientific studies used
to derive and verify it. This second letter is a further attempt at
clarification so that interested readers might objectively judge
the facts for themselves. Since upwards of 25 million people suffer from these disabilities, it is imperative that they and the
medical community know what the latest research says and how
it might direct treatment.

Leading researchers in ADD such as Dr. Paul Wender have reported that up to 50 percent of subjects with ADD have dyslexia
or LD *as well as* balance and coordination neurological signs
and symptoms. This repeatedly confirmed clinical observation
triggered the following questions: Might not an inner-ear disorder cause—and thus explain—the above-mentioned relationship
and resulting symptoms? Would not this inner-ear theory explain
why the stimulants and related medications traditionally used to

treat ADD successfully also stabilize inner-ear functioning and prevent motion sickness; why combinations of these very same antimotion-sickness stimulants and antihistamines are used by all astronauts before space flights; and why antimotion-sickness antihistamines were found useful in ADD?

To validate the inner-ear hypothesis, I administered sensitive and sophisticated tests to thousands of patients. Approximately 90 per cent of those with ADD were *also* found to have dyslexia or LD (and the reverse) as well as balance, coordination, and related neurophysiological evidence diagnostic of inner-ear dysfunctioning. These data significantly corroborated Dr. Wender's findings and the inner-ear theory of ADD and dyslexia or LD. Additionally, Sir John Eccles, Nobel Laureate in cerebellar neurophysiology, and a leading group of renowned inner-ear specialists (neurotologists such as Drs. Kenneth Brookler, Howard House, Wallace Rubin, etc.) have publicly supported these findings and conclusions, including the diagnostic use of my 3D Optical Scanner.

All the above data and a wide array of corroborating scientific references supporting the inner-ear basis and treatment of ADD and dyslexia or LD can be found in a series of recently published research papers, including my paper on "The cerebellar-vestibular basis of learning disabilities in children, adolescents and adults: hypothesis and study," in the *Journal of Perceptual and Motor Skills*, and my forthcoming book entitled *Total Concentration—Understanding and Treating ADD* (M. Evans & Co., Fall 1990).

Harold N. Levinson, M.D.
Clinical Associate Professor of Psychiatry
New York University Medical Center

Additional Insights

A patient of mine called after reading Dr. Silver's book and hearing him speak. She thought he might have changed his mind about occupational therapy and the inner-ear system—and perhaps even my research. And another parent heard of this lecture and wrote to him for clarification. Following are her letter to Dr. Silver and his response:

October 5, 1992

Larry Silver, M.D.
Georgetown University Medical School
Department of Psychiatry
3800 Reservoir Road NW
Washington DC 20007

Dear Dr. Silver:

I am the mother of two delightful, active boys. The older one, age 9 years, is having increasing difficulties in school. He cannot concentrate well in class, reads very slowly, uses his finger to keep his place on the line, and makes many spelling errors although we practice a lot at home. Also his balance and coordination (especially in sports) leaves much to be desired. In trying to find some answers, I checked out your book *The Misunderstood Child* from the library and read it with great interest. In fact I had heard you on a radio show several years ago talking about hyperactivity.

Because I respect your opinion and expertise, I am writing to you for understanding on a point that confuses me. In the first edition of your book and also in the revision, I note that you seem skeptical about Dr. Harold Levinson's work with dyslexia and the inner ear connection. I live very close to Dr. Levinson's office and have several friends who have brought their children to see him— all with very good results. About a month ago I traced (through another friend) a parent in Michigan who had heard you speak at the state-wide LD Association conference last November. She said you had stated very positively that cerebellar-vestibular dysfunction was now a known cause of dyslexia. What confuses me is that in your recent edition of *The Misunderstood Child* you don't seem any more favorably inclined to Dr. Levinson's theory about the cerebellar-vestibular relationship, despite what I understood you to include in your lecture in Michigan. Perhaps I misunderstood her, or she misunderstood you?

Before our family spends the money and invests the emotional "hope" in a chance for help through Dr. Levinson's office, I was writing to ask your opinion. My own pediatrician is "sitting on the fence" about this. I would very much appreciate you taking a few minutes to let me know your thoughts about Dr. Levinson. Our family would happily consult with you in WDC—if only we lived closer!

Thank you so much.

Sincerely,

Christine Schmidt

Dr. Silver's Response

Georgetown University

Department of Psychiatry

Child and Adolescent Psychiatric Services

School of Medicine

October 22, 1992

Dear Mrs. Schmidt:

May I try to answer your questions. In the first edition of my book, *The Misunderstood Child*, published in 1984, I reviewed the literature on Dr. Levinson's theory and treatment and concluded that his approach was controversial and not supported by any research (he did none of his own). In the second edition of my book, published in 1991, I update the research on his theory and treatment and again conclude that there is no evidence to support his concepts. In addition, over these years he wrote three other books. Each is less clear and each has no research data. I also note that if he were correct about the cause and treatment for dyslexia, why is not anyone else in this country or the world using his treatment? And, why has no one else been able to get the same results as he claims he gets?

At no time have I stated anything except what is above. Thus, I do not know how anyone might have quoted me as doing so. I do mention Sensory Integration Therapy in my talks. However, this is not a form of cerebellar-vestibular therapy.

I would encourage you not to waste your money or time on Dr. Levinson's treatment. The treatment for Learning Disabilities, as I discuss in my book, is slow and long term. But, it does work. I would stick with special education.

Sincerely,

Larry, B. Silver, M.D.
Clinical Professor of Psychiatry;
Director of Training in Child and Adolescent Psychiatry

Further Clarifications

I should like to clarify a few points so that readers may better understand not only my critics, but also dyslexia and the "controversial therapies" that work vs. the traditionalist medical void. But before getting on with this task, I'd like to present you with a Silver-quote for a rapid analysis of reality: "In the first edition of my book . . . I reviewed the literature on Dr. Levinson's theory and treatment and concluded that his approach was controversial and not supported by any research (he did none of his own)." Is this fact or fiction? And if fiction—what is motivating it?

In addition, the sensory-integration therapy that Dr. Silver mentions in his letter is also known as vestibular (inner-ear or CV) stimulation or enhancement therapy. This therapy and its basis clearly and concisely supports both my inner-ear hypothesis and treatment of dyslexia. So why does Dr. Silver state, "I do mention Sensory Integration Therapy in my talks. However, this is not a form of cerebellar-vestibular therapy." Is this statement correct? Obviously not. Might it reflect either ignorance of the topic and/or bias? Thus, for example, for years most traditionalists, Dr. Silver included, referred to sensory-integration or vestibular therapy as "controversial" and refuted its use and efficacy. And his discussion to this effect, "The 'Magical Cure'," in the *Journal of Learning Disabilities* (1987) as well as the informed rebuttal by a vestibular therapist, Teri Wiss, speak for themselves (see Appendix C in Book II).

In retrospect, although Dr. Silver showed only a superficial awareness of the dyslexia-related subjects he so eloquently criticized, he must be given credit for sincerely attempting to help and thus save dyslexics, albeit he appeared to be saving them from me and other "controversial" therapists.

Had any of you considered the reasons that motivated the traditionalists—like Silver—to attack nonsensically *all* non-traditional therapies? And what led him to claim *that vestibular stimulation or sensory-integration therapy has nothing to do with the use of medications to enhance or stimulate inner-ear or vestibular or cerebellar functioning.* Hopefully the reasons are by now obvious to all. But let me attempt to put your thoughts down on paper—just to make sure our reasoning is similar.

The primary reason that most traditionalists who believe in the thinking-linguistic brain theory of dyslexia refute sensory-motor integration, ocular-motor exercises, tinted lenses, etc.—and the use of antimotion-sickness medications in dyslexia was really quite simplistic. They reasoned as follows: Dyslexia is assumed (and really concluded) to be of a thinking-speaking brain origin. Therefore, any therapy that does not improve this assumed thinking-linguistic dysfunction can't help dyslexics.

It never dawned on these "experts" to consider an alternate hypothesis: *If, indeed, these "controversial" therapies help dyslexics, albeit to varying degrees, might this data suggest that dyslexia may not be of a thinking-linguistic*

*cerebral origin? And since all the controversial therapies—
including auditory perceptual training—improve inner-ear-
related functioning, do not these therapeutic benefits suggest that dyslexia is inner-ear-determined?*

Obviously, this realization escaped Dr. Silver and his
many cohorts. Were they not too taken and perhaps even
"blinded" by their club sanctioned convictions? By the way,
should Silver have recently changed his mind about the
value of sensory-motor integration in dyslexia, I would consider it a plus. However, from his writings it appears that
Dr. Silver's views remain unchanged, but their sound may
have been diplomatically softened by his Washington experience and thus misinterpreted by some hearing his dyslexia-related lectures on "magical cures."

Dr. Silver's "The 'Magic Cure'": A Review of the Current Controversial Approaches for Treating Learning Disabilities[1]

Although Dr. Silver's stated purpose in this article is "to review the significant literature in an effort to assist parents
and professionals in assessing controversial approaches to
treatment," *because of his apparent traditionalist bias and
neurophysiological background, he seemed to have had difficulties doing so objectively. Add to this his apparent lack of
first-hand on-site experience and his mistaken comments become more readily understandable. Indeed, his title, "The
'Magic Cure'," is a dead give-away.*

Accordingly, I felt obliged to review *"The 'Magic Cure'"*
and assess Dr. Silver's critical views and their underlying
motives. Thus, for example, Dr. Silver justifiably links my
research with that of Jane Ayre's contribution to the *vestibular* basis of sensory-motor integration *here* (1987)—*although denying it in his letter to Mrs Schmidt* (10/22/92),
where he states: "I do mention Sensory Integration Therapy

[1]*Journal of Learning Disabilities* 20, No. 8, Oct. 1987.

in my talks. However, this is not a form of cerebellar-vestibular therapy." Since vestibular stimulation is a form of vestibular or CV therapy—as all must readily agree with—what motivated Silver's 1992 denial? And upon analyzing Silver's review, it became readily apparent that his understanding for both Jane Ayre's and my CV medication therapy appeared regrettably inadequate, thus defeating his stated purpose.

In any event, Teri Wiss' intelligent and informed response to Dr. Silver's apparent misunderstanding concerning occupational therapy and sensory integration in children with developmental and learning problems was as helpful as her review of the scientific literature. And in a similar manner, I will attempt to highlight a few points that transparently reveal Silver's apparent confusion regarding my research:

1) He claims that my colleague Dr. Jan Frank and I, as well as De Quiros, did not provide specific information about the caloric testing or ENG procedure—so that our "direct evidence for nystagmus cannot be evaluated." Quite the contrary. Exact details are described in *A Solution to the Riddle—Dyslexia* (especially Appendix D), a medical text he states to have read and reviewed.

2) In discussing my blurring-speed test, in which a moving series of elephants are accelerated until blurring occurs, Dr. Silver once again claims, "It constitutes visual stimulation, not vestibular." Incorrect! Anyone with a neurophysiological background knows that a moving visual target will trigger cerebellar-vestibular (CV)-determined reflex fixation and tracking movements so as to preserve *clear vision*. And so *visual blurring* serves as an endpoint measuring maximum adaptive cerebellar-vestibular-determined fixation and tracking capacity. As is clinically apparent, dyslexics invariably manifest let-

ter, word, and sentence ocular fixation and tracking problems ("word blurring")— most often requiring a compensatory slower reading speed and need for a pointer or marker. And as this impairment is due to CV-determined "clumsy" eye movements, it stands to reason that inner-ear dysfunctioning patients with dyslexia will "blur-out" a moving visual sequence much faster than people with normal inner-ear function—unless, of course, learned compensatory tracking and processing mechanisms occur over time. (This blurring-speed technique will be described and illustrated in greater detail in Book II.)

All this is clearly described in *A Solution to the Riddle—Dyslexia* and *Smart But Feeling Dumb*, which Dr. Silver claimed to have read, and in a series of published research papers which were denied. Might unwitting bias mechanisms and their analysis help explain these "errors"?

3) Since rotation studies are typically used by most researchers, including NASA, to test for inner-ear induced nystagmus (a reflex pattern of rapid to-and-fro eye movements), and as Ayres used this test in a lighted room with eyes open, Dr. Silver claims this "provides both visual and vestibular stimulation; thus, it may not be a valid test of vestibular function."

Although this sounds logical, Dr. Silver apparently has neither *personal* nor neurophysiological experience with this test. When rotated, people develop an inner-ear-determined nystagmus and get dizzy. And when spun sufficiently, the rate and intensity of the induced inner-ear nystagmus cannot be inhibited or blocked—even when the eyes are open and testing is done in a lighted room. Thus the detectable inner-ear-determined nystagmus, even if less than would be present were it measured electronically with the patient's eyes closed while in a darkened room, is still inner-ear-determined!

For this reason, the rotation and caloric studies performed at the Medical Dyslexic Treatment Center use closed eyes and darkness to maximize the detection and measurement of inner-ear (CV)-determined nystagmus. Since this is also discussed throughout *A Solution to the Riddle—Dyslexia*, it seems strange that Dr. Silver failed to mention it in this critical article!

4) Finally, Dr. Silver uses *rotation studies* by Helene Polatajko (*Developmental Medicine and Child Neurology*, 1985) to refute the vestibular basis of dyslexia or LD. Once again, he and Polatajko appear to conclude that one or two rotation test parameters of vestibular function are capable of completely defining and measuring the functioning—and thus dysfunctioning—of the entire cerebellar-vestibular system as well as their interrelationships with all other vital brain functions. This makes as much sense as saying that the simple knee-jerk test that physicians use to examine neurological functioning is fully capable—by itself—of encompassing total brain function and dysfunction. [And for readers interested in greater detail, this critique is reviewed in my research paper "The diagnostic value of cerebellar-vestibular tests in detecting learning disabilities, dyslexia and attention deficit disorder" (*Perceptual and Motor Skills*, 1990)].

In many ways, this all-or-none thinking is reminiscent of the way the traditionalists conceptualize dyslexia—as a severe reading disorder. It doesn't seem to bother them that: 1) dyslexia is much more than a reading disorder; 2) a majority of dyslexics do not have—or overcome—severe reading disorders and yet still experience typical dyslexic reading, writing, spelling, math, memory and related symptoms; 3) nystagmus is just *one of many, many* neurological signs and symptoms of an inner-ear (CV) dysfunction, and not the only one; 4) not all nystagmus is inner-ear determined; and 5) not all tests detecting inner-ear dysfunctioning will be abnormal in any given patient or sample. Hopefully, this brief review as well as Teri Wiss' response will give the reader a clear and objective view of Dr. Silver and his fellow traditionalists.

A word of caution: Do not be frightened by Silver's deliberately chosen title: "The 'Magic *Cure*'." There is *no cure*, just help. And there is *no "magic"* about treatment responses. They can all be clearly understood by any dyslexic, even those with severe reading disorders (see Chapter 13). Just remember: Any help and improvement is better than none—even if this help bothers the traditionalists. Even if they didn't discover the method, or even prescribe it. Clearly, the traditionalists use "magical" *scare* tactics to frighten away those in need. They pretend to be your friend and savior while doing so, all for their own purposes. Unfortunately, the traditionalists have no medical way of diagnosing and treating dyslexia—a century-old fact they keep forgetting to tell their listeners and readers, while attacking all "controversial" others who attempt to help.

In retrospect, I was forced to wonder: Is it not strange or paradoxical that concepts and therapies that work are labeled "controversial," whereas the traditional theories leading nowhere during the last 100 years are considered accepted, proven, or "non-controversial"? Is scientific reality not only denied, but reversed?

Another Case In Point

Before ending my analysis of Silver's "The 'Magic Cure'" and his refuting the efficacy of vitamins and related substances in dyslexia, I'd like to present a *parent-physician's observations* regarding the use of Deaner (DMAE) which I use in addition to the antimotion-sickness medications. Although only about 5-10% of dyslexics report improvements on this substance, and fewer on vitamins and related preparations such as Lecithin, *I consider any improvement better than none.*[1] *However, since Dr. Silver and his traditionalist colleagues have been used to* no *neurophysiologically-derived improvements for the last 100 years, I guess they have difficulty coping with a change in their 0%. As a result, they must be inwardly driven to reject all medical improvements greater than theirs.* And you all know what that means— that *any medically based or related improvement* of dyslexic symptoms must appear to them "magical" and a "cure."

May 15, 1983[2]

Dear Dr. Levinson:

Just a note to bring you up to date on the progress of my daughters, Paula and Robin.

Paula is a student at the Ethel Walker School in Simsbury, Conn. She had been having a difficult time increasing her reading speed and comprehension in spite of intensive extra help from a reading skills professional at school for one and one-half years. When she was placed on Deaner (DMAE) in addition to Meclizine her roommate noticed that she was completing her homework in much less time. When she came home for spring vacation we went to Italy for two weeks of touring and skiing. I was

---

[1]Gary Chapman reported dyslexia-related improvements from vitamins and analogous substances (Chapter 7). And Ann Dixon, a 16½-year-old, experienced significant improvements in balance from multivitamins and lecithin (Chapter 1-B). Just remember, even a 1-2% improvement rate is infinitely greater than 0%—especially for those experiencing the improvement. And so results are maximized when all helpful methods—controversial or not—are holistically combined.

[2]This real-named case dating back over ten years was presented to dramatize the power of the traditionalists, and thus their ability to have blocked similar treatment responses for years and years.

amazed to note that during that time she read the *Thorn Birds*, a feat that would have required a whole summer to complete the year before. I asked the reading skills teacher to retest Paula to see if there was any change in her reading ability since she was placed on Deaner (DMAE). The results showed a jump from the 13th percentile to the 48th percentile which she (the teacher) thought was amazing and difficult to explain.

This year her grades went from the 4th quintile to the 1st quintile (high honors). She has been accepted to the University of Vermont, which was her first choice.

Robin has been doing well on Deaner as well. I wasn't sure at first, but when she ran out and I was slow to get some more to her, she noted difficulty maintaining her level of scholastic achievement.

Sincerely,

Norman J. Zeig, M.D.

A "Common Sense" Reviewer

Finally, I would like to mention a book by Dr. Anne Huston, *Common Sense About Dyslexia* (1987), favorably reviewed by none other than *Dr. Silver* as "both informative and practical . . . important reading for all concerned about this problem . . . especially helpful to individuals who are dyslexic and their families." At the time, Dr. Larry Silver was director of the National Institute of Dyslexia.

No doubt you are wondering what this book and review have to do with me. As you will note, Huston couldn't grasp the essence of what my research had demonstrated: (1) that dyslexia is an inner-ear syndrome and that some with this disorder compensate well for reading, spelling, etc., and (2) that the medications I use often help improve speech-related symptoms as well as auditory discrimination and processing difficulties for words and sentences heard, even in those that also have auditory acuity difficulties when tested with mere beeps rather than words. Thus, Dr. Huston states (p. 122): *"Levinson reports that some of his 'dyslexics' have been excellent readers and spellers. . . . He even claims that his medication has cured deafness and stuttering as well as dyslexia."*[1] And in her criticism, following these distortions, she condescendingly emphasizes in italics: *"Dyslexics cannot do their work at the expected grade levels—much less perform well above average."*[2]

Considering Dr. Silver's expertise in dyslexia and eminent position, should he not have corrected these nonsensical comments? Unless, of course, he also shares these views and underlying motives. Perhaps the book's title should have been *"Nonsense About Dyslexia"*? Had Silver and Huston read and understood my writings, they would have come across innumerable dyslexic patients with delayed and scrambled auditory (and visual) input problems as well as those responding favorably to medication. Have there not been significant numbers of dyslexics presented indicating that stuttering and speech symptoms as well as auditory processing improve on inner-ear-enhancing medications? Indeed, these very same symptoms were spontaneously observed to intensify during ear infections or when the compensatory antihistamines were stopped.

There's even more to be said here, but enough is enough. You can read professor Silver's other comments of a similar nature concerning *all* the non-traditional therapies shown thus far to be helpful in dyslexia and LD. But rest assured that I will be objective and fair with the traditionalists. And so in the next chapter I will clearly and

---

[1]By now, the reader has "seen" and "heard" many favorable responses of dyslexics in which improvements ("cures") were reported in auditory discrimination and processing as well as speech—stuttering included.

[2]Hopefully Dr. Huston and all the other traditionalists will benefit from the insights to be derived from one of my successfully treated, gifted patients (see Chapter 10, A Dyslexic Without "Dyslexia").

completely summarize all the traditional medical therapies developed and initiated since 1896.

Last is Best

Oops. I almost forgot two of Dr. Silver's most important comments. And I instinctively saved them for last. Thus, for example, in his "critical" letter to Christine Schmidt (10/22/92) he states: "If he [Dr. Levinson] were correct about the cause and treatment for dyslexia, why is not anyone else in this country or the world using his treatment? And, why has no one else been able to get the same results as he claims he gets?"

Although this expert-sounding and scary criticism is by now familiar, I thought it appropriate to answer Silver by presenting you a letter recently received from a physician in South Africa. Hopefully its content and intent will be helpful to Drs. Silver, Ente, and the rest of the "club" members. It is typical of others reported to me over the years.

March 26, 1993

Dear Dr. Levinson:

I am a General Medical Practitioner in private practice in Durban, South Africa who has, through your book, become aware of your theory and approach to dyslexia.

I am happy to report that I have tried combinations of Cyclizine and Imipramine in about five children, all of whom have reported dramatic improvement. All the parents have bought your book!

I do realize that you probably get many inquiries of this kind, but, nevertheless, I would be most grateful if you could answer my following questions:

1. Have you any literature or references; especially on the use of the various medications?

2. I would like to assess my patients objectively and scientifically. Do you have any suggestions or is there perhaps a specific pro forma in use at your Center?

3. You do maintain that an ordinary audiogram is often not very helpful. What does your ear evaluation involve— also, what exactly is the role of your 3-D Optical Scanner in your management of cases? How does it work?

I, together with some of the mothers, am thinking of getting a group together in order to help the children better and also to promote your theories as a solution to a very big problem.

I really appreciate your help.

Yours faithfully,

R.P. Perold, M.D.

And believe it or not: Professor Silver's NIH consultant, Dr. Martha Denckla, highly critical of my cerebellar research, recently substantiated the cerebellar role in ADHD and ADD while Silver states (pp. 186-187): *"No other researcher or research team has found his [Dr. Levinson's] claimed cerebellar-vestibular (inner ear) dysfunction as the probable cause of these [ADD, ADHD, Dyslexia] syndromes."*[1]

Thus, within his book on ADD (1992), Dale R. Jordan, Ph.D., notes: "In 1991 Martha Denckla reported results from . . . children with ADHD and ADD. *Magnetic Resonance Imaging (MRI) research at the Johns Hopkins School of Medicine had revealed immature, incomplete function within the cerebellum.* This defect in cerebellar function triggers such problems as poor organization and poor inhibition of impulses. The result is behavior that is never well organized and is usually impulsive."

---

[1]Since both Denckla and Silver presented at the very same 1991 Chicago LD Association National Conference, the confusion characterizing Mrs. Schmidt's 1992 letter to Silver (pp. 193-194) became readily understandable. However, the experts' confusion and savioristic needs required additional analysis. Interestingly enough, the name of Silver's [February 27, 1991] paper presented was "Attention deficit-hyperactivity disorder: If it is for real, why all of the confusion?"

CHAPTER 9

Equal Time

Because my "controversial" medical treatment of dyslexia as well as all other "magical cures" (eye exercises, occupational therapy, tinted lenses, etc.) have been significantly criticized by the Ortonians and their many and varied saviors, I thought it only fair to devote an entire chapter to presenting all contrasting traditional medical therapies for dyslexia—especially as my critics in the past have demanded *equal time* from the "Today Show" and "Donahue" following my appearances with successfully treated dyslexics (see Chapter 6).

Perhaps modesty has thus far prevented the traditionalists from documenting their own medical success stories as I and my fellow "controversialists" have. Or perhaps the reader might be interested in learning a lesson I taught my daughter Joy when she was very young: *"Sometimes it's what people don't say that's most important—not what they do say."*[1]

---

[1]When Joy was 9 years old and considering summer camp, my wife and I had a representative come to the house and show us a "camp film." As soon as it was over, Joy pulled my wife and me aside and quietly but definitively whispered: "I'm not going to that camp!!!" Shocked, we asked Joy, "Why? The camp film looked beautiful." Her reply: "They showed you beautiful bunks and grounds. But they don't have bathrooms. Do you remember what you once told me about looking for what's not shown you? The film didn't show any bathrooms."

So here goes. The following *symbolic graph* is a complete and thorough review of *all the traditionally accepted and reported medical breakthroughs to date:*

A Symbolic Graph

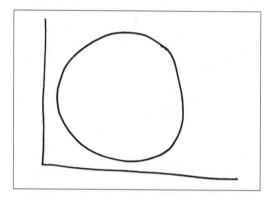

Figure 1   The traditionalists' zero medical progress—diagnostically and theraputically—over the past 100 years.

No, I'm not joking. In fact, I'm dead serious. Do you recall how often I've repeated that the traditionalists live and thrive in their diagnostic/therapeutic medical vacuum? Well, now you can clearly see it for yourselves—in all its "graphic splendor."

Tragically for millions of dyslexics and their families, this thorough review might be the shortest "progress report" in medical history. After reviewing this chapter, perhaps you all might better understand:

- the traditionalist experts and their criticism;
- their "silent modesty" concerning mention and comparison of their own medical therapies (and diagnostics) vs. mine and others;
- the chutzpa of the traditionalists referring to *my* diagnostic/therapeutic research as "controversial"—"unsupported or unproven"—when in fact they have nothing medically to show in the way of progress over the last 100 years and no explanation or even apology;

- the oversized "scientific egos" characterizing the dyslexia traditionalists, considering their *zero progress curve* and the confusion and denial characterizing their expertise.

And their diagnosing dyslexia as a "pure" disorder in which reading scores must be at least two years below peers and/or potential is also invalid, and thus deserves a zero rating as well.

For those skeptics—professionals and others—still remaining, I encourage you to review carefully Dr. Larry Silver's "The 'Magic Cure'" and related content and then ask yourselves: What is most important? What he said or what he left out? Or might both be equally vital and thus reflect underlying bias-determinants similar to those I've already mentioned?

Part B

Dyslexia ≠ "Dyslexia"

CHAPTER 10

A Dyslexic Without "Dyslexia"

To highlight the deadly error leading traditionalists to equate the syndrome of many and varied symptoms called dyslexia with only severely impaired reading scores, also mistakenly referred to as "dyslexia," I thought it essential to present you with the informative case in point of a gifted woman named Joan Sparks. And because Joan is a typical dyslexic without "dyslexia" who responded dramatically and favorably to medical therapy, her study also illustrates that dyslexics with and without "dyslexia" require equal hope and help: treatment.

Although these rather simple points are absolutely vital to solving the many diagnostic and therapeutic riddles characterizing dyslexics and their disorder, no traditionalist expert to date was able or willing to listen. Perhaps they will listen and learn from Joan—as I have. Hopefully dyslexia experts will now recognize that the vast majority with this syndrome are dyslexics without "dyslexia"—rather than "lazy," neurotic, or worse. Hopefully they will belatedly recognize Joan's many personal and "controversial" attempts at compensation, including the use of eye exercises, tinted glasses, and inner-ear-enhancing medications. And finally, assess for yourselves if Joan needed or would have benefitted from Ortonian tutoring.

By carefully reading through Joan's self-report of symptoms and favorable therapeutic responses (and those of others to follow), I hope you will develop an insight into dyslexia as well as the benefits of medical treatment that cannot be obtained in any other way—certainly not by the infinite number and variety of test scores (reading, writing, spelling, math, IQ) provided by hands-off and aloof experts in place of hands-on understanding, empathy, and help. And I hope you will be able to understand and judge the confusion and denial characterizing the traditionally accepted dyslexia definitions and conceptualizations. Hopefully you will be as inspired by Joan as I was. Indeed, were it not for the immeasurable inspiration provided me by the often "life-saving" favorable therapeutic responses of thousands of similar dyslexics, I would have never been able to *easily* endure, understand and complete *A Scientific Watergate—Dyslexia.*

Favorable Responses to Medication

Because patients know themselves so well—infinitely better than physicians such as myself can—I decided to let Joan describe her improvements and symptoms uninterrupted, except for footnotes. These notes have, via a separate dialogue, enabled me to highlight points of interest and contrast between the reality of dyslexia and the traditionalists' theoretical fantasies. In addition, Joan's improvements on inner-ear-enhancing medications as well as the other so-called "magical cures" presented throughout this work highlight and symbolize the therapeutic medical void characterizing the traditionalists described in Chapter 9. Joan's improvements more than speak for themselves and my critics.

Joan Sparks

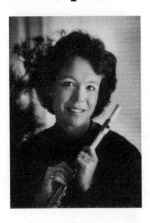

Two months ago, I was diagnosed by Dr. Levinson as dyslexic, and I began the program of medications and vitamins that he prescribed. The change has been and continues to be profound. I kept a diary of each medicine and its effect as they were added to my daily routine. Each addition or increase in medication had a specific effect, and continue in combination to have a cumulative positive improvement. The following is a summary of my experience as a patient of Dr. Levinson.

1 July 1992. Appointment with Dr. Levinson. Took part in a blind study in which I was given a pill and was told that it was either a placebo or an antihistamine. About 20 minutes later, I went into the Ladies Room and noticed *that the floor tiles were not in motion as they had been earlier in the day.*[1] As I later learned, I had been given the antihistamine.

2 July. Began first medication, an anti-emetic, antihistamine. I began, as with all medications prescribed by Dr.

---

[1]Are not movement illusions also speed-related and thus timing illusions? Do they not improve on medications? Note these time-related symptoms characterizing Joan's case since they will be relevant in Chapters 17 and 18. To highlight these symptoms, I have italicized passages where they are described.

Also, Joan's spontaneously written content clearly highlights that "double-blind" studies were conducted at the Medical Dyslexic Treatment Center, although the results have not as yet been published.

Levinson, with ¼ of a tablet. I noticed the next morning as I did my usual three mile walk/run, that the *objects around me did not bounce around as much with every step.* I felt as if I were in a movie, since *all of the things around me (trees, houses, the roadway, etc.) now moved smoothly and in a controlled manner. As I increased the dosage, the effect continued to increase, until I had a still horizon at all times.* Until this point (as in the case with all the other medications) I had no idea that this was part of being dyslexic. The other benefit of this first medication is that I am no longer dizzy after exercising (I run and swim).

12 July. Began the vitamins. No significant improvement noticed at first. After two months, I find that my hair, skin and nails are healthier.

30 July. Began the second antimotion-sickness pills. Immediately my peripheral vision was more in focus.[1] I could see in stereo; objects had depth. I could look at a tree in the distance and see definition in the leaf and branch formations. I could also see depth into the leaves and branches. In general, all objects as well as my depth perception began to take on more clarity. I began to write more neatly without trying, and I wrote in a straighter line. Perhaps the most surprising event was the first time I went to the grocery store. I again experienced the phenomenon that the objects around me moved when I did, and in an orderly manner; I felt as if I was gliding down the aisles (I had previously hated to grocery shop and only went in desperation).[2] The objects I wanted were where I expected them to be. I left the grocery store and realized that

[1]Contrary to the research of Geiger and Lettvin published in the *New England Journal of Medicine* (1987), most dyslexics experience impaired (rather than enhanced) peripheral vision which improves on inner-ear-enhancing medications. Also their front/back vision or depth perception improved—reflecting an inner-ear-determined "flat" perception in untreated dyslexia. Similar phenomenon occur in auditory and tactile perception—as will be described by Joan.

[2]These symptoms often trigger shopping phobias or agoraphobia. (See my work entitled *Phobia Free* [1986].)

I was not dizzy and confused as I had always been before. Later that day as I was balancing the checkbook I again realized that I was not tense, dizzy and confused as I had always been in the past when working with numbers.

As time went on, I noticed an improvement in my night vision. The letters on directional signs were no longer blurred-out, but were clear and crisp. Street lights and the headlights of oncoming cars no longer had halos around them. I found that I would work at the PC longer without tension, and the words were much more quiet on the screen. In general any information that was acquired through reading, whether words or music, was more available, my eyes were tracking better than before: better than when I had worn Irlen lenses, or after the two courses of vision therapy I had taken in previous years.[1]

1 August. Began the next vitamin. No noticeable change.

2 August. Took my seven-year-old son Christopher to see Dr. Levinson. I had long suspected that Christopher and I shared similar perceptual problems. After my diagnosis, I realized that the best thing to do for Christopher was to have his problems diagnosed early. This is his first-grade year, the year he learns to read, and especially important. As it turned out, my instinct was correct. Christopher is beginning the same medication regimen as I. One incident at the appointment was particularly poignant. Christopher and I were in the nurse's office, waiting to be briefed on the routine. We were given release forms to sign, giving consent to make data available to Dr. Levinson from Christopher's appointment. As I pointed to the three lines for his signature, Christopher said, "Mom, you'll have to show me each one, one at a time. The letters and lines are bouncing around so much I can't tell where you

[1]Contrary to the opinions of Dr. Silver, these so-called "controversial therapies" and "magic cures" work—by enhancing inner-ear functioning. Where are the traditional medical cures? Additional insights regarding these lenses will be provided in Chapters 13 and 15.

said to put my name." I replied, "You know, I was just remembering the first time I was here. The lines and letters
were bouncing around for me then too. But today, since
I've been taking the medication Dr. Levinson told me to
take, the letters are still." He said, "That's why I'm here!"

7 August, driving to Maine. My personal panorama became larger and more well-defined. As I read road signs, I
could feel my left eye begin to cross over, and then snap
back into place. The left eye always crossed when I concentrated on an object (It also was near-sighted, and I
have noticed that it is much less nearsighted, with the improvement dating from the addition of the antimotion-sickness drug). The guard-rail supports did not blur-out as
they had before. I realized that I had always avoided looking at them because the blurring-out would make me uncomfortable.[1] The same was true with the lane dividing
lines, when they were on new, black pavement, and were
newly painted. I began to not have to squint any more to
focus on the road, signs, or anything else I needed to
read. Words were clear, and it took much less effort to
take them in.

One day, while on vacation, I forgot to take my afternoon dosage of medicine and vitamins. The next morning I
got up early to go and buy donuts as a special treat for the
kids. This meant a drive of six miles. As I drove, I realized
that I was gripping the steering wheel tightly, and was feeling anxious about where I was going. I have been vaca-
tioning at the same spot once a year for eighteen years

---

[1]Because dyslexics report blurring while fixating and tracking, it seemed
logical to develop my 3D Optical Scanner to measure these inner-ear
phenomena. Note how the medications improve this function. Since the
inner-ear controls muscle tone and the alignment of the eyes for focusing
and tracking, the latter functions are often impaired in dyslexics and so
contribute to strabismus or "eye crossing"—especially when fatigued—
unless compensated for by inner-ear-enhancing medications. In addition,
via eye exercises, the underlying and related inner-ear circuitry can be conditioned—thus resulting in reading and related concentration improvements.

now. The trip to Congdon's Donut Shop was a ritual. As I drove into the lane back to the house (with the requisite dozen donuts of various flavors) after nearly turning down the wrong lane (there are two close together off the county road) I realized that I had not taken my medicine the previous afternoon. This was how I had felt all the time prior to July 2. I took the morning dosage, and within a half an hour, I again felt the improvements I had come to enjoy.

22 August. Began the final addition to my regimen, which is another anti-emetic and antihistamine. To my astonishment, I see even more clearly. *Now the letters on any page are entirely still.* I had feared that even with Dr. Levinson's prescription, words would never be entirely still on the page. They are now. In fact, information is now not only more available, it is aggressive. It is with amazement that I now see words pop out at me, with ease and clarity. My peripheral panorama is greater than ever before.[1] The periphery of my vision is organized, no longer chaotic. I find I can look with comfort at things I had always avoided, such as MAC [automated banking] machine screens, the computer screen, plaid, hounds-tooth, or striped patterns on clothing and furniture, oriental rugs, floor tile patterns, escalator steps, and most importantly to me, music.

I have not mentioned other sensory improvements, because in some ways these improvements are more subtle. The improvement in my hearing is most important to me as a professional musician [flutist]. I have always had a good ear; my sense of pitch is often called "perfect pitch," and even though it could be capricious, it still could hold me in good stead, especially when sight reading (which for

---

[1]These sensory improvements on inner-ear-enhancing medications and the corresponding symptoms initially led me to recognize the role of the inner-ear (CV) system in processing the total sensory input as it does the total motor output. In addition, the improved auditory (and visual) processing clearly highlights the ignorance behind Dr. Anne Huston's criticism of (1) my "curing the deaf," and "dyslexia," and thus (2) my view of reading-score-compensated dyslexics.

obvious reasons had always been the area of most concern for me). Since I have been taking the program prescribed by Dr. Levinson, I have noticed a far greater acuity
in my hearing. I can now hear three- and four-part coun-
terpoint as all four voices moving at once. Before, I had always been forced to segregate one voice and follow it. In
fact, I had to make a firm rule for myself at the time of the
final medication addition: I could not listen to classical music on the car stereo, because it was so beautiful and so
clear, and too distracting. I have been enjoying a tremendous improvement in reading music in general. My
eyes track the notes clearly and at fast tempi. The notes
no longer blur-out. *My sense of rhythm is better. Complicated rhythmic patterns come more quickly.* I no longer
need to constantly check patterns of musical notes, or
even repeated notes, because they stay put. They are
where I remember them to be. The same sense of depth
and stereo I have visually is improved aurally as well. *I
hear, with greater distinction, fast technical passages
when I or others play them.* I can hear the quality of
chords, and identify them. There are improvements in
terms of tactile facility.[1] Certain musical technical passages and trills which were always particularly difficult for
me are easier to learn and retain.

In general, I seem not to have to make the extra effort
it always took to do any of the tasks that involve analytical
use of my senses. As mentioned earlier, information is now
not only more available, it is aggressive. As a consequence, I no longer feel mentally numb at the end of the
day, or even at mid-day. I can read for longer periods of
time, and retain more of what I read. I skip lines much less
when I read, and can find my place readily when I look
away from the page.[2] My memory is better. I have noticed

[1]Note the improvement of "tactile facility"—adding to the improvement
in total sensory-motor processing.

[2]As repeatedly stated by me, dyslexics without "dyslexia" still have
reading symptoms which often improve on medications.

improvement in such things as remembering a phone number after seeing it only once, or remembering people's names. I spell better. Background noise is not as distracting. *I don't have to take time to process what I have heard in order to respond,* so that now I can come up with witty repartee and fast answers in meetings and discussions. I enjoy conversation with groups of people much more. *I can process others' words and respond with a speed that was previously unknown to me.*[1]

Finally, I am writing this at my PC, typing without looking down at the keyboard. This is a first for me.[2]

There are some considerations that need to be mentioned, not necessarily as negative, but in terms of cautions. I have learned to eat a much larger breakfast, and have had to incorporate a 3:00 snack into my schedule. I did gain about five pounds at first, but now that I have adjusted to a new (and healthier) pattern of eating, I have lost it. I cannot drink alcohol with the same abandon as before. One glass of wine is about it at social occasions. One glass has the effect of three. I also notice fatigue, in terms of not enough sleep, and have had to be more careful to approach an eight hour sleep schedule. I cannot let myself become too hungry. The one symptom that prevails when I am not cautious of the above mentioned items is that I feel groggy, and have the sense that I am indeed taking medications. Otherwise, I have no sensation that I am taking anything other than vitamins.

Yesterday, I took an audition for the first time since starting Dr. Levinson's program. *I took the audition for the*

---

[1]Similar observations of rapid improvement in all sensory-motor functions and the underlying corresponding impairments led me to initially develop 3-D Optical, Auditory, and Tactile Scanners as well as motor (balance and coordination) tests for dyslexics.

[2]The ability to know where fingers and body parts are in space is part of a sensory function called proprioception—neurophysiologically reported to be controlled by the cerebellum. Its improvement by use of inner-ear-enhancing antihistamines resulted in corresponding improvements in Joan's typing skills.

sole purpose of determining how well my visual acuity would stand up under pressure. I purposely chose one of the most difficult concertos in the repertoire, and prepared the orchestral excerpts at a faster tempo than is required. In the morning, as I drove west on the Pennsylvania Turnpike, and as the adrenaline started to kick in, I noticed that the landscape was clear and sharply defined. Before the medication, my peripheral vision would become even more chaotic with nerves. This time the periphery was clearer than earlier in the day, and more available. The highway divider supports were absolutely distinct and not blurred-out, and I read words on highway signs clearly. As I warmed up before the audition, *I could, clearly and with control, track the music, without experiencing the blurring-out that had always happened when I was nervous.* I went into the audition and, during the playing of the concerto, realized that I was more nervous than I needed to be. I saw everything. It was there on the page. All I had to do was play. As the audition progressed, I was able to let go of the nervousness and achieve a greater degree of control than I ever had before, *allowing me to finesse such things as speed and amplitude of vibrato*, the tonguing patterns I was using, and the loudness of my breathing. I "nailed" each one of the treacherous orchestral excerpts, for the first time, using an assertiveness I had never attained before.

In conclusion, the most important and least understood aspect of dyslexia is its subtlety, and myriad effects.[1] I had considered my collection of symptoms little more than charming (and not-so-charming) idiosyncrasies. The range and depth of the improvement has indicated to me that dyslexia is a disorder which impacts the dyslexic to a greater degree than even the dyslexic can comprehend. I am grateful that my son, with all his talent and intelligence,

---

[1] If only the "experts" understood this. Joan's improvements in sensory-motor timing or temporal processing will be continued in Book II.

will be able to assume his role in society (and he will be a person who will make a contribution) without the struggle to simply keep up. He will be able to realize his full potential, which is his and every child's right.

Joan Sparks' Dyslexic Symptoms: Historical Data

Although this history of symptoms was presented by Joan Sparks last in her self-report, I took the dyslexic-inspired liberty of shifting its original position, as I thought these symptoms would be better appreciated by the reader following a thorough review of their disappearance on medications.

Sunday, March 14. Called my friend Anne and others to request permission to use their names and statements for this article. The reading teacher was especially supportive. She was thrilled to see such a dramatic improvement in Christopher since the conference. She knew how very intelligent Christopher is, and was glad to report that he is now working up to that potential. "You know," she said, "I gave him two hugs last week, and drew stars on his hands. I wanted him to know how well he had done."

One person I spoke to today remarked that it was difficult for her to think of me as having a problem such as dyslexia. She said that I had always been very well organized, happy, and had a successful career in *music* of all things! As I explained to her some of my past, I realized that it would be helpful for readers of this article to know what I experienced prior to treatment.

I was not a good student. In the second grade, I read at the sixth grade level, but could not spell. So I was only allowed to check out books at the second grade level from the school library. My sixth grade yearbook lists as my motto, "Wake up and read." I read constantly, and yet continued to have trouble with spelling and *grammar. I frequently received "D's" in math.* I had a terrible temper, sometimes resorting to throwing things. I had tantrums well past the terrible twos. I was sensitive to sounds and confusing situations. *I was clumsy*, affectionately called "the klutz" by my family. *I was forgetful, absent minded.* I required much more sleep each night than my sisters and brother.

I graduated from high school with a 2.5 grade point average. The guidance counselor advised me not to expect to graduate from college. My report cards were filled with comments such as: *"She does not work up to potential." "Her hand cannot keep up with her mind when she writes." "She is careless, lazy." "She daydreams through much of the day."* I remember when I began to print instead of write: I consciously decided I would do better if I slowed down enough to be able to think of each letter of each word as I wrote.

I would begin each new school year thinking that this year would be different. The new clothes, books, supplies would inspire me to try even harder. Somewhere during the first month I would realize that this year was to be like every other, and I gave up. Specifically, it was exponential notation in the seventh grade which led me to the conclusion that it mattered little how hard I tried: it was no use. So I flung myself into swimming and eventually music.

My grade point average for my undergraduate degree was a 3.2. Earlier I explained how I had found an efficient way and place to study. I further developed compensatory skills in graduate school, where I earned a 3.9 for my masters, and had a 3.9 for the first portion of my doctorate. The dramatic change in my graduate work had to do with a process of synthesis which I followed for each course. By the time of the final exam, all of the information from reading, lectures, and research for the term would be in the form of an outline on one piece of paper. Each statement of the outline would trigger the memory of the details of what I had read or heard.

During graduate school, a portion of work for music-
ology courses was harmonic analysis, which can be
thought of as the mathematical aspect of music. On many
of my research papers, the professors would puzzle at the
excellent work I had done in all respects except the harmonic analysis, which was very bad.

I had an undiagnosed eating disorder during my undergraduate years. I would alternately starve myself, or binge/
purge.[1] I remember thinking that I could not justify being
well fed when so many in the world were starving, and
that many of those people were undoubtedly more deserving to live than I. Although diminishing in severity, the eating disorder persisted, finally resolving when I became
pregnant with Christopher. I was, in retrospect, clinically
depressed. There was a time when it took a conscious effort to swallow. I had to carefully gather saliva in my
mouth, move it back on my tongue, allow it to start to flow
down my throat, and finally gag in order to swallow. I was
afraid that soon I would not be able to breathe without the
same conscious effort. I remember looking at people and
wondering how it was that they were able to get through
each day. I would use my imagined motivations of those
people to enable me to get through my day.

At that time, I met the man who has been my husband
for eighteen years. Falling in love ended the depression
crisis, but I always knew that it was still there, held at bay.
I would easily slip into what I called to myself the "gray
zone." I would feel as if I were numb, that I had no feeling
at all, that nothing could touch me emotionally.[2] These
episodes lasted at most a day or so, without any pattern

---

[1]Increasing experience suggests that CV dysfunction and the resulting
primary and/or secondary symptoms may predispose some to eating
disorders (A CV diagnosed and successfully reported case study is
presented in Book II).

[2]Feelings of depersonalization are also present in patients with ADD.

which I could determine. Through an infertility crisis which lasted for five years, I was counseled by a wonderful therapist, who helped me develop self-confidence. Had it not been for her help, I would not have been able to recognize symptoms that I later learned were dyslexic.

Other characteristics I experienced may be helpful to those who aren't sure of their symptoms. Thought patterns, mental as opposed to spoken, were fragmented, and I would perseverate. My thought patterns would seem to me to spiral, the same thoughts going around and around without resolution. I was constantly mentally checking and rechecking those things for which I was responsible. Worst case scenarios were carried out to extremes in my imagination, to the point where an innocent slip on my part would be seen to result in catastrophic events. For a while, I would check and recheck my weight often after each meal, to make sure I was in control. I would end the day mentally numb, sometimes feeling that the effort to express myself was too difficult to attempt.

Perhaps the most difficult aspect was the knowledge that I was smart. The trouble was that I had difficulty with those things that others most commonly used to measure intelligence. I would sit through meetings, discussions, and conversations having solved those problems at hand long before others could, but not having the where-with-all to speak up. I was frustrated every time I heard another flute player who had a more successful career than I, but who clearly did not have the grasp of the abstract concepts of tone, pitch, line and expression that I did. And yet they could play more of the correct notes than I could. It simply did not make sense, and the harder I tried, the more remote the possibility of solving the mystery became.

Now that I am aware of the disorder dyslexia, I am aware of its presence in others. I have recommended that two of my friends consult with Dr. Levinson, and my unofficial diagnosis was confirmed. I have come to realize that the initial indication of dyslexia is a wide disparity between types of intellect. If a person has a very high verbal skill combined with a low non-verbal skill, I suspect that there is a probability of dyslexia. During my own decision to be diagnosed and treated, I found reading Dr. Levinson's progress reports to be very helpful. The first time I read them, I was amazed to realize just how many of the statements were true about me. Things I never before had associated with dyslexia, or even considered to be anything remarkable or treatable. Finally, I began to realize that there may indeed be an explanation for the mystery.

As I enjoy the incredible benefits of treatment, I find I would like additional assistance in the remaking of the brain pathways that control spelling and handwriting. I still do not see my spelling errors, even with SpellCheck. Maybe they should invent SyntaxCheck!! SpellCheck does not pick up "form" as a misspelled word when the sentence should read "from." When I write things by hand, it is as if I must go slowly enough to think of every letter in a word, while my brain by that time is at the end of the paragraph. I also notice that whenever I start a new word with the same letter or two as the previous word, I skip that letter. As in "new word," I would write "new ord." Often I do not catch a mistake like that during proofreading. However, I do notice that new information really stays with me. I know now with confidence that "receive" has an "ei" in the middle, not an "ie." Also the word *squirrel*. I always had to look up that word in the past, and now I spell it with glee.[1]

In conclusion, the overwhelmingly most important change I have enjoyed while being treated by Dr. Levinson is the ease in which I now go through each and every day.

---

[1] As can be seen, new words learned while the patient is on medication are correctly retained and spelled. Accordingly, the difficulty with old, previously misspelled words is having to learn to erase incorrect imprints.

I have lost the anxiety that has surrounded even simple tasks. I feel as if my brain can now function at its full potential. In fact, in general, I do function at a level now which I had only glimpsed before. I enjoy life to a degree never before possible.

The enclosed tape is a progress report—in a format I am sure you don't expect. It is a live concert I played February 12. I can hear the difference and thought perhaps you could too.

You might be interested to know that Christopher's first grade teacher, Barbara Tucker, has made an appointment with you on April 12 for both of her children.

While I am happy to speak with any prospective patients yet unsure of plans to consult with you, I am concerned that several have asked me medical questions for which I am not qualified to advise. Perhaps an open letter from me, citing my perspective both as a patient and parent of a patient would be helpful to those seeking that kind of information. . . .

If I can be of any further assistance, please let me know. If any of those who doubt your program would like to test me or hear from me, I would be happy to do so. I refer here to other "professionals" in the many fields who regard dyslexia as their province. Perhaps, as I experience such vast differences of perception when not taking the medication as opposed to when I do take it, I may be of some interest to them. It occurs to me, however, that they would rather study someone whose symptoms coincide with their theories and treatment.

Nonetheless, I continue to marvel at the improvement Christopher continues to enjoy. Many, many thanks.

Sincerely,

Joan Sparks

CHAPTER 11

Understanding Dyslexia

Because Dr. James M. Murphy[1] has a degree in history rather than in fields related to dyslexia or learning disabilities, he apparently read and reviewed *A Solution to the Riddle—Dyslexia* with a calm, cool, neutral perspective. As a result, his clarity and objectivity contrasts sharply with that of the traditionalist experts. It is also representative of a host of positive reviews which could not be presented here because of space restraints.

Of all the critiques of my work reported here and elsewhere, Murphy's came nearest to restating what I said and meant—completely devoid of bias, distortion, and egoism. As a result, I chose to present his review from the *International Schools Journal* in its entirety. It's well worth your reading. And it's certainly easier than tackling *A Solution to the Riddle—Dyslexia.*

[1]Dr. James M. Murphy did his graduate work in history at Columbia University in New York, and has recently retired from the U.S. Department of State after many years of service in Europe. Unhampered by any particular background in the technical world of neurological research, Dr. Murphy seemed an ideal person to judge whether this new and important work was accessible to the general reader.

Book Review

Understanding Dyslexia: A Story of Scientific Detection
by James M. Murphy

"Teachers in international schools will be particularly interested," Dr. Murphy writes, "in the author's claim to have developed a technique for diagnosing dyslexia independent of reading scores . . ." thus opening the way for early identification of this condition in non-English-speaking children. But this is only part of the absorbing story of research and discovery recounted in the following review.[1]

The Historical Perspective

Very few teachers today are unfamiliar with the concept of dyslexia; fewer still have not at some time encountered its puzzling, even bizarre, indications in the reading and written work of children, particularly in the early grades. In recent years, dyslexia sometimes seems to have taken on the aspect of a fashionable disability and more than one teacher knows parents who could not conceal their relief to find that their child's failing performance resulted from a genuine handicap—one which did not carry the life sentence of inadequacy implied by a "low IQ," or worse, the traumatic suggestion of "minimal brain damage." It does not take much imagination, moreover, to appreciate that such early difficulties in learning to read can have pervasive and very damaging effects upon children as they move from grade to grade and must master an ever-increasing volume of reading in order to keep pace. Such children are progressively schooled in a sense of their own incompetence and educated in a web of anxiety, frustration and failure whose origins they cannot even dimly understand. One can only speculate how many generations of "behavior problems" have thus been unwittingly cultivated— how many children have grown up pitted in confrontation with parents and teachers who, perhaps understandably, have had recourse to the easy, moral diagnosis of "laziness" or "inattention" to explain away a performance whose causes, even whose nature, they were no more able

[1]*A Solution to the Riddle—Dyslexia,* by H. N. Levinson, MD, Springer-Verlag, Heidelberger Platz 3, Postfach, D-1000, Berlin 33, Germany. 398 pages. US $40.00. 1980. ISBN 3-540-90515-4. (This book is currently available through Stonebridge Publishing, Ltd, Great Neck, New York.)

to grasp than were the children. With this background in mind, one can easily understand the very human tendency to derive comfort merely from an ability to give a name to such a mysterious and frustrating disability.

Yet dyslexia is by no means a new discovery: it was first recognized as a learning disability in 1896 by two English physicians, Kerr and Morgan, who gave it the name "word blindness," by which it is still known in some areas. Nor has the ability to fix a name on this condition meant, by any means, that its nature or origin was understood. On the contrary, definitions of the condition have multiplied over the years (Dr. Levinson has counted some thirty-five recorded in the literature) and a lengthy list has grown of good descriptive diagnoses meant to enable the doctor or teacher to recognize a dyslexic when he found one. In the prevailing confusion of diagnosis, and given the inability to pin down specific mechanisms which underlie what we recognize as dyslexic performance, some educators have even taken the view that the condition does not exist as such, that its characteristic reading and writing difficulties are simply aspects of slow learning and developmental lag. For all the burgeoning literature, and for all the growing awareness among teachers and parents of the existence of specific handicap, one was left with little more than a name, a collection of symptoms, and some tantalizing, often maddeningly contradictory, neurological clues—the ingredients of a classic scientific riddle.

Dr. Levinson's book is a record of his fifteen-year scientific effort to penetrate this riddle and unravel the complex clues that identify the primary neurological origins of this condition. As the title of his work indicates, Dr. Levinson believes that he has succeeded in arriving at a diagnosis of what dyslexia is, not merely another description of its symptoms, and in reaching certain conclusions which could have revolutionary implications for the ability of schools and teachers to work with students afflicted with this disability.

Perhaps of even greater significance, the technique which he has developed to diagnose the neurological dysfunction which lies at the heart of dyslexia can be used also to detect this disability in the many other children who have been able to compensate for it, to one degree or another, and whose reading and writing is sufficiently corrected to place them with the "normal" population. The existence of such masked or "hidden" dyslexics must raise the thought-provoking question of how far unevenness in school performance ultimately reflects not simply the commonly accepted inequalities of "native intelligence" but subtle and varying degrees of both neurological dysfunction and the ability of some compensatory mechanism to deal with it. Going beyond the immediate diagnostic problem of dyslexia, moreover, Dr. Levinson has found room for intriguing speculation on the role which the complex neurological interplay he analyzes may play in promoting pathological states that normally have been considered psychogenic—the possibility that compulsions, phobias and a host of other personality disorders may well stem, in some measure, from undetected disorders in the nervous system itself, and not in the patient's mental history or development.

Locating the Origin of Dyslexia: Cortical and Cerebellar-Vestibular Explanations

Dr. Levinson's search began against a background of uncertainty about the nature of the dyslexic condition, a "diagnostic void" which he has summarized in a quotation from two recognized authorities in the field:

> The obvious criterion of reading-retardation is that a child is not able to score at the reading achievement level proper to its age and years of instruction. It is a simple matter to identify reading retardation, but far from simple to make a differential diagnosis of specific dyslexia.

> The fact of the matter is that no one has yet devised a foolproof way of diagnosing specific dyslexia. . . . To a significant degree the problem hinges on the fact that no one has as yet uncovered any telltale sign or group of signs that are exclusive to the syndrome of specific dyslexia and are not to be found in other conditions of reading retardation.

This assessment was echoed in the words of yet another researcher:

> The definition (of dyslexia) has to be a descriptive one since one does not have one single symptom nor one

straightforward objective finding on which to base the diagnosis. On this point, there is no difference from the kind of delimitation one is obliged to adopt with other psychic disorders where a descriptive diagnosis has to be used.

The absence of a diagnostic base to account for the manifest symptoms of reading difficulty did not mean there was an absence of speculation about what the root cause of dyslexia was. Behavioral problems—anxieties, frustrations, and so forth—were often noted in connection with severe reading retardation. In the absence of more specific and hard neurological indicators—perhaps, more accurately, in the face of so many conflicting and complex neurological findings—it is not surprising that some took flight into the somewhat less austere and often agreeably self-validating hypothesis that dyslexia was psychogenic in nature, that the cause of reading problems, like those of personality or behavior dysfunction, was to be looked for in the psyche rather than in the nervous system itself. As one panel quoted by Dr. Levinson put it:

> Some unpleasant and painful experience may have occurred during the earlier efforts of the child to learn and, as in cases of arithmetical disability. . . the child becomes conditioned against reading. Reading may be the one subject stressed by a hated and severe parent. The child, unable to express his antagonism to the parent openly, does so indirectly through refusal to learn to read. Reading is the acquiring of knowledge through looking. If a child has been severely inhibited in his "peeping" activities, all acquisition of knowledge through looking may come under the ban of the child's superego.

And so forth. But was this somewhat robust assumption of psychological stress borne out by follow-up examination of dyslexic children? Dr. Levinson, a psychiatrist with psychoanalytic training, found that it was not. What is more, he showed an admirable scientific objectivity, not a commonplace in the fraternity, by stating that such a psychogenic explanation of dyslexia was clinically inadequate and therapeutically unsatisfactory.

There remained the generally accepted belief that in some unknown and unspecifiable way, dyslexia was the result of an impairment or dysfunction in the cerebral cortex—the part of the brain in which is localized our ability to grasp or comprehend what the sensory nervous system reports of the world around us. The literature on this point is as complex, and the evidence as elusive, as one might expect to be the case in subtle differential diagnoses of neurological disorders. Some researchers found points of similarity between the impaired directional sense displayed in dyslexia and that manifested in Gerstmann's syndrome, and thought such parallels sufficient to argue that the former, like the latter, must therefore be an impairment of the cortical area. Other authorities disagreed on the relationship of this symptom with dyslexia or of dyslexia with Gerstmann's syndrome.[1] But there remained a general consensus that the dyslexic condition, after all, resulted from some form of cortical impairment: the child *saw* but did not *comprehend* the words and letters before him; his disability arose in that final and somewhat mysterious step by which we "make sense" of the data which our senses provide.

It was at this point that Dr. Levinson's line of investigation took a critical turn, and, as is so often the case with classical scientific detective stories, it began by a questioning of assumptions. Was it correct to relate dyslexia to a dysfunction in the cortical area? He could find no accompanying evidence of cortical impairment in dyslexics—none of the "cortical signs" which one would expect. On the other hand there were other indicators present in most dyslexics which pointed to a dysfunction in a different portion of the brain—the cerebellum, which sits on top of the spinal column and modulates the motor nervous system—as well as the vestibular circuits relating to the balance mechanisms found in the

[1]Gerstmann's syndrome or tetrad: Finger agnosia, acalculia, agraphia, right/left confusion; a cluster of four symptoms defining a disorder within the dominant cerebral cortex. This cerebral syndrome was mistakenly equated with dyslexia despite the fact that: (1) alexia is not part of the syndrome, (2) the remaining symptoms in Gerstmann's syndrome are analogous—but not identical—to those in dyslexia and, (3) Critchley denied the existence of this syndrome in children (see discussion in *A Solution to the Riddle—Dyslexia*). In other words, the identity of dyslexia with Gerstmann's syndrome represents another traditionalist attempt to force an inner-ear-determined syndrome (dyslexia) into a cerebral cortical alexic mold.

inner-ear. Signs of malfunction in the cerebellar-vestibular (CV) system, such as balance and coordination problems, tendency to motion sickness, and so forth, had been noted before, but given the general acceptance of a cortical origin of the impairment, they tended to be dismissed or put to one side as puzzling discrepancies, epiphenomenal findings that did not bear upon the principal source of the problem. Putting the case so simply, and in such a rapid summary, it may now seem obvious that research into the possible CV role in dyslexia would be a fruitful line to take. It is therefore important to stress here that a brief review can hardly do justice to the complexity of the questions involved, the great influences exerted by received ideas on those working in the field, and the subtle diagnostic problems which arose as the research went forward. Then too, retrospection tends to invest all good ideas with the appearance of being obvious, although, of course, this is never really the case. Knowing the answer enables us to see the problem in a certain way and subsequent thinkers benefit from a measure of clarity and order which the solution itself imposes on a disordered and uncertain base of unprocessed data—what Dr. Levinson described very aptly in this case as a "clinical stew."

> In the absence of a clear understanding of the psychological and physiological origins of dyslexia and related learning disabilities, victims of these disorders are often subjected to "shotgun" diagnostic batteries of psychiatric, neurological, psychological, educational, optometric, ophthalmologic, and pediatric tests and examinations. Most often, the children, families and researchers are overwhelmed and flooded with a volume of reports and a mass of names, numbers and test scores, which at times appear contradictory and inversely proportional to the medical-educational-diagnostic-therapeutic yield. Retrospectively, one was forced to wonder if this testing compulsion and accompanying data collection were not symptomatic reflections of a defensive attempt at dealing with urgent patient needs as well as scientific anxieties over innumerable uncertainties.

Dyslexia as a CV Impairment

Following up a retrospective study of the records of 1000 children in the New York school system who were selected as severely retarded in reading (two years below grade level), Dr. Levinson went on to test his hypotheses in several other programmes of research with other groups of normal and dyslexic children. In one "blind" neurological examination series, the examining physicians detected a 97% incidence of CV dysfunction and 6% of cortical impairment in referred dyslexics; in another the figures were 96% and 6%. As the results of these programmes accumulated, Dr. Levinson became convinced that his earlier insight had been justified, that the condition called dyslexia did indeed arise from impairment of the CV system. But this conclusion, in turn, led to a further theoretical problem: how to explain the manner in which the CV system interferes with, or scrambles, the signals being received by the senses.

Two analogies are offered by Dr. Levinson to explain the interaction between the balance and directional or "compass" sense of the vestibular system and the cortical circuits which are associated with comprehension. The scanning electron beam which, in a sense, writes out the picture we see on a television screen is modulated or controlled by, among other influences, electronic regulators for vertical and horizontal "hold." The proponents of a cortical interpretation of dyslexia liken this condition to a man who sees a clear picture on his TV set, but does not comprehend what it signifies or means. In Dr. Levinson's analogy, the devices within the set which control the vertical and horizontal "holds" are malfunctioning: the viewer is watching a scrambled signal which he cannot make sense of. Again, this balance and coordination function of the CV circuits can be compared to the complex systems built into naval gun emplacements which permit the gun to remain fixed on the target despite the continuous movement of its platform. Celestial guidance systems, which "lock on" to a star for navigational tracking in flight, involve a similar principal of compensation, adjustment and tracking of a stationary object from a moving receptor. It goes without saying that even these most elegant direction-seeking gadgets of our "space-age" technology are, in their turn, like flint axes when put alongside the tens of millions of patterned neurological circuits humming with reciprocal energy and reverberating to the unheard harmonies of biological inner space.

Reading Scores Alone are No True Test of Dyslexia

Having reached conclusions about the neurological origins of dyslexia, Dr. Levinson turned to the job of developing techniques of diagnosis and, ultimately, of treatment. In this summary of his account, one can do little justice to the difficulties which this task presented, much less to the ingenuity with which Dr. Levinson and his research reduced them to manageable and solvable dimensions. Not the least charm of Dr. Levinson's book is his readiness to share with the reader the disappointments, the apparent inconsistencies and the clinical paradoxes that he encountered along the way—an account which reminds us once again that the progress of scientific inquiry in unknown territories is seldom the predictable, continuous process which classroom demonstrations later tend to make it appear. In order to test out his hypothesis of CV malfunctioning, it became necessary for Dr. Levinson to create more refined devices for detecting otherwise unrecognized or "subclinical" nystagmus, or eye movement, which he had come to feel was a CV "sign" for dyslexics. This process was by no means an easy one, and readers are led through a description of the refinements, both in equipment and in conception, which were necessary in order to resolve the statistical inconsistencies which emerged from the raw data. In essence, the technique involved a "3-D Optical Scanner" which could project either a moving line of letters or objects against a stationary background, or a moving background to stationary figures or letters. The speed at which the subject found the images to blur out of recognition represented the level of the patient's capability for ocular tracking—his "blurring speed." As might be expected, the clinical examination of patients was not as simple as that; the technology of measuring blurring speed had to be refined and improved; different types of blurring speed had to be accounted for, and—most complex of all—puzzling contradictions in the data had to be rationalized. It is not possible here to retrace the steps by which Dr. Levinson achieved his results, but the reader will find that these chapters will repay the careful and attentive reading they require. For it was out of this highly complex investigation that Dr. Levinson found it possible to elaborate on a conception, not only of the neurological origins of dyslexia, but of the crucial importance of compensation for this dysfunction, a correction which can and does take place in many dyslexics with sufficient frequency to render reading ability insufficient in itself as an indicator of dyslexic impairment. Dyslexia, in effect, is a dynamic condition—one in which a central CV malfunction, in complex interaction with other brain centers, is one element in a combination of dysfunction and compensation which, together, shape the student's reading performance.

The implications of this recognition are obvious and far-reaching. What Dr. Levinson calls the "fallacy of reading-score-dependent definitions of dyslexia" is simply the failure to see that, while all (or at least most) children with severely retarded reading ability will display the neurological symptoms of dyslexia, many others, no less neurologically impaired, will have been able, in some measure, to compensate for their handicap and obtain "normal" reading scores. Teachers of both younger children and adolescents must find such a conception very thought-provoking. And not only teachers; for, as Dr. Levinson speculates:

> Reading-score-compensated dyslexics were often found referred to psychiatrists and neurologists for the evaluation of such non-reading symptoms as enuresis, headaches, abdominal pain, insomnia, school phobias, height and motion phobias, obsessive-compulsive neuroses, temper outbursts, acting out and/or delinquent behavior, as well as writing, spelling, math, memory, directional, and balance and coordinational difficulties. Most often, the underlying CV dyslexia basis of this symptomatic complex remained completely hidden or subclinical—resulting in unwitting misinterpretations and diagnostic-therapeutic scrambling. The dedicated search for only primary emotional determinants often resulted in fallacious psychoanalytic formulations and such iatrogenic complications as a faulty therapeutic alliance and negative-transference/counter-transference acting-out.

Occasionally, he points out, young dyslexic children with intact or compensated-memory function or high IQ are able to perform well when starting out in school. As the volume of reading material to be mastered increases, however, they tend to stumble and fall behind. All too often these children— whom he describes as showing "clinically-delayed dyslexic symptomatic patterns"—are referred for psychological evaluation rather than for diagnosis and treatment of dyslexia. Dr. Levinson quotes another authority in the field, McDonald Critchley, who notes:

> In the case of the "cured" dyslexic (i.e., one who has compensated sufficiently to raise his reading score to grade level) defective writing and spelling may continue to appear long into adult life. . . . As the reading of the dyslexic improves, he and his teachers become increasingly aware of, and concerned with, his conscious inability to spell correctly. The time may come, especially in a teenager or adolescent, when the original delay in the acquisition of reading has been forgotten. . . . The problem now presents itself as an intelligent scholar who is handicapped in his written work by its untidiness and atrocious spelling.[1]

A New Insight Into an Old Problem

In developing a diagnostic technique which goes beyond apparently "normal" reading scores to detect subclinical signals of hidden dyslexia, Dr. Levinson's work adds a further dimension to our understanding of what "normality" involves. One result of such an approach is a new and intriguing line of thought concerning possible causes of emotional or behavioral problems, which had seldom been taken into account before. Going beyond even that level of speculation, Dr. Levinson notes that the CV circuits which plot position and direction are a link between our minds and the gravitational forces that regulate the equilibrium of our physical world—indeed of the universe itself.

In the present review, concerned with those aspects of his work of interest to teachers, such larger considerations may be put to one side. It

[1]Note, when reviewing Dr. Gold's "blind" neurological data within Chapter 16 and Appendix A, that this "simple" reading-score-compensated concept of dyslexia is denied. As a result, dyslexics with and without "dyslexia" are diagnosed completely different—despite having identical neurological (cerebellar) signs and dyslexia-related symptoms.

is only fair to say, however, that readers of Dr. Levinson's book, whether they agree with the author or not, will surely find his philosophic reflections not only fascinating but somewhat chastening: they force us to think again about the easy acceptance of "what everyone knows."

As for teachers, even the rapid and selective summary above, inadequate as it is to convey the breadth and detail of Dr. Levinson's work, should be sufficient to show that A Solution to the Riddle—Dyslexia is a study of major importance—indeed, required reading—on an educational problem which Dr. Levinson's research indicates is probably far more pervasive and more recalcitrant than is generally thought. In summarizing the fruits of his fifteen years of research on the problem, Dr. Levinson lists a number of successes or conclusions, a few of which follow. He has:

- correlated and proved dyslexia and related learning disorders to be due to a primary CV dysfunction, with secondarily related emotional and cortical manifestations;

- hypothesized and proved that the visual reading symptoms of dyslexia are due to a CV determined ocular fixation, tracking, and processing dysfunction;

- developed a 3-D Scanner and blurring speed methodology capable of a rapid and accurate diagnosis and prediction of CV induced fixation and tracking dysfunction in dyslexia;

- determined the incidence of CV dyslexia to be approximately 15-20% of a middle class population;

- demonstrated that the blurring-speed diagnosis between male and female subjects, as well as between right- and left-handed, is identical, thereby suggesting that sex and handedness may be independent of dyslexic variables;

- speculated on the genetic and constitutional origins of dyslexia as well as the possible etiologic role of infectious, allergic, toxic and traumatic CV factors occurring during early childhood;

- highlighted the vital, dynamic role of CV compensatory mechanisms—leading to the discovery of reading-score- and blurring-speed-compensated dyslexics;

- recognized that the dyslexic CV disorder need not be defined in terms of IQ and reading score impairment;

- demonstrated the therapeutic efficacy of the antimotion-sickness medications in improving dyslexic symptomatology;

- developed new methods of facilitating compensatory processes and minimizing emotional and educational traumatization and scarring.

Teachers in international schools will be particularly interested in Dr. Levinson's claim to have developed a technique for diagnosing dyslexia independent of reading scores. His method will obviously be a most welcome new tool in analyzing the educational needs of many children who are not speakers, much less readers, of English, and who cannot adequately be tested for reading competency in their own language. Of importance on a more general level is Dr. Levinson's reference to techniques and equipment he has developed for assisting dyslexics in compensating for their handicap. Teachers of remedial reading in particular will want to know more about such developments; no doubt we shall be hearing more of them as they come into wider use and are subject to more detailed evaluation. Any readers familiar with Dr. Levinson's treatment of dyslexics will be aware of the good results he has achieved with antimotion-sickness drugs. The efficacy of such medication, of course, bears directly on Dr. Levinson's hypothesis of a vestibular factor at the heart of the dyslexic condition, and he devotes some coverage to the part such drugs can play in its treatment. Here again, we may hope that further research and refinements of pharmacology may yield improved and even more specific medication for use in helping children overcome this disability.

As one might well expect a record of long, serious research to be, Dr. Levinson's book is one for the library table (and definitely for the teacher's workroom), but not for the bedside table; readers must be prepared to read carefully and attend to the text, for Dr. Levinson makes no concession to the layman in presenting this account of his work. No concession, that is, save one—and that, the most important one of all: the use of clear, intelligible and jargon-free language. There are, of course, a fair number of technical terms that are necessary to a discussion of the subject, but no reader equipped with a dictionary should find this too much of a difficulty.

Dr. Levinson is not without his critics, and apparently hostile ones at that. With ingratiating candor, he devotes a full chapter to their objections and marshals arguments in rebuttal, and while an unqualified layman would be foolhardy indeed to arbitrate professional disputes on such an advanced and technical level, it is only fair to acknowledge that in their scope, reasoning and straightforwardness, Dr. Levinson's research and conclusions are very persuasive indeed. There can be little doubt that his careful and highly professional work well deserves a close look, particularly from all those in the field of education who are, after all, the first to confront this little-understood handicap in children, and best placed to help its victims overcome it.

CHAPTER 12

Demystifying the Experts

While thumbing through the pages of *Harper's Bazaar* one November morning in 1988, I came across an article referring to my research entitled, "The Dyslexic Dilemma."

Another explanation points to a lack of eye coordination and spatial relationship skills. Dr. Harold Levinson, Associate Professor of Psychiatry at New York University Medical Center, NYC, postulates that the answer to the riddle lies in the cerebellum and inner ear. "The inner ear controls motion, eye movements and tracking, and balance—all needed to read effectively. A dyslexic has something wrong with the pathway between the cerebellum and the ear, which causes a form of motion sickness that makes the letters seem to jump around." He prescribes ordinary traveler's drugs and claims that up to 75 per cent of his patients have improved.

As I continued to read this article, I stumbled across another traditionalist insulting me and my research as follows:

Dr. Frank Vellutino, professor of psychology and educational psychology at the University of Albany, where he heads the Child Research and Study Center strongly disagrees. *"No one takes Levinson's work seriously. It's unfortunate that some parents get taken in by this type of thing."*

Dr. Vellutino takes quite a different approach. He maintains that dyslexics see like everyone else. Rather, it is their linguistic capability that suffers. "They're not able to perceive words analytically (from their meaning) so they miss what should be obvious because of a sentence's structure. For example, within the context of a sentence, the recognition of the words 'was' and 'saw' should be automatic." The child's knowledge of phonetics also tends to be weak. "Quite possibly, there is some brain dysfunction," he suggests, "but it could also be due to sheer lack of experience or because of basic difficulty with whatever it is that allows us to learn language."[1]

This is supported by recent research at both the University of Colorado at Boulder and at Harvard Medical School in Boston. Experiments suggest that dyslexics' right brain (responsible for nonverbal functions) is better developed than their left. In some cases, the right brain was even found to be superior to that of normal readers.

Scientists haven't ruled out the possibility that the disorder is hereditary. "In studies done with twins, we've learned that if one has it, the other almost always does too," he notes. "Boys also have it more often than girls."[2]

Treatments for dyslexia are as varied as the speculation about its causes. "It's very important for the child to get one-on-one tutoring to suit his or her particular symptoms and weak points," says Vellutino. *"There's no trick solution."*

Here We Go Again

You're right! That's exactly how I felt! But what would you do? Would you quickly write an editorial response? Or would you just use your reactive energies and adrenaline

---

[1] Do you really understand this? I wonder if Vellutino does. It sounds like something he memorized and is parroting. Compare my explanations in Chapter 13 and in my children's book, *The Upside-Down Kids*.

[2] Although there is much to criticize about Vellutino, let me ask: How can you perform reliable genetic studies on dyslexia when the definitions and concepts of this disorder are erroneous? Also, my studies and those independently confirming them by Shaywitz and colleagues at Yale (1990) indicate that gender and handedness are unrelated to dyslexia!

to effect more therapeutic responses such as those presented throughout this and other works?

Obviously, you're right again. Had I spent all the time needed to respond appropriately to critics, especially those whose arrogance matches their bias, I would be writing defensive letters continually. So instead, I just filed the article and memo away and forgot about it—at least partially.

And as chance would have it, several years ago Vellutino's name suddenly reappeared in a letter I received from Lisa Nomer, a former dyslexic patient of mine who had just graduated from law school.

May 29, 1991

Dear Dr. Levinson:

Enclosed is a copy of a report from Frank R. Vellutino, Ph.D., of the State University of New York at Albany, consultant to the Connecticut Bar Examining Committee. Dr. Vellutino is asked to evaluate prospective candidates for the bar as to whether or not they are dyslexic (or learning disabled) and make recommendations for any special treatment they should receive.

As you can see, yours is one of the reports documenting the validity of my dyslexia and my requirements for special accommodations. Upon reading Mr. Vellutino's report, you will see that *he does not understand the nature of dyslexia and invalidates all other professionals and the tests they administer as not competent*. He bases the outcome of his remarks to the Bar Commission on the Woodcock Reading Mastery Test and the Woodcock-Johnson Psycho-Educational Battery, *never personally interviewing and testing any of the applicants himself.*

I find his report offensive to myself in that he repeatedly insinuates that I have and continue to conspire to somehow defraud the bar as a "malingerer." In addition to your valuable testing, *I have overwhelming evidence from my school record and tests performed over the years to prove*

that I am dyslexic and truly deserving of the special accommodations which you have recommended for me in
your report. I also feel, as I'm sure you will see is quite
evident, that *Mr. Vellutino is implying that you are either
not a competent professional or that I am an incredible liar
or both.* Therefore, I ask your assistance to *help me overcome yet another obstacle in my long and protracted
battle against an insensitive and uneducated educational
system.* Please write or fax a letter to the Connecticut Bar
Examining Committee. If you send a letter, make sure you
send it return receipt requested, so that your letter is not
simply lost. Please note that they meet on June 8 to decide my ultimate fate. Therefore, time is of the essence!
Thank you again for your help.

Sincerely,

Lisa Nomer

No doubt, you'd want to read expert Vellutino's letter—
just out of curiosity, if nothing else. Rather than reprint
Vellutino's lengthy statement to the Connecticut Bar Examining Committee, I have reviewed the essentials.

In Vellutino's letter to his friend "Dave" (David Stamm,
Administrative Director, Connecticut Bar Examining Committee) concerning Lisa Nomer, he states:

- Anyone can claim to be an expert in diagnosing a learning disability such as dyslexia, and there are no inherent controls over
  incompetence, fraud, or even quackery. . . . And the number of
  such incompetent experts are "legion."

- None of the three experts examining Ms. Nomer (Dr. Levinson
  included) reported any evidence of a "severe reading problem.". . . Anyone with a severe reading disability ["dyslexia"]
  can't possibly read as well as Ms. Nomer—just ask any expert
  who really knows what they're doing. And to reduce "the
  chances of malingering" among law students, specific reading
  tests and cut-off scores are vital. . . .

- As a result, it is "mystifying" how clinicians can diagnose dyslexia in someone without a severe reading-score disability ["dyslexia"].

- In addition, the vestibular basis of reading problems has "little credence"—and the same holds for occupational therapists who "advocate a similar theory."

- As a result, it is also "mystifying" how "diametrically opposed prescriptions" for the same "inferred" [dyslexic] disorder can "cure dyslexia": *dramamine*, which helps motion sickness and decreases dizziness vs. "vestibular stimulation" or occupational therapy which triggers dizziness.

- Furthermore, people with a "specific language disability" which causes a "reading disability" cannot have "strengths in language based skills. . . . "

- And since Ms. Nomer evidences neither a severe reading nor language disorder, it is apparent that she does not have "a reading disability or dyslexia if this term is preferred." And thus the need for her obtaining extra time and related accommodations on the bar exam is rejected.

Vellutino closes his comment to Dave with his esteemed title: Frank R. Vellutino, Ph.D., Professor, Departments of Psychology, Educational Psychology and Linguistics, Director, Child Research and Study Center.

Attached to this letter were Ortonian articles critical of my cerebellar-vestibular research and books.

An Initial Question

After reading Vellutino's original letter, I was impressed by its erudite style as well as the expert's academic title. His understanding of dyslexics such as Lisa, however, left much to be desired. And I couldn't help but wonder: How could one explain professor Vellutino's letter to his friend Dave—especially its condescending tone, erroneous content, insinuations, and even accusations? One can't—not yet. But let's attempt an objective analysis of the situation.

Analysis of Vellutino's Content and Intent

The Problem

A well-known traditionalist expert on dyslexia espousing the standard linguistic-thinking (alexic-aphasic) party line attempted, for reasons in question, to prevent one of my dyslexic patients who graduated law school from taking the bar exam *with extra time.*

Incompetent Experts and Malingering

Although expert Vellutino repeatedly claimed to be "*mystified*" by how dyslexics can be dyslexic and still read decently and many other common sense phenomena, his biggest concerns were that: *(1) "Anyone (besides himself of course) can claim to be an expert in diagnosing and treating a learning disability such as dyslexia, and there are no inherent controls over incompetence, fraud or quackery," and (2) people can take advantage of the "extra-time" provision given dyslexics by "malingering."*

Who in their right mind can argue about either one of professor Vellutino's concerns? *As a result of his first concern, I was forced to write* A Scientific Watergate—Dyslexia. *And although his second concern is valid, it makes absolutely no sense in the context of this specific patient and her alleged "superior reading scores" on testing—by testers who still diagnosed her as dyslexic.*

My point is very simple, since as a psychiatrist I must often consider malingering as a possibility—especially where legal and compensation issues are concerned: *Were this patient malingering, why wouldn't she deliberately score lower on reading tests? What would stop her—except her conscience? And certainly psychopaths are seriously lacking in this respect. And who reviewing her test scores—expert Vellutino included—would know whether she really or deliberately scored lower than capable on reading and related tests?*

In fact, her higher than expected reading test scores prove she wasn't a malingerer or a psychopath! And if she was sincere and all other "experts," Vellutino aside, consider her to be dyslexic and thus extra time (and writing aids so as to compensate for her associated dysgraphia or impaired writing) would be helpful and appropriate, why should Vellutino object?

In the absence of God-like absolute powers and knowledge, shouldn't we all, as educators and healers, give patients such as Lisa the benefit of the doubt? If this is so, then this forces us to recognize another question: *Why is professor Vellutino being so adversarial—even accusatory? Or might he really consider his diagnostic powers to be supreme and thus feel perfectly justified in attempting Lisa's "mental crucifixion"—as Lisa experienced and called it? Might the reverse be true? Could his dyslexia concepts have been threatened and so he reacted defensively—offensively? Have his theoretical feathers been unwittingly ruffled?* And if so, why and "who done it"?

Traditionalist Misconceptions

As noted, Vellutino was "mystified" as to how someone with a severe reading disability ("dyslexia") could read as well as Ms. Nomer. Dogmatically he states that "It just does not happen" and that experts who really know what they're doing will readily agree with him. (Completely untrue—as recently confirmed by Shaywitz and colleagues [January 1992] and as my dyslexic patients indicate.)

Vellutino then states that the clinicians testing Lisa's reading skills claimed she had "a severe reading disability. . . This is mystifying to say the least." (They never said Lisa had a severe reading disability. They merely said she was dyslexic. *Are not the two statements completely different?*)

Obviously, Vellutino believes *dyslexia = alexia* and so *equates* the disorder or syndrome called dyslexia with severe degrees of its variable reading-score parameter ("dyslexia"). And since professor Vellutino equates the syndrome of many and varied symptoms called dyslexia with "severe reading disability," he winds up *mystified.* By analogy, one would be just as mystified if diabetes were equated with comatose blood sugar levels. How then could we explain diabetics showing below comatose blood sugars and even below normal blood sugars? (See Chapter 2.)

Refuting the Vestibular Theory and Treatment of Dyslexia

In refuting the vestibular basis of dyslexia, expert Vellutino also denies both the efficacy of vestibular stimulation (occupational therapy) and motion sickness drugs (i.e., Dramamine) "as the cure for dyslexia."[1]

Once again, this erudite-sounding expert condescendingly claims to be *mystified*—as if the problem couldn't possibly lie within himself. *He also can't understand why Dramamine, which prevents dizziness, and vestibular stimulation, which produces dizziness, should both be helpful.* Should he not have asked me—if he really wanted to know? Or did he merely assume that if he didn't know, no one else would either?

I somehow feel comfortable that the reader can *demystify* professor Vellutino. But let me put your questions and thoughts down on paper. Thus, for example: *Why are the astronauts trained via vestibular stimulation?*

---

[1]Note how expert Vellutino sees a similarity between the inner-ear (cerebellar-vestibular [CV]) system and occupational therapy as well as that of my own diagnosis and therapy. However, Dr. Larry Silver indicates this same relationship in his "magic cure" article in *The Journal of Learning Disabilities* and denies it in his letter to *Christine Schmidt* in Chapter 8. Is Dr. Silver perhaps slightly confused—and confusing? Or have I misinterpreted his stated comments?

And why are the astronauts also given Dramamine or similar inner-ear-enhancing medications before space flights?

Might the neurophysiologists within NASA also be incompetent, or quacks! Perhaps not! Let's not accuse too easily. There may be a method to their madness—even if it completely escapes and thus mystifies expert Vellutino. And as anyone who thinks in depth knows, there are often simple explanations for seemingly paradoxical data. Simply stated: *Vestibular stimulation conditions the inner-ear circuitry to tolerate greater and greater degrees of vertigo-triggering motion stimulation—thus making the system stronger and less apt to trigger dizzy reactions than before. And inner-ear-enhancing medications like Dramamine also strengthen the inner-ear's capacity to tolerate destabilizing influences—using a chemical vs. physical stimulus and correspondingly different compensatory mechanisms.*

Are there not many other seemingly opposing therapies to compensate for one and the same underlying disorder? Thus, for example, did expert Vellutino ever hear how some allergies are treated: *desensitization vs. antihistamines?* Surely he must have—but had he never connected the two?[1]

And what about *infectious* disorders? *Does not exposure and even immunization trigger compensatory immunity responses while antibiotics attempt to kill?* What about the treatment of phobias? Has expert Vellutino ever heard of: *(1) desensitization via exposure to the frightening stimulus, (2) anti-anxiety medications attempting to "kill" or dampen the anxiety response at its inception, and (3) the most effective treatment—the simultaneous use of both "mystifying" methods?*

---

[1] By the way, difficulty in integrating two variables or steps at a time is a typical dyslexic or inner-ear characteristic. Thus, President Ford was said to have difficulty walking and talking at the same time. And as previously noted, President Bush was alleged to have similar problems integrating his thoughts and speech output (verbal and nonverbal) at the same time.

Language Skills vs. Dyslexia

Professor Vellutino is also mystified "that a person (like Ms. Nomer) with a reading disability caused by a specific language disability typically does not demonstrate strengths in language based skills. . . ." Might there be a very simple solution to Vellutino's apparent confusion? *What if reading disability or dyslexia were not due to a specific language disability (or aphasia)?* Indeed, what if the reverse were true? What if the disorder responsible for dyslexia may only occasionally impair language functioning—thus also explaining the large number of dyslexics with normal and even superior language skills?

Obviously, professor Vellutino never even considered this alternative hypothesis—*despite his extensive review of my CV-based research.* Had he never examined or read about verbally gifted dyslexics—such as those I presented here and elsewhere as well as dyslexics with superb acting (verbal) abilities, e.g., Cher and Tom Cruise? And what about the excellent verbal skills of Olympic dyslexics Bruce Jenner and Greg Louganis? Were not Einstein, Edison, Patton, daVinci, etc. also stated to be dyslexic? I do not recall any traditionalist expert refuting their dyslexia or being "mystified" by their language abilities! Strange?

Even Dr. Per Udden—the gifted physician, entrepreneur, benefactor, and organizer of the Rodin (Dyslexia) Society (discussed in Chapters 17 and 18) claims to be dyslexic, despite superior verbal skills. And to my knowledge, he even completed medical school without untimed tests. Yet not one of the many language-dyslexia traditionalists comprising his vast scientific entourage ever doubted his dyslexia or considered that he might be malingering dyslexia. Indeed, I've even read that the father of neurosurgery, Dr. Harvey Cushing, was dyslexic. And I'm almost positive I read this in the Ortonian literature.

Surely Cushing's reading scores weren't severely deficient and it is highly improbable that his language skills were worse than Ms. Nomer's.

No doubt you are wondering what all this means. Simply stated, it means that expert Vellutino and all the other traditionalists are in error concerning the language (aphasic-alexic) origins of dyslexia and dyslexics, and that these experts failed to integrate and properly correlate the clinical facts and reality of dyslexia with their theoretical fantasies.[1]

The Traditionalists' Denial

In retrospect, only the massive denial of verbally normal or gifted and reading-score compensated dyslexics (as well as the denial of their CV-based disorder and responses to CV-enhancing medications) can sustain Vellutino's language-dyslexia convictions and resulting confusion. Have not all the traditionalists been in a similar state of denial? Had not resolving this "scientific denial" and the circular logic sustaining the cerebral-language dyslexia theories for the past 100 years resulted in the breakthrough CV-based insights and therapies characterizing *A Scientific Watergate—Dyslexia?*

No doubt I can go on and on to attempt professor Vellutino's demystification. But I have a simpler method. Let him read *A Scientific Watergate—Dyslexia* with plenty of extra time for proper assimilation and understanding, considering his preexisting conflicting views. And so before concluding here, I will ask the reader a simple question. *If the evidence proves, beyond a reasonable doubt, that Lisa Nomer is not malingering and that professor Vellutino is in error, might we, in turn, raise another question:* What is the clinical and research background or basis for professor Vellutino's dyslexia expertise?

[1]Perhaps readers will understand better the need to highlight the theoretical nonsense leading traditionally-minded experts to view President Bush's alleged speech symptoms to be evidence of aphasia.

Beyond A Reasonable Doubt

Lisa Nomer was initially examined by me July 1, 1983 at the Medical Dyslexic Treatment Center when 19 years old. She was diagnosed as dyslexic with severe dysgraphia and medically treated *eight years before taking the bar exam.* Enclosed is an extract from a letter written by her father, Rev. Charles J. Nomer.

July 6, 1983

Dear Dr. Levinson:

Words are inadequate to express to you my profound gratitude for the time you took to see my daughter, Lisa. Our visit with you and your diagnosis explained many problems that Lisa has encountered in the learning process. She knows herself better today and has more self-assurance in her ability to cope with the gift of life. I marvel at the basic goodness of people and how this was generously expressed by you to my family.

Tom Palmer loaned me your book, *A Solution to the Riddle—Dyslexia.* I have not read much of it yet. My attention was drawn to page 316, the second paragraph which states: "In retrospect, man could neither have contemplated nor accepted cosmic, organismic, and inanimate mind in other than the religious concepts of God and Heaven." Truly we are spiritual brothers who exist and function in creation because of a concerned God. I have believed for a long time that science and religion are headed in the same direction. When we finally reach the mountain top, our common goal will be God who has made everything possible.

Once again, I am truly grateful to you for your concern and generosity.

Thank you,

Fr. Charles Nomer

Following is Lisa's progress report from August 30, 1983:

On Medication—The basic reading I've been doing this summer has been church related. It's generally small print and tough reading material. The first couple of weeks I seemed to zip right through the material with complete understanding.

It was the same with memory and speech, both were clearer and came more readily (same with spelling mistakes too).

Doc, what happened was none of the local druggists had the Meclizine you prescribed. He told Mom (who was filling the prescription) Bonine was the same thing and to use that til he ordered the other stuff. The Bonine worked great. I made steady progress on it and got up to two whole tablets a day. On the Meclizine I got irritable, etc. I'm down to a ½ tab a day and have reverted to normal (dyslexic). Could it be there's a difference in the two drugs? I'm going back on Bonine til further notice.[1] Any chance you might put me on Vasopressin. I've read it does incredible things for memory.

Other Correspondence

Because of Lisa's dyslexia and severe difficulties with writing (dysgraphia), she asked me to explain her condition and special needs to her college dean. Note our concerns over Lisa's dyslexia then—and how it was handled. Obviously this letter was written long before Lisa even contemplated law school.

November 28, 1983

Dear Dr. Philips:

Dyslexia is a syndrome of many symptoms which may impair reading, writing, spelling, math, memory, speech, sense of time

---

[1] I have often found that chewables vs. other forms of the same chemical are differently absorbed and so have different effects. Were this a placebo effect, both pills should have had identical results!

and direction as well as related functions, grammar, concentration/distractibility/activity, mood, anxiety levels, balance and coordination, etc.

According to my research, this disorder is caused by an impairment within the inner-ear system and tends to scramble various sensory-motor signals—depending on the specific circuits impaired. By analogy, the inner-ear is similar to the vertical and horizontal TV knobs. Channel drifting results in signal scrambling and thus difficulties in processing related inputs and outputs.

A regime of inner-ear-enhancing medication has been prescribed for Lisa which should help correct her difficulties. To further facilitate improvement, the following is recommended:

- The use of taped content: of textbooks/required reading—to be listened to in conjunction with the reading of the same material. The auditory reinforces the visual input.

- The use of a tape recorder to tape lectures—they can be played over and over again as required and avoids writing—which is difficult for Lisa.

- The use of cards, like flash cards, for facts that must be memorized.

- The use of printed material that has dark, large, bold lettering—small print, closely-spaced tends to blur together and make reading more difficult and tiring for the eyes.

- The use of untimed tests—since the dyslexic needs a longer amount of time to assimilate and comprehend incoming information as well as compensating for poor graphomotor functioning or dysgraphia. The added pressure of completing a written or oral test in a timed situation tends to create anxiety and blocks in recall.

- The use of a multi-faceted approach which incorporates all five senses greatly facilitates the learning and recall processes of the dyslexic—since some input and output channels are blocked and require others for compensation.

Needless to say, the understanding and cooperation of the faculty is very important and germane to any overall improvements and success. I hope this information proves helpful to you.

Sincerely,

Harold N. Levinson, M.D.
Director, Medical Dyslexic Treatment Center

An Important Question and Concern

Because Lisa was diagnosed to have dyslexia in 1983—long before contemplating law school—and because her college dean understood this diagnosis and helped her accordingly: Why in the name of heaven should a pastor's daughter be accused (even indirectly) of malingering dyslexia by an esteemed expert in 1991 when in fact this diagnosis of dyslexia was confirmed and treated *eight* years before? Might not her reading scores and related symptoms have improved over the years, albeit not "cured" as traditionalist experts claim?[1]

Is there not a reasonable doubt that Lisa was truly dyslexic—and so merely another victim of the 100-year-old traditionalist vacuum? Should Lisa have been "mentally crucified," as she referred to this experience, for allegedly malingering dyslexia just because her symptoms didn't conform to the traditionalists' expectations and standards? Have bias, denial and defensive ignorance once again triumphed over truth? Was God asleep—or did He know that this initially traumatic and overwhelming experience would catalyze Lisa to succeed beyond all expectations?

Since Vellutino never met or interviewed Lisa or her father, he certainly had nothing personally against them.

---

[1]McDonald Critchley, a well-known and truly gifted neurologist actually described dyslexics with compensated reading scores as reading "cured"—despite his awareness that other symptoms of the disorder persisted [Critchley, 1969]. (See *A Solution to the Riddle—Dyslexia*. Also refer to Chapter 11.)

And yet Lisa and even nondyslexics read and interpreted Vellutino's report to his friend Dave (as well as his quote in *Harpers Bazaar*) similarly: as insinuating that she might be a liar and malingerer and that I was an incompetent expert and thus malingering as well. Thus all wondered: Might the CV-based dyslexia concepts have triggered Vellutino's responses? Might Lisa's language and reading score-compensated abilities have also threatened Vellutino's traditionalist concepts? Might Vellutino have been interested in impressing the *administrative director of the Connecticut Bar Examination Committee* with his own abilities, defensively attacking all "controversial" and related others? Needless to say, only a proper traditional analysis of professor Vellutino's content and intent—with his direct help—seemed capable of providing objective understanding and insights.

Since definitions and diagnoses of dyslexia are dependent on clinical-theoretical considerations, conflicting opinions often arise even among unbiased experts with just differing points of view. Accordingly, I thought it essential to summarize *My Inner-Ear Concepts vs. The Linguistic View*—a view shared by Vellutino and others. And while at it, I thought it vital to also explain the "magic cures" as well as most other helpful therapies in dyslexia.

Part C

Additional Insights

CHAPTER 13

What's in a Theory?

Since the reader has witnessed critical experts like Vellutino, Silver, Huston, Denckla, Jansky, Gold, and so on espousing linguistic theories or claiming that dyslexia is part and parcel of a cerebrally determined language disorder, I thought it important to explain the differences between their linguistic dyslexia theories and mine. Hopefully the following three segments will clearly portray a traditional language theory which can only explain "dyslexia" in dyslexia vs. an inner-ear or CV theory which can clearly account for every symptom characterizing the dyslexic syndrome as well as the therapies or "magical cures" reported as helpful.

A

The Linguistic-Thinking
Brain Theory

The linguistic theory of dyslexia is very simple. It assumes an impairment within a specific language center of the dominant thinking brain, resulting in the inability to interpret visual and phonetic reading symbols. In other words, the signals reaching the impaired area are fine—they just can't be interpreted. And if words can't be interpreted or "analyzed," this theory mandates that the ensuing reading disorder be severe, and its prognosis over time very poor.

This theory is completely inconsistent with:

(1) the reality of the mild and moderate reading symptoms characterizing dyslexia, as well as the favorable prognosis of most dyslexics, providing they're not educationally and psychologically traumatized by misguided experts,

(2) the cerebellar neurological signs found,

(3) the inner-ear-enhancing therapies that help,

(4) the acquired inner-ear impairments that can create dyslexia or its symptoms, permanently or transiently,

(5) the complete absence of localizing neurological signs substantiating a defect within the thinking-linguistic centers of the brain, and

(6) the need, scientifically, to explain the vast majority of reading and non-reading symptoms and their intensities characterizing dyslexics and dyslexia.

Since my CV theory of dyslexia was derived *entirely* after listening to and analyzing the symptoms reported by thousands and thousands of dyslexics, I would be very surprised if this patient-based inner-ear theory did not fit *all* the facts characterizing the reality of dyslexia. As a result, I felt it important to present the stories of as many dyslexics within this book as possible so that readers might independently test out these opposing theories and their respective abilities to encompass and explain *all* the symptoms presented and *all* the therapies found helpful.

By contrast, the linguistic theory was derived entirely *from a fantasied analogy of dyslexia with alexia*—the latter resulting from a proven deficit within the thinking-language center of the cerebral cortex. Since *all* alexics have severe reading conceptual impairments, they cannot understand the meaning of written letters and words, and so their ability to compensate is very, very poor, no matter what you do for them.

Now step back a moment before continuing and reflect: Does the linguistic theory explain and encompass *all* the variable and diverse dyslexic symptoms and therapies thus far presented? And will it hold for those to follow when you look back? I seriously doubt it for the reasons given—and those to follow. But don't let me talk you into anything that doesn't make sense. Let's wait and see—especially for those who are justifiably skeptical of "controversial theories" like mine and "miracle cures" such as those attributed to me by traditionalist experts.[1]

---

[1]Refer to Chapters 15 and 18 for further discussions on the cerebral vs. cerebellar theories of dyslexia.

B

My Cerebellar-Vestibular (CV) or Inner-Ear Theory

Since 1973 I have postulated that there exists a cerebellar-vestibular or inner-ear-determined visual fixation, tracking and processing impairment underlying the visual reading symptoms characterizing dyslexics. Among these visual symptoms are: continual skipping over letters, words, and sentences; reversals; word blurring and word movement; double-word vision; reading headaches, nausea and/or dizziness as well as related visual concentration/distractibility symptoms; light sensitivity or photophobia; visual memory impairments for words read; visual word perseveration (the eye sticks to a word and requires blinking to unglue and proceed); lags in visual input reading so that it takes much longer to interpret words seen; head tilting and preferred reading positions.

In other words, I theorized that the inner-ear system was akin to vertical and horizontal TV stabilizers. When they go awry, then the brain's "TV channels" that process visual letter and word symbols drift—resulting in letter, word, and sentence blurring, drifting, movement, reversals, scrambling, and the other problems listed above. And similar "stabilizers" regulate "phonetic" signals. Thus this impairment may result in corresponding auditory-related input dysfunctioning and symptoms as well as problems in the links integrating the visual-auditory and motor components of the reading process.

As a result, the thinking-linguistic centers of the brain receive temporal and spatially "deformed" or scrambled signals. And the thinking brain's resulting or *secondarily-determined* difficulties will depend on the degree to which these signals are deformed vs. its ability to descramble and reinterpret them.

Eventually I postulated that the inner-ear or CV system modulates all sensory-motor and related functions. And the resulting conceptualizations simply and readily explained every single known reading and related dyslexic symptom found characterizing over 25,000 patients that I've meticulously examined clinically, many of whom have been treated and have responded in a manner similar to the cases presented, and those to be presented. Moreover, this concept is consistent with the presence of CV or inner-ear signs in dyslexia, and the complete absence of thinking-linguistic brain localizing or *primarily-determined* neurological evidence. In addition, it readily explains why the severity of the "typical" reading, writing, spelling, math, memory, and other impairments in dyslexia appear completely unrelated to the presence and/or intensity of speech and language difficulties.

In fact, it is not unusual to find severe non-readers who are linguistically gifted, and the reverse. Were dyslexia part and parcel of a linguistic disorder of the thinking brain, as believed by Vellutino and all other traditionalists, one would expect to find linguistic difficulties (severe) in all or most dyslexics and certainly a corresponding relationship between the intensity of speech and reading symptoms, since the prognosis or compensatory abilities of alexia and aphasia are very, very poor.

Moreover, the inner-ear theory of reading and related dyslexic symptoms can readily account for the varying ranges of symptomatic intensity and their fluctuations over time as well as the onset or intensifications following ear infections (inner-ear difficulties) and their improvements using inner-ear-enhancing therapies (i.e., eye exercises, vestibular or sensory-motor therapy, CV-enhancing medications, tinted lenses, auditory training, etc.). And since the compensatory range for inner-ear-determined dyslexic symptoms is as significant as it is symptom-specific—mirroring the way medications often target and thus improve some symptoms more than others—it is easy to explain the variations in symptom-combinations and symptom-intensities that characterize the reality of dyslexics and dyslexia.

Explaining All Dyslexic Symptoms

To understand the generalized cerebellar-vestibular or inner-ear mechanisms that I found to characterize and thus explain the vast majority of symptoms and helpful therapies among dyslexics, I decided to update and edit material taken from *Smart But Feeling Dumb*. Hopefully, you will see the difference in explanatory power between my concepts and those of the traditionalists.

Simply stated, the inner-ear serves the following ten crucial functions:

1. *The inner-ear acts as a guided-missile computer system—guiding our eyes, hands, feet, and various mental and physical functions in space and time.*

Thus a disorder within this system may deflect our eyes while they reflexively and automatically fixate and sequentially track letters, words, and sentences while we read. As a result, the dyslexic's reading process is characterized by letter, word, and sentence fixation and tracking difficulties, requiring compensatory slow reading, finger pointing, the use of cards, etc. What's more, the resulting visual scrambling will trigger the insertion and omission of words, the illusion of new words formed from word-parts separated by unseen distances, etc. Frequently words will seem blurred or in movement, requiring compensatory blinking and squinting in order to restabilize the drifting input. (See Figure 1 for the visual fixation and tracking errors characterizing the reading process in dyslexia.)

Error Diagram

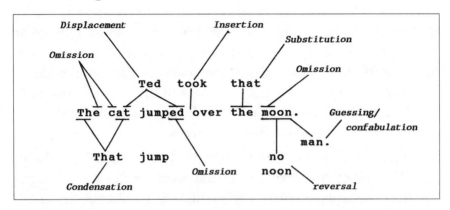

Figure 1 The "typical" dyslexic errors and mechanisms triggered when a sample of reading-disabled patients attempts to read the sentence, *The cat jumped over the moon.* By means of an error analysis and diagram, the mechanisms underlying the dyslexic reading performance are reconstructed: omissions, insertions, displacements, condensations, rotations/reversals/scrambling, substitutions, guessing, confabulation.[1] Taken from *A Solution to the Riddle—Dyslexia*, p. 31.)

Inasmuch as the tracking in dyslexics is coarse and jerky, the reading process becomes tiring and unpleasant. Often these dyscoordinated or clumsy eye movements, mistakenly referred to as apractic rather than dyspractic, keep retargeting the same words in a sentence over and over again, a process clinically labeled ocular perseveration.[2]

[1]Upon completing my psychiatric and Freudian training, I was initially struck by the resemblance of the mechanisms responsible for the dyslexic reading errors to those primary process or subconsciously determined dream, neurotic, and psychotic mechanisms such as displacement, condensation, reversals, omissions, insertions, etc. In this respect I found it curious that spatial-temporal and even gravitational representations appear to have little or no logical significance to the dreamer or to dream content in general. Are we not dyslexic in our dreams? And in our unconscious? Considering also that the traditionalists' initial denial of reality characterizing Freud's discoveries of "the unconscious" appeared to mirror those triggered by my CV-dyslexia research, I wondered if the CV circuits are not related to those modulating subconsciously determined mechanisms, etc.?

[2]Apraxia is a severe disturbance in motor planning and execution of cerebral origin whereas its mild dyspraxic counterpart is of inner-ear origin. And in ocular perservation, the eye remains glued to a letter or word, often requiring blinking or medication for compensation.

If our hands, our feet, or our speech mechanisms are not accurately guided in space and time, a wide range of dyscoordinated, clumsy acts or "Freudian slips" ("dyslexic slips") will occur. If the hand holding a pen is misguided in space and time, our writing will look discombobulated or dysgraphic. Most often the writing will drift off the horizontal if unlined paper is used and if concentration and effort are not used to extraordinary degrees.

Perhaps a slight "illustration break" here will be helpful. The following written samples of dyslexics to copying and dictation clearly highlight the graphomotor, spelling, grammatical, and related memory errors characterizing the CV-determined dysmetric dyslexic and dyspraxic (DDD) disorder. Also, the greater the number of coexisting functions (spelling, grammar, memory, conceptualization, etc.) required for the written task, the more corresponding and overall errors will be made—since compensatory concentration and related integration mechanisms will be stressed and overloaded. And these errors in writing coordination obviously mirror those in reading coordination.

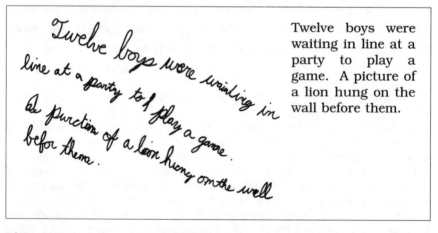

Twelve boys were waiting in line at a party to play a game. A picture of a lion hung on the wall before them.

Figure 2 An 11-year-old dyslexic was instructed to read and then copy several printed sequences into script. The writing drifts significantly from the horizontal. Letters are poorly formed and spaced, as well as inappropriately omitted, inserted, and condensed. Occasionally, letters from successive words are fused or condensed. Grammatical details such as crossing t's are intermittently and carelessly omitted.

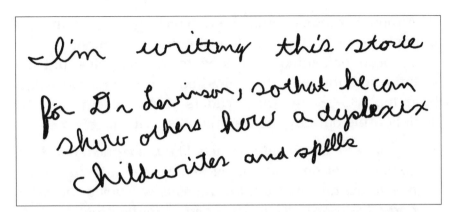

Figure 3 Graphomotor spelling errors of a bright 10-year-old dyslexic girl. A neurodynamic analysis of the spelling errors suggests a dysfunction in the visuo-motor memory of letter sequences and the use of compensatory phonetic recall. Letters and letter pairs are repeated (perseverated), and at times inappropriately fused or condensed. Moreover, the spelling is complicated by graphomotor incoordination, drifting, and the omission of grammatical details. Interestingly enough, this girl's oral spelling was found to be superior to her graphomotor spelling, suggesting that the motor channel utilized to test spelling may significantly alter the performance.

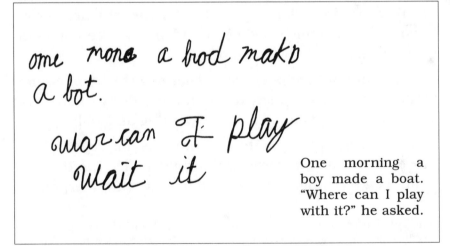

One morning a boy made a boat. "Where can I play with it?" he asked.

Figure 4 Spelling performance of an 8½-year-old dyslexic girl asked to write a few sentences she just read. Her visual-motor memory for sequential letters is severely deficient. Letters and syllables are omitted or substituted for one another, and guessing or confabulation is determined by randomization plus phonetic cues.

Although thousands of these typical and even atypical examples exist within my clinical records, some having already been presented, I decided to use samples and descriptions contained within *A Solution to the Riddle—Dyslexia* (pp. 36-38) so that readers might also judge the denial of this data by the traditionalist critics.

2. *The inner-ear system also acts like the vertical and horizontal holds on a television set. It fine-tunes all motor (voluntary and involuntary) responses leaving the brain and all sensory responses coming into the brain.*

If voluntary motor responses leaving the brain are improperly fine-tuned, one's motor functions become dyscoordinated and imbalanced. This may result in delays or difficulties in fine, gross, and rhythmic motor activities. Specifically, the following symptoms may occur: problems with crawling, sitting, walking, tying shoelaces, buttoning, zippering, holding and using writing implements and scissors, as well as playing various sports.[1] Also speech delays and/or symptoms such as stuttering, stammering, articulation errors, Freudian slips-of-the-tongue, etc. are not infrequent, mistakenly considered evidence of a cerebral language vs. inner-ear dysfunction.

If involuntary motor responses leaving the brain are improperly fine-tuned, then toilet training delays may arise as well as such symptoms as bed-wetting and soiling.

If the sensory input to the brain is improperly fine-tuned, then this input will drift or scramble. The thinking brain, however bright, will have difficulty with interpreting,

---

[1]The correlation of motor delays (i.e., crawling) with learning disabilities has led some investigators such as Delacato to assume that patterning will reverse the disorder. Delacato's theory is significantly incomplete; the benefits observed occur because the exercises improve inner-ear function. Blyth and McGlown (1979) had also recognized the organic (inner-ear) basis of neuroses and learning disabilities and designed therapeutic motor exercises.

remembering, and concentrating on a drifting, scrambled input. If the drift is 180 degrees, then reversals occur for both incoming and outgoing signals.

Even a genius watching and/or listening to a drifting input (or a drifting TV channel) will have great difficulty remembering and concentrating on the picture seen and heard. Variations in the drifting will account for variations in the degree of clarity. Some segments will be seen and heard clearly, while others will be only partially seen and heard. And some will be completely blurred, resulting in compensatory guessing and even illusions.

This very same person, if asked about the content of what he observed on the TV show, will not be able to answer too many questions. And if this genius is unaware that his difficulties are due to the TV image's drifting, then he will instinctively feel stupid, regardless of his IQ. In fact, the smarter he is the more frustrated he will become and the dumber he will feel.

For this reason, most of the time compliments make bright dyslexic kids feel worse. These kids know they are not able to grasp, remember, and reproduce information as well as their classmates or as well as their instincts and feelings tell them that they should. Reassuring these children that they are smart when they instinctively feel frustrated and stupid often makes them feel worse. They feel they are being lied to in order to make them feel better, to make them feel less stupid. Thus they conclude that they really *are* dumb; otherwise, the compliments and reassurances would not be necessary.

In other words, bright dyslexics are instinctively aware of the many difficulties they have, and therefore react with feelings of stupidity. *Although reassurance does not reverse feeling stupid—and, in fact, may seem to heighten it—it is nevertheless crucial because it keeps dyslexics going and striving until compensation occurs—if it occurs.*

Criticism, on the other hand, is felt very deeply, for it reinforces their gut feelings of stupidity, resulting in a deeper sense of inadequacy.

How can a teacher help but view these children as stupid, indifferent, and defiant, especially if she is viewing this same content from a separate, clear TV channel? If the teacher does not see the drift, she will naturally assume that the child is also watching a simple, clear TV picture. Thus she cannot comprehend the resulting errors and learning disabilities. Moreover, the child watching the drifting TV channel will lose his concentration and become distracted and restless. He'll want to get away from this frustrating input and shift TV channels.

This experience is very similar to how one reacts to motion sickness. Instinctively one wants to eliminate the input, either by fight or flight. If a child can't play hooky or change his channel in school by means of distracting mechanisms, he will fight. If his anger and fight are inwardly directed, he will become depressed and give up. If his anger is acted out, he will be viewed as a behavior problem with disruptive tendencies. Children will sometimes unconsciously behave in a manner that provokes authorities to suspend or expel them from school, thus attempting to get out of a most frustrating and humiliating situation. At other times, underlying guilt associated with feeling stupid and inadequate will trigger mechanisms that invite punishment and consequently alleviate guilt—a most unfortunate cycle. If, on the other hand, children try to avoid the frustrating drifting channel altogether, they'll be labeled "school phobic."

In order to understand all the variations and complexities of the dyslexic disorder, one has to carry the TV analogy a few steps further. Picture the brain as a giant TV set with millions of specific channels. Imagine each separate event as being independently processed on its own wavelength or TV channel. Thus one channel may drift while another remains fine-tuned. One channel may drift mildly while another is completely blurred out. One channel may drift vertically while another drifts horizontally. One channel may drift from right to left while another drifts from left to right. On and on the possibilities go, accounting for the diverse combination of symptoms seen from patient to patient and from sample to sample.

Furthermore, the fine-tuners may vary in function from moment to moment, depending on a series of known and unknown variables and circumstances. Spontaneous variations in the fine-tuning mechanisms may result in corresponding variations in symptoms from time to time, most often beyond the individual's control. Allergies of various kinds may trigger signal drifting, accounting for regression in spring and fall or when sugars and dyes are present in the diet.

3. *The inner-ear is also a compass system. It reflexively tells us spatial relationships such as right and left, up and down, and front and back.*

If this compass system isn't working efficiently, then one must devise such consciously directed compensatory methods as wearing a ring or a watch on one hand, or recalling which hand has a scar or was broken or was used to pledge allegiance. Related difficulties in sensing, knowing, and even understanding east and west, and north and south may also occurr, triggering anxieties about getting lost.

The compass system directs all body functions: sensory, motor, speech, thought, even biophysical patterns. Moreover, one sequence may be misdirected or scrambled while another remains unaffected or compensated for and is seemingly unaffected.

4. *The inner-ear also acts as a timing mechanism, setting rhythms to motor tasks.*

A disturbance within this system may result in difficulty in learning to tell time and sensing time. Frequently, dyslexic children do not know *before* from *after* and can't sense whether a minute, an hour, or several hours have gone by. As a result, dyslexic individuals may become "compulsively" late or early. Speech timing may be off, resulting in slow or rapid talkers and even dysrhythmic talkers or stutterers. The inner-ear also serves to inhibit or modulate the speed of the various sensory-inputs. Accordingly, dyslexics experience visual, auditory, tactile and related inputs as being faster, and thus they blur out these sensory sequences at lower thresholds than do normal subjects.

5. *The inner-ear also serves as a dynamic filter, significantly blocking out maladaptive sensory-motor and mental backgrounds.*

Impairments or "holes" within this filtering system account for the sensory-specific distractibility symptoms (visual, acoustic, etc.) of dyslexics as well as the internal or subconscious "leaking" of thoughts and impulses resulting in daydreaming, stealing, hitting, obsessions and compulsions, etc. Similarly, background motor movement must be inhibited or filtered out in the interest of smooth, rhythmic and goal-directed or foreground action; otherwise, clumsiness and dyscoordination result.

6. *Integration of sensory-motor functioning is also inner-ear related.*

As a result, dyslexics not infrequently experience a breakdown in integrated or composite movement patterns as well as sequenced sensory-input experiences. Thus, for example, klutzy individuals must slow down movement patterns into individual steps—an inner-ear impairment called *decomposition of movement.* And they compensate consciously by attempting *a reintegration or recomposition* using slow *secondary or compensatory* cerebral or thinking-brain mechanisms. Similarly, dyslexics characteristically experience tunnel vision during reading—often seeing only one or two letters of a word sequence at a time. They are then forced to look at and sound out each letter of a word sequence—one at a time. Then they must attempt a conscious reintegration or recomposition of the total sequence so as to complete the reading task. And often central and peripheral visual mechanisms are decomposed so that dyslexics use one or another rather than both together.

Sound sequences are also decomposed among some dyslexics—explaining their auditory input processing lags as well as a need for repetition before speech is "sequentially heard," compensated for, and thus understood. By analogy, *aphasics* hear the verbal sequences clearly—they just can't interpret them.

This same disintegration phenomena may decompose the simultaneous processing of visual-acoustic-proprioceptive-motor processes during reading—thus resulting in the various "types" of reading difficulties characterizing dyslexics as well as their special compensatory styles. Although many an "expert" has unwittingly fragmented dyslexia into various types—mirroring their disintegration tendencies—it seems more logical to view dyslexia as one disorder with various impairments in underlying mechanisms similar to those presented here.

7. *The inner-ear, via its connection to various mood, anxiety and motor-energy centers of the brain, modulates these various functions.*

   Accordingly, a failure in these various functions may result in secondarily-related and interconnected anxiety, mood, impulsive and activity disorders—symptoms characterizing ADHD.

8. *The inner-ear serves as a gyroscope to the brain,* thereby maintaining a stable visual alignment relative to the positions of the head, neck, and body.

As a result, dysfunctioning in this mechanism readily explains such dyslexic symptoms as seeing written print on an angle as well as the compensatory need for head and body tilting so as to effect a neurophysiological realignment. Similar repositioning is experienced during writing— for analogous reasons.

9. *The inner-ear processes muscle tone and gravity signals.*

Impairments in muscle tone not infrequently lead to "double jointedness," slouching, or head and shoulder drooping, even facilitating scoliosis and flat feet (pes planus) in those physiologically predisposed. Indeed, tonal imbalance may contribute to strabismus and "jelly legs" when the eyes and feet are respectively affected. Improper gravity processing may contribute to the sensations of falling, being pulled to one side, and even irresistible feelings and fears of being pulled to the ground when looking down from heights.

10. *The inner-ear is also assumed to facilitate the processing of starting and stopping functions.*

Thus, for example, it is not unusual for inner-ear dysfunctioning dyslexics to have difficulty stopping and re-starting or continuing a motor sequence—thus resulting in the repetition or perseveration characterizing their reading, stuttering, and writing errors. And as repeatedly observed, inner-ear-enhancing medications and even corrective conditioning often improve this impairment.

C

Understanding the "Magical" and Related "Cures"

To date, the traditionalists cannot explain the various therapies reported helpful in dyslexia using their cerebral theories. And instead of changing their theories so as to explain the therapies found helpful, the traditionalists refuted or denied the efficacy of these treatment modes by condescendingly referring to them as "magical cures." Similarly, instead of modifying their 100-year-old language theories to encompass the many and varied symptoms found characterizing dyslexics, they denied the entire complex syndrome in favor of the oversimplified equation: *dyslexia* = *"dyslexia."*[1] As a result, the traditionalists were unwittingly forced to assume that all "nondyslexic" or non-reading symptoms characterizing the dyslexic syndrome were due to separate brain dysfunctions, i.e., minimal brain dysfunction, diffuse brain dysfunction, static encephalopathy, etc.

By contrast, I listened carefully to my many dyslexic patients and their loved ones and so attempted to explain how each of the "magical cures" works and even why they might fail. And by doing so, I found that my insights into dyslexia were greatly enhanced—resulting in the first and only comprehensive understanding of a holistic treatment approach.

[1]Paradoxically, they have also fragmented or decomposed the unitary origin of the CV-determined dyslexic syndrome into a complex mass of alleged separate disorders mistakenly considered to be of corresponding distinct origins. And thus to encompass all these overlapping syndromes such as "dyslexia", ADHD, mood and anxiety disorders, etc., the traditionalists were forced to reintegrate or recompose them under such frightening umbrella terms as diffuse brain damage or dysfunction, minimal cerebral dysfunction, static encephalopathy, etc.

Medical Treatment

As previously discussed, I discovered that dyslexia is due to a dysfunction in the inner-ear system and realized that antimotion-sickness medications helped strengthen the inner-ear's capacity to handle motion input and balance/co-ordination output (thus alleviating the various sensory-motor symptoms characterizing motion sickness). I then reasoned that these very same medications may indeed improve the ability of the inner-ear system to fine-tune and process the *total sensory input* as it does the motion input, and the *total motor output* as it processes the balance and coordination difficulties noted in motion sickness. Indeed, this reasoning was clearly and decisively validated when dyslexics were treated with a variety of antimotion-sickness antihistamines and related medications, and their favorable responses were carefully recorded. A series of typical medication responses have been presented so that these various sensory-motor and related improvements could be noted.

The wide range of expected and unexpected improvements due to my medical treatment more than justifies my theory of the inner-ear system as the fine-tuner for the brain's entire sensory input and motor output. Furthermore, the observed medication-triggered improvements have clearly highlighted the inner-ear-determined and related mechanisms previously noted to be responsible for creating the diverse symptoms characterizing the dyslexic syndrome.

Now that you better understand why and how various medications I use help dyslexics, you must be curious about the mechanisms underlying the favorable responses reported by allergists and nutritionists, occupational therapists, optometrists, psychologists and psychiatrists, chiropractors, dentists, and educators. Until now, most theories unwittingly confused and reversed hidden dyslexic causes with the resulting symptomatic effects. For example, the emotional symptoms and poor self-image triggered by, or resulting from, the dyslexic process were mistakenly assumed to be the cause of dyslexia. And the reading and speech symptoms triggered by the underlying inner-ear dysfunctioning in dyslexia were mistakenly thought to be part of a primary language disorder of cerebral-cortical or thinking-linguistic origin. Also, most theories were insufficient to explain and encompass the total symptomatic and therapeutic realities characterizing dyslexia—despite the repeated cry for a holistic approach.

Accordingly, an understanding of why various therapies work or do not work may significantly contribute to every professional's ultimate aim: a meaningful multidisciplinary cooperative approach. It is anticipated that this understanding will lead to new and better ways of helping dyslexics, regardless of the professional's title or the name of the therapy.

Nutritional Treatment

Inasmuch as dyslexia was found to be caused by an inner-ear disturbance, and in view of the fact that niacin, related B vitamins, and minerals were reported to sometimes improve inner-ear-related dizzy and balance symptoms, the findings of nutritionists in dyslexia became readily understandable.

Dr. Ben F. Feingold, a noted allergist, recognized that sugars, dyes, and various other allergenic substances may aggravate such dyslexic symptoms as hyperactivity and distractibility. Accordingly, the elimination of these substances leads to a corresponding improvement in symptoms. In my experience, allergies merely magnify or intensify dyslexic symptoms. They typically do not cause dyslexia—unless the allergic attack is of a severe enough magnitude to damage inner-ear mechanisms and structures.

Generally speaking, any harmful process or substance, whether stress-related, allergic, metabolic, infectious, or toxic in nature, may impair or disrupt inner-ear functioning, aggravating a dyslexic disorder.

Occupational and Optometric Treatment

Occupational therapists and optometrists have reported academic as well as coordination improvements when dyslexics perform various motion-related and/or eye-training exercises. Inasmuch as the inner-ear controls body and eye movements as well as motion-related activities, and in view of the fact that repetition leads to improvement in the specific motor task repeated, it seems reasonable to assume that practicing motor skills could result in an improvement in the inner-ear mechanisms governing them. However, one must still account for the reported academic improvements when only motor exercises are performed. In other words, why will a child given eye exercises and asked to participate in various balance and coordination tasks read, write, and concentrate better? The answer is not very difficult to obtain if one goes back to my previously described concept of dyslexic mechanisms and functioning.

Transfer of Function:
Specific vs. Generalized Improvement

If repetitive motor tasks indeed improve underlying inner-ear mechanisms, and if we assume that this improvement extends to, or is transferred to, neighboring inner-ear circuits or channels, then we can readily explain the generalized improvements that sometimes occur when specific "TV" circuits are strengthened by repetition, practicing, or conditioning.

For example, if repetitive eye-tracking techniques help fine-tune and condition its underlying "TV" circuit, or channel e, and if this conditioned or improved effect is transferred to neighboring and interconnected circuits, then channels r, w, m, c, t, etc.—reading, writing, math, concentration, and tennis—will correspondingly improve. However, in most circumstances transfer of functional improvements to neighboring circuits does not often occur, or is significantly restricted, accounting for the limitation of the above therapies.

When astronauts and other experimental subjects were readied for space and spun in various directions, an interesting observation was noted: Rotating someone repeatedly in a counterclockwise direction most often led to an improvement in his tolerance for counterclockwise rotations. However, it did not frequently lead to improvement in tolerating clockwise and other types of directional rotations. This observation clearly indicates how the body *specifically* adapts or changes in order to respond to correspondingly *specific* stimuli and conditions.

Athletics Improves Concentration and Cognition

Fortunately, transfer of functional improvements to neighboring circuits does occur at least in certain contexts. In my practice I've repeatedly noted the existence of an initially puzzling and strange phenomenon: Dyslexic athletes often do best academically when in training, despite the limited study time they have. Upon termination of their sports activities, due to either a changing season or an injury, a significant number of athletes report a corresponding decrease in their concentration, memory, and overall academic functioning.

At first glance, one might mistake this correlation as an excuse conjured up by athletes to justify their training time. This was not the case, however, for most often it was their parents who reported this fascinating but puzzling correlation. It therefore appeared that sports activities and exercises resulted in a transfer of function to neighboring underlying inner-ear circuits, which in turn resulted in an academic improvement. Cessation of practice led to a regression in underlying functioning, and the transfer of function was in turn eliminated. The unexpected observation that physical exercises in dyslexics may result in increased mental capacity is in accord with the adages "Practice makes perfect." and "Sound body, sound mind."

Conditioning experiments in humans and animals follow a very similar pattern. If not continuously reinforced, conditioned functions and improvements disappear with time.

Over my long research career, I have repeatedly tried to understand and explain seemingly paradoxical data. I have learned that confusing events—or events occurring opposite to my expectations—invariably result in significant insights if enough time is spent looking for an explanation. By contrast, important insights remain hidden when confusing or contradictory data are denied or swept under the scientific "rug." As a result, I have disciplined myself to record and attempt to explain contradictions or criticism. When criticism is valid and constructive, surmounting it carries research a significant step forward. When criticism is destructive, it points out hidden flaws in the critic—flaws of which the critic and his audience are most often unaware, once again highlighting areas requiring additional attention and explanation.

The analysis of flaws, in oneself or in one's critics, has provided me with answers crucial to solving the riddles characterizing dyslexia and dyslexic research. As a result, I have devoted Chapter 13 in *A Solution to the Riddle—Dyslexia* to the investigation and analysis of this phenomenon. And correspondingly, Chapter 13, here, in *A Scientific Watergate—Dyslexia* attempts to summarize those resulting insights.

Chiropractic and Dental Treatment of TMJ Syndrome

Patients have occasionally reported to me some symptomatic improvements arising from chiropractic manipulation and/or dental corrections of their temporomandibular joint (TMJ) syndrome. Needless to say, these observations are as valid as any other type and must be accounted for rather than "criticized" away. It is well known that many dyslexics will tilt their head, neck, and body in order to read, write, and concentrate better. The neck is an important integration point for the inner-ear circuitry. Perhaps the chiropractic adjustment of these and other positions serves a similar purpose to that performed instinctively and reflexively by dyslexics from within.

Dental problems affecting the temporomandibular joint may often lead to headaches, dizziness, impaired concentration, and dyslexia-like functioning. To explain these symptoms, I have assumed that an inflammation or misalignment of the temporomandibular joint may be transferred to the neighboring inner-ear system, thus either mimicking or aggravating dyslexic symptoms.

Educational Therapy: How it Works and Fails

Educational therapy is as complex as it is crucial. Specific memory functions are characteristically impaired in dyslexia. Thus repetition of specific inputs is crucial if any improvement is to result. As stated earlier, specific channels of information invariably drift in dyslexics, leaving their victims relatively "blind" or "deaf" to certain inputs.

Thus, the task of educators is to find and utilize clear, open channels, as well as channels that drift very mildly, so that they may be used to impart crucial information. This teaching-learning process is very similar to what we do for the deaf and blind. In view of the fact that the majority of dyslexics are neither deaf nor blind, however, it is vitally important to improve the drifting channels via repetition or conditioning while simultaneously utilizing and stimulating open channels—thus also explaining the efficacy of visual and auditory training.

If a given sensory input drifts, the corresponding message to the thinking brain is blurred, reversed, or scrambled, rendering it difficult to remember and/or understand. Moreover, these drifting or blurred imprints are frequently wiped out or erased because they are perceived as faulty. Repetition and conditioning frequently force an adaptation in which these drifting inputs are finally "imprinted" or accepted for storage and memory retention. In other words, the underlying inner-ear-related mechanisms processing sensory inputs have been triggered to compensate in a manner similar to the way repetitive motor tasks force an underlying improvement in the specific circuits that process these tasks.

Just as repetitive motor tasks lead to an improvement in the underlying controlling mechanism, as well as a possible transfer of function to neighboring circuits, the repetition and stimulation used in teaching with a multisensory approach (visual, auditory, touch, proprioceptive) may also lead to both underlying and transferred functional improvements.

Tinted Lenses

Recently, the use of tinted lenses was recognized to be helpful in minimizing or compensating for the various reading symptoms characterizing dyslexia. Since inner-ear dysfunctioning subjects may be light-sensitive or *photophobic* due to impaired light-wave-specific filtering, then it appears reasonable that tinted lenses may be as helpful for some dyslexics as is increasing the print size in reading material for others. Also color and increased target size enable the eye as an inner-ear-directed guided missile to better hit its target.

Each therapeutic approach has its own corresponding theory. I have tried to harmonize the successes and failures of all treatment techniques with those of my own, so that patients and professionals will have a choice as to which combination of therapies may best suit specific needs. I have saved the medical (neurologic and psychiatric) theories and treatment approaches for last.

Psychotherapy vs. Neurological Referrals

Until very recently, psychoanalysts, psychiatrists, and related professionals believed child-rearing and emotional disturbances were responsible for many learning, emotional, and behavioral symptoms that characterized dyslexics. Consequently, a host of very specific subtheories and psychological mechanisms were formulated in order to account for each of the many dyslexic symptoms. Invariably, psychotherapy was advised in an effort to cure or alleviate the emotional factors deemed *primarily* responsible for the dyslexic symptoms.

The fact that psychotherapy often alleviates a dyslexic's symptoms does not prove that psychological factors caused the disturbance. Indeed, psychotherapy merely alleviates the stress and secondary feelings of stupidity, frustration, and helplessness, factors that further complicate and destabilize an already impaired fine-tuning system. My research has clearly indicated that the psychological symptomatic fallout of dyslexia is caused by a physiological disturbance within the inner-ear system. In other words, the surface psychological and behavioral symptoms are *secondary reactions* to the dyslexic's inability to function and compete normally.

The traditionalist neurological approach to dyslexia was significantly guided by the mistaken belief that this disorder was due to a *primary* dysfunction within the cerebral cortex—the thinking, speaking brain, the seat of the intellect. This "cortical theory" has led clinicians to misdiagnose dyslexics as having minimal brain damage, minimal cerebral dysfunction, static encephalopathy, or cerebral developmental delay, despite the *complete absence* of tangible neurological findings supporting a diagnosis of *primary* cerebral dysfunction. Clinicians still clinging to this outmoded point of view openly admit that they can neither diagnose this disorder properly nor treat it medically.

Following a rather stereotyped but traumatizing diagnosis of cerebral dysfunction, the neurologic treatment most frequently consists of *referrals*. Thus, patients are sent to any one or combination of therapists, often in a biased, helter-skelter fashion.

Indeed, the cortex or thinking brain *is* impaired in dyslexics. However, it is *only secondarily* impaired. For example, if our thinking brain, regardless of how bright and intact it is, receives a drifting, blurred, scrambled, or reversed input, it cannot deal effectively or efficiently with the content it receives. Thus, even the cortical dysfunction theory of dyslexia is consistent with my conviction that dyslexia is due to an impaired inner-ear system. The "cortical" theorists merely confused the *primary* (inner-ear) site and cause of dyslexia with its *secondary* effects on cortical function.

In retrospect, psychiatrists and neurologists were similarly misled. They confused the *secondary* fallout of the dyslexic disorder with its *primary* underlying cause in the inner-ear. Psychiatrists mistakenly assumed that a *primary* psychological or mental dysfunction explained the behavioral and emotional symptoms of dyslexia. And neurologists mistakenly assumed the presence of a *primary* cortical dysfunction to explain the presence of intellectual and speech symptoms in dyslexia. Each and every specialty unwittingly held onto its prior assumptions tenaciously—perhaps even using the same perseveration mechanisms characterizing dyslexics.

Invariably, misdiagnosed patients are returned to educators with either no helpful information or outright misinformation. Thus, educators have been given a near impossible task, one that requires a Herculean effort of patience and intuition. In the final analysis, educators are ultimately responsible for the education and treatment of the children and adults before them. They are forced to assume the total burden of the psychiatric, neurologic, pediatric, and optometric specialties, without the benefit of any meaningful medical understanding. They are forced to help, or attempt to help, millions and millions of dyslexics in the dark. Many accomplish wonders under the circumstances. Some are not equal to the task.

A Dynamic Concept of Symptoms

By carefully studying the improvements in dyslexia, regardless of the therapies triggering them, a unique and dynamic understanding of the symptoms and forces characterizing this syndrome materialized. And interestingly, this dynamic concept paralleled that initially discovered by Freud to explain mental events and their corresponding symptoms. As previously discussed, any combination of inner-ear mechanisms may be impaired among dyslexics. Similarly, any mechanism may be compensated for, or even overcompensated for. By recognizing that the impaired mechanisms underlying dyslexic symptoms are in a dynamic equilibrium with compensatory factors, a concept of symptom formation evolves in which each symptom is viewed as a resultant of opposing forces, dysfunctioning and compensatory. If gifted functions are also taken into consideration, as are self-corrective versus regressive forces, then we have truly arrived at the concepts needed to understand dyslexics and their fascinating disorder.

The above-described inner-ear mechanisms and concepts have resulted in the first comprehensive explanation of *why* and *how* the various theories about dyslexia and their corresponding therapies, including my own, work or do not work.

A Final Question

Now that the *traditionalist cortical theory vs. my inner-ear concepts* of dyslexia have been presented and compared, I encourage readers to judge which explanation best encompasses all the symptoms, neurological signs, and treatments characterizing dyslexics and dyslexia! Quite frankly, had I been satisfied with the explanatory capabilities of preexisting theories, I would never have been *forced* to develop my own.

CHAPTER 14

Scientific Denial:
Dyslexics without "Dyslexia"

Contrary to ordinary expectations, denials of reality have occurred rather frequently in science, invariably *masking and resisting* major breakthroughs. For example: 1) The denial of cosmic reality resulted in "fantasies" that the earth was flat and the center of the universe. 2) The denial of our evolutionary animalistic origins led to the belief that man was a unique and supreme form—independent of all others. 3) The denial of subconsciously active sexual and aggressive instinctive (animalistic) drives and resulting conflicts, as discovered by Freud, led to the mistaken conviction that conscious and logical mental determinants were sufficient to explain *all* our thoughts, feelings and actions. And as analyzed within *A Solution to the Riddle—Dyslexia*, man's subconsciously determined egoistic need to view himself as "master of the universe" appeared to readily explain all of the above denials and supporting theoretical fantasies.

As previously discussed, the study of dyslexia led me to recognize yet another traditionally accepted fantasy: *dyslexia = "dyslexia."* And to sustain this nonsensical belief scientifically, the vast majority of dyslexics—those without "dyslexia" or severely impaired reading scores were denied, as was the following common sense reasoning:

- Everyone—expert and nonexpert—will readily agree that you can't *define and equate* the complex syndrome or disorder called diabetes with *only* severe degrees of *only* one of its highly overdetermined variables—very high or coma-triggering blood sugars—also considered "diabetes" by traditionalist experts many, many years ago before they knew what diabetes was really all about.

- Similarly, you can't define and equate the complex syndrome of many and varied symptoms (such as those typically illustrated by many inner-ear dysfunctioning dyslexic patients and improved by inner-ear-enhancing medications) *called dyslexia* by *only* severe degrees of *only* one of its many and varied overdetermined variables—severely impaired reading score levels (two or more years below peers and/or potential), also *called "dyslexia."*

Despite the above logic, *all* esteemed and gifted dyslexia research experts have to date repeatedly defined the *whole* dyslexia syndrome by only the severe "tip" of one of its many, many, many parts. Since critics often refer to my elephant test or blurring-speed measurement of inner-ear function and dysfunction, might I raise another analogy and question: *Can you conceptualize and define an entire elephant by only the size of just the tip of its tail? I can't! But obviously the traditionalists can and do.* And they do so via denial—for it cannot be done by any other means.

So why are you being repetitive, the reader must be thinking. We're not stupid—we get your point. We've read about reading-score-compensated dyslexics repeatedly by now. In fact, your patient—Joan Sparks—was a perfect example. And you went through all this then, too.

Don't be insulted. I'm sure that readers do fully understand what I'm saying, as do my patients and their loved ones. Just listen to them. In fact, the only ones that don't understand the difference between dyslexia and "dyslexia" are the traditionalist experts—*despite my having repeatedly written about this over and over again for the past twenty years.* As you've read, Vellutino was "mystified." So were experts Denckla and Jansky—*angrily.* And professor Richard Allington, Vellutino's colleague at Albany, was *also* mystified. Thus his critical review of my medical text, sarcastically entitled, "Dyslexia has little to do with reading: a riddler's solution," triggered my responding critique, "Allington's Folly." (See *The Review of Education,* 7 [2], pp.153-158.)

And if you refer to repeated footnoted and related comments throughout this text you'll note that a very gifted Yale group led by a solid and thorough researcher— Shaywitz—appeared similarly misled by dyslexia and "dyslexia." Thus, for example, this group recently confirmed that the reading scores of many young dyslexics improve and even approach normalcy over time. In fact, their research was considered so important and new that it was published as a lead article in the *New England Journal of Medicine* (1/92), entitled "Evidence that dyslexia may represent the lower tail of a normal distribution of reading ability."

There was only one major problem with the above study. Instead of recognizing that dyslexics may not have "dyslexia" or severely impaired reading scores, the researchers stated *"that dyslexia may not exist as a discrete diagnostic entity."* In other words, they also *completely* equated the disorder called dyslexia with its severe reading score impairment, also called *"dyslexia."* And so they erroneously reasoned *that one couldn't exist without the other!* Even these esteemed researchers couldn't recognize and thus conceptualize *dyslexics without "dyslexia"!*

In fact, the reverse is possible too: You can have a severe reading score impairment of non-inner-ear (psychological or educational) origin without having the disorder called dyslexia. And so *"dyslexia" may even exist without dyslexics*— if we utilize the reading-score-based definitions and conceptualizations of my esteemed critics.

No doubt you are all thoroughly bewildered by the *experts' confusion*—especially since the points repeatedly made are simple. In all honesty, I was at first mystified too. But upon reflection and the examination of thousands of dyslexics such as those presented in this book, I *demystified* myself. And since these comments have been repeated over and over again by this author here and elsewhere, it seemed strange that *traditionalist experts refuse to admit to this simple reasoning and the supporting clinical data— data they condescendingly refer to as merely "anecdotal," rather than quantitative or objective.*

To understand the "expert confusion," I reasoned as follows: *The experts must never have examined enough dyslexic patients in the detail I presented to you here and to others in my prior books and papers to have demystified themselves.* But this reasoning seemed insufficient to explain their denial of simple logic as well as its defensive intensity—just a part. There had to be deeper and much more important determinants explaining Vellutino's and Allington's and Dr. Denckla's *mystification.* Here's my analysis:

- If dyslexics can read, then their prognosis is good. *So they can't be like alexics—who can't read at all.* (*Alexia* is a severe reading disorder resulting from a proven defect within the thinking-speaking brain— the dominant cerebral cortex.)

- And if dyslexia is not similar to *alexia*—where the prognosis is very, very poor and thus alexics remain unable to read, *then might dyslexia not be of a thinking-brain origin?*

That's it! Sure sounds right! That had to be a prime reason for the above-noted denial by traditionalist experts of the reality about dyslexia and "dyslexia" (or a severe reading score impairment of more than two years below peers and/or potential). It certainly seemed logical. And it clearly and simply explained the intensity with which the traditionalists denied—and still deny—what's always been right before their eyes: *Dyslexics without "dyslexia"* and of course *"dyslexia" without dyslexics.* But I couldn't help but wonder: Might the incidence of reading-score-compensated dyslexics be far higher than realized? Might many of my critics be subconsciously driven to deny the compensated dyslexia within themselves—and so recognize only the severest "dyslexia" forms? In other words, do they unwittingly attempt to define themselves as non-dyslexic? It would certainly help explain their scrambled and intense responses to my simple clinically-based reading-score concepts of dyslexia.

Perhaps now you will understand my repeated attempts to drive these *dyslexia vs. "dyslexia"* points home. But as you see, the critical experts were too biased and defensive to listen to reason—certainly from a mere clinician who happened not to be a member of their "club."

A Triple-Blind Study

And for those interested and curious readers, a review of one of my research papers ("Dramatic favorable responses of children with learning disabilities or dyslexia and attention deficit disorder to antimotion-sickness medications: four case reports" [12/91]) will clearly indicate how and why another group of dyslexia researchers were once again misled by the nonsensical equation *Dyslexia = "Dyslexia."*

Although an interested researcher, Joel Fagan, M.D., came to my clinic, observed our diagnostic-therapeutic methods, and allegedly read all my scientific literature as well as being told all the pitfalls of double-blind studies performed *"triple-blind"—without clear insights and concepts*, he nevertheless fell right into the traditionalist dyslexia trap.[1]

---

[1]In a double-blind drug study, neither patient nor physician knows whether real or sugar pills are used. And I call a "triple-blind" study one in which the researchers and their design are also "blind."

Despite a wide range of drawbacks to their study (*a very small sample of treated dyslexics, approximately half of them unwittingly given demonstrated toxic doses of meclizine, and too short a re-evaluation time to measure any significant changes in reading-score improvements*), Fagan and colleagues demonstrated:

- *that the dyslexics, prior to treatment, had a cerebellar-vestibular-determined fixation defect—using a testing parameter similar to that measured by my 3D Optical Scanner (Raymond, Ogden, Fagan, & Kaplan [1988]—clearly validating my CV diagnostic methods and conceptualizations of dyslexia;*

- *that meclizine, in both single doses and over a three-month interval, resulted in improved ocular fixation and balance.* However, as could have been expected had Fagan read and understood my suggestions, reading scores didn't improve over three months in dyslexics comprising their rather small sample. As a result, these traditionally trained researchers erroneously concluded, "The failure of antimotion-sickness medication to improve reading in developmental dyslexia: results of a randomized trial" (Fagan, et al., 1988).

Even a cursory review of this paper's content clearly indicates their confusion over *dyslexia* = "*dyslexia*." And since in this study *meclizine* only helped *dyslexics* but not their "*dyslexia*"—especially since the doses were toxic and the re-evaluation time too short for too few cases treated—these researchers completely and unwittingly misconstrued the significance of their data.

Considering the massive denial "blinding" *all* dyslexia experts, it became apparent that all were probably motivated or driven by common subconscious forces. Hopefully the remaining chapters of this work will present a clearer dissection and understanding of the factors triggering the above scientific denial in dyslexia research.

CHAPTER 15

What's in a Color?

Because the Ortonians had demanded equal time on "Donahue" ever since 1981 and as I had published *Smart But Feeling Dumb* in 1984 and didn't mind an open and honest scientific debate, the Phil Donahue show finally scheduled a conflicting TV situation: *The Ortonians vs. Levinson.* Once again, the deck was stacked.

Dr. Drake Duane, a Mayo Clinic neurologist and *the leading* spokesperson for the Orton Society, appeared on the show with me. But he had two other critics to help him: Ortonian tutor, Betty Osmond, and a complaining Floridian mother of a child who was seen only once by a colleague at my dyslexic treatment center.[1]

---

[1]Even at the time, it seemed strange that she should have any complaints about our office: (1) since the fee was $600.00 for *all* 2½ hours worth of medical testing and all ensuing follow-up time—and as she was at least 80% covered by insurance, (2) since her airfare to New York was completely paid for as an airline employee, and (3) since she never once called or sent in a progress report that she was requested to return—especially as *all* the *call-in-time* was free and ready-made progress reports were given her in *colored* envelopes so that my staff would recognize—and answer—them as rapidly as possible.

So what did she complain about? She appeared upset: (1) that our office delayed sending a *medical* consultation report to her son's school— a report intended for and probably readable by only physicians, and (2) that her son was tired—and so she stopped the medications on her own without even bothering to make even *one free* call to our offices.

Negotiations

My only ally was Sue Stafford—the dyslexic and teacher I co-dedicated this book to. But she was *positioned* by one of Donahue's producers, whose son was taught by Ortonians, offstage and down at the audience level. And this was a major concession, since this producer initially refused to have Sue or any of my patients with me until I refused to attend. Thus the producer had no choice, since it was my book—*Smart But Feeling Dumb*—and it was my concepts that had any meaning and interest to Donahue's audience. And as usual, all the Ortonians had was criticism. So I was given this token concession. But this time I was better prepared than at the Ortonian scientific set-up in 1975 (see Chapter 5).

The Show

In any event, Betty Osmond's red dress and smiling Ortonian facade eventually caused Donahue to redirect his staged attack from me to Betty: "What are you smiling about," he said. "We're talking about a serious topic—that affects the very lives of millions of children." So she suddenly stopped smiling. And her red dress didn't seem as red as before.

The Audience's Favorable Response—Thumbs Up

Before getting to the main point, I'd like to reassure my readers that I didn't have to say a word in defense of myself. The audience saw right through the Ortonians' facade, and they came right to my aid, claiming: Why are you all attacking Dr. Levinson and his treatment when you (the Ortonians) have *nothing* to offer yourselves?

The audience was obviously impressed with Susan's description of her improvement—as noted following the dedication, as well as what I said about dyslexia and the way the inner-ear tracks and processes visual and related sensory information. Why, the audience asked me, was your fee so low—considering the time and effort put in?

My response: As you all *feel*, my primary aim is to make this new or breakthrough diagnosis, understanding, and treatment affordable to all. Could you imagine the criticism if I *really* charged what I could have—just to get rich? Even the critics were amazed at my "low" fees. Theirs were more or certainly equivalent.

The Party Line

Before millions of television viewers, Dr. Drake Duane repeated the standard or traditionalist Ortonian line—that dyslexia was a language disorder. But that's it. There was nothing offered of any substance. And so the audience saw right through him. And Donahue heard the audience. So Donahue reversed himself and sided with the audience—who sided with me.

By the way, Dr. Duane seemed interested when I displayed Dr. Gold's "blind" cerebellar findings before the TV conflict began—as did Donahue's producer. But it never influenced their format. Nor did they say a word about it again during the entire show. Nor would they allow me to present the graphs highlighting Dr. Gold's "blind" cerebellar findings in dyslexia—the ones in *A Solution to the Riddle—Dyslexia* and in Chapter 4.

Naturally, I disagreed on TV with the Ortonian view. And unfortunately, much real and meaningful information was lost to the audience watching a staged dispute.

Follow-up—One Year Later

And Dr. Duane once again repeated his dyslexia convictions when contacted by the *Morning Star* (4/12/85) after I gave a lecture at Kuntztown University:

> "*Dr. Drake D. Duane*, a Mayo Clinic neurologist who sat opposite Levinson on the "Donahue" program three years ago, *said*

the accepted theory is that dyslexia is a central nervous system disorder related to the way the brain processes language. He said it is supported by anatomical studies that dyslexic behavior stems predominantly from the left half of the brain."[1]

The Convert

Dr. Drake Duane appeared to completely reverse his language-dyslexia position in 1992 when contacted by the *New York Times*. The reporter was reviewing Harvard researchers' Margaret Livingstone's and Albert Galaburda's allegedly new visual processing theory in dyslexia. According to Duane:

> *"This is the first observation that the visual system may be involved in dyslexia*, and it is extremely important," said Dr. Drake Duane, an international authority on dyslexia and learning disorders at Arizona State University. "It reinforces the idea that the nervous systems of those who are dyslexic are atypical."
>
> "Dyslexia, a broad term that includes a number of disorders affecting people's ability to read, is believed to affect 4 to 5 percent of the population, or some 12 million Americans. The new finding gives theoretical support to one method of treating dyslexia, through the use of *color filters* in reading. If validated, it is also likely to suggest novel kinds of therapy," Dr. Duane said.[2]

[1]Although these brain studies by Harvard researcher Albert Galaburda and colleagues initially reported cellular abnormalities in one case just where the traditionalists expected it to be, later studies found these alleged "cellular abnormalities" all over the brain. Recently, they were even "found" in the "magnocellular layer"—refuting the language theory. (This topic will be discussed further in Chapter 18.) But just think about the following few simple questions: Is it really possible for bright and gifted dyslexics to have such abnormalities all over their thinking brains and still compensate? And if these abnormalities are allegedly prenatal (occurring before birth), how can dyslexia and all typical symptoms be acquired *after* birth—following ear infections and damage to the inner-ear? And how can spinning trigger dyslexic symptoms and the cosmonauts develop "space dyslexia" at zero gravity? Surely these latter triggers do not result in so-called cellular abnormalities of the brain! And do inner-ear-enhancing medications and therapies which improve dyslexic symptoms result in the disappearance of these "cellular abnormalities?"

[2]Once again, note how the media completely *accepts* the validity of what traditionalists say without searching for an opposing opinion. Do they assume there are no opposing opinions since "club" members fear voicing them?

So what's wrong with Dr. Duane changing his mind? Nothing at all! Just that his comment in the *New York Times* states that this visual processing theory was *new*. Nonsense! Dr. Duane attempted to refute my visual processing theory of dyslexia—dating back to 1973. He did so again on "Donahue" before millions in 1984. And he repeated this refutation again in 1985. *So this visual theory wasn't suddenly new to Dr. Duane* when proposed by Harvard researchers Livingstone and Galaburda—although the latter still clung to a theory based on a cerebral and / or magnocellular origin vs. my cerebellar origin.[1]

Even Dr. Galaburda, formerly a leading spokesman for the Orton Society, appeared to significantly change his theory—all for the good.[2] But he was not quoted as changing theories in the *New York Times* or elsewhere. Why? I don't know. I've changed theories many, many times throughout this research effort. And I've stated so in writing, for each change catapulted me a giant step forward.

The Switch Hitters

Does not Dr. Duane's switching to a *visual theory* sound opportunistic? Why did he never mention being a leading proponent of the language theory until just prior to the *New York Times* interview? And the *Times* article in question very clearly states that the visual theory tends to cast doubts on the language theory. *Where were all the language experts and why weren't they defending their language theory? Where were Drs. Denckla, Silver, Vellutino, Allington . . . ? Where was Dr. Duane?*

Do the traditionalists fear challenging views they disagree with? Obviously not! So might they fear or avoid

[1]On Livingstone's and Galaburda's theory and the term magnocellular, refer to Chapter 18.

[2]Thus, the Ortonians—including Dr. Duane—describe Galaburda's prior anatomical studies and *use* them to validate their otherwise defunct cerebral language theory.

challenging club members? Obviously so, since they must feel it *politically* advantageous to be on the winning side, right or wrong. Or might there exist a self-serving unwritten club code that sounds something like this: You cover me and I'll cover you. And thus they all thrive happily ever after—albeit the status quo remains. Thus, for example, *the same* "covering" phenomena occurred when a Yale group led by Shaywitz (1990) confirmed what I have been stating for twenty years: that handedness and gender are unrelated to dyslexia. These data further refuted the basis of Orton's theory.[1] Yet no Ortonian dared challenge these Yale researchers!

All the Colors—"60 Minutes" (1988)

Interestingly, in many respects this alleged "new" visual processing theory just mentioned was based on the color findings of another "controversial" maverick—Helen Irlen. "60 Minutes" showed how her "colored lenses" enabled dyslexics to see and thus read letters and words better. And so she instantly was put on the dyslexic map—despite the critics and their club. And they've really been trying to "club" her for many, many years.

As a result of these "colored" insights going back some time, Irlen was harassed and criticized by the very dyslexia-language experts now using her data for their own

---

[1]Although Harvard researcher and Ortonian Norman Geshwind, M.D. had been extremely puzzled by the frequency of clumsiness and dyscoordination in his article, "Why Orton Was Right", since this inner-ear symptom refuted Orton's theory, I'm sure you readers are not. By contrast, my prior research had shown *why Orton was wrong* and even *why Geshwind was wrong*. And despite Geshwind's dyslexia confusion, a memorial prize was established by the Rodin Dyslexia Society in his honor (see Chapter 18, Acceptance Without Reference).

Might Geshwind's memorial prize highlight an attempt by the traditionalists to solidify their crumbling conceptual base? And so by honoring Geshwind, are they not also honoring themselves and their own language-based concepts of dyslexia?

purposes—no doubt including Dr. Duane who mentioned the use of "colored filters" in the *New York Times* article *without referring to Irlen*. I know what was going on because I heard the traditionalists attacking her behind her back at dyslexia meetings. And they seemed also to be counting the money they fantasized she was rolling in. In fact I told them: What does money have to do with whether or not the treatment works? A lot! Money triggers sour grapes. And these grapes then get very, very sour! As a result, I was the only physician who stuck up for her when she needed to defend herself from a scientific near-lynching.

Why Was Irlen Attacked?

Was Irlen attacked because her "colors" worked or because they didn't? Once again the intensity of the criticism, even more than its content, signalled the presence of bias. *And those initially most critical of her views and method now took and used these very same concepts—without so much as a thanks, or even a reference. And none of the other club members called attention to this blatant attempt at what bordered on scientific plagiarism.*

Why the Antagonism from Traditionalist Experts?

In many respects, the antagonism to Irlen's publicized controversial findings were similar to those afforded me. Until the "60 Minutes" publicity, the traditionalists were able to significantly block her views and "cures" from the public and so attempt to preserve their own traditional turf and "dyslexia monopoly."

Consciously, the traditionalists initially reasoned as follows: If dyslexia is due to a language impairment within the thinking-speaking centers of the cerebral cortex, how can "colored" lenses or transparencies help? However, were the traditionalists once again able to consider an alternative possibility—even if it meant giving up turf—they could easily have solved the seeming paradox. *If colored lenses do help improve the reading ability of dyslexics, then might dyslexia not be of a thinking-linguistic brain origin?* As just presented, some of the club members are beginning to switch from a language-oriented theory to a visual one— albeit proper references as to scientific originality seem to have been overlooked. And they appear to have no better understanding of dyslexia than before—for each of their theories appears capable of explaining only a very small segment of the syndrome.

Why Color Works

In many, many ways, my research had predicted and explained Irlen's color-related finding in dyslexics years ago. In fact, the explanation is referenced in my 1989 scientific paper ("Abnormal optokinetic and perceptual span parameters in cerebellar-vestibular dysfunction and related anxiety disorders") and in *Smart But Feeling Dumb* (1984). In these works, I emphasize the benefits of color and large print on facilitating the eye's fixating and tracking letters and words during the reading process. And finally, the explanation for the benefits derived from colored lenses was so simple that it was offered to children in my book, *Turning Around—The Upside-Down Kids* (1993).

One of the criticisms I've often heard about Irlen is: How can her treatment work if she can't explain it? This is nonsense. But at least Helen Irlen was honest enough to admit that the therapeutic mechanism of action escaped her. But there were simple inner-ear-based explanations for the benefits of "color" in dyslexia. Thus, for example, my research with the 3D Optical Scanner or "elephant test" showed: (1) that colored elephants are often fixated easier and tracked better than black ones; and (2) that the same held for certain size/space/darkness parameters— the larger and darker, the better, up to a certain size. So the print size/space/darkness relationship in *The Upside-Down Kids* was scientifically designed to facilitate reading. And all of us know that advertisers use *colors* to catch our eye for the same reason. In fact, might Ortonian Betty Osmond have dressed up in *red* to better attract the audience's eye on "Donahue"? And there you almost have the answer to the color red and *what's in a color.* Almost.

But there's more to why colored lenses work. And all the reasons clearly support the inner-ear dyslexia theory, while refuting its traditionally-backed thinking-linguistic origin—thus accounting for the quality of the traditionalists' often defensive and offensive attacks.

As I've repeated many, many times in scientific forums and in Chapter 13 here, *filtering* is among the many important functions of the inner-ear. If motion isn't properly filtered, we get motion-sick and even motion-related anxiety and phobias, e.g., fears of moving elevators, escalators, cars, trains, buses, etc. And if sounds, touch, and visual signals aren't properly filtered, we get corresponding forms of these sensory overloading phenomena, i.e., "visual overloading" or "visual sickness" and even touch-sensitivity and related phobias and avoidance (see *Phobia Free*).

Clinical experience with thousands of inner-ear or cerebellar-vestibular dysfunctioning dyslexics has clearly shown that many are prone to "photophobia" or "light avoidance." And diagnostically, this term reflects inner-ear impairment when there's nothing wrong with the eye itself. Often this light sensitivity is wave length or color specific. Even flickering and/or fluorescent lights may trigger similar photophobic responses. And now we really have most of the explanation needed: *Inner-ear dysfunctioning dyslexics—with and without* "dyslexia"—may be light-wave sensitive and thus predisposed to visual overloading. Therefore, cutting down or cutting out these wave-specific visual triggers facilitates greater amounts of visually-related fixation and tracking compensation and thus decreases visually-related symptoms amongst dyslexics, e.g., blurring, word movement, reversals, etc.

Hopefully, you can now readily understand my intent: to use the criticism and its analysis in *A Scientific Watergate—Dyslexia* constructively so as to facilitate understanding and acceptance of *A Solution to the Riddle—Dyslexia*. Hopefully my dyslexic patients have shown you how these colored glasses help—as do other inner-ear compensatory therapies.

Summary

In retrospect, there was nothing of medical or neurophysiological significance behind the Ortonian *Color Red* on "Donahue." By contrast, there was something behind the colors on "60 Minutes": *another "controversial treatment" that worked and one that further disproved the traditional or Ortonian view while substantiating the inner-ear or cerebellar-vestibular theory of dyslexia and related disorders.*

Before concluding, I'd like you to think about the following questions that follow patterns similar to those described by authors Broad and Wade in *Betrayers of the Truth.* Why were "club members" presenting visual data refuting the linguistic and related Ortonian views not attacked or labeled "controversial"? Why do the traditionalist "switch theorists" often neglect to explain their changed viewpoints nor properly reference them? Is it not chutzpa?

CHAPTER 16

Chutzpa

I'm sure most of you have heard and know the Yiddish expression chutzpa—regardless of your background. And those who don't will intuitively figure it out by the content presented.

The title *"Chutzpa"* was chosen here to highlight the *significance* of Dr. Arnold Gold's continuing to find and document *cerebellar neurological signs and deficits in dyslexia*, as well as his public and private denial of these very same data. Accordingly, I considered the following rhetorical question: Were critical experts like Dr. Arnold Gold honestly able to read and acknowledge their own data, then would they not have, by themselves, discovered the solution to their riddles about dyslexia? And these riddles are: *(1) How can dyslexia be of a thinking-linguistic brain origin in the presence of only cerebellar neurological signs and in the absence of localizing cerebral signs? (2) How can cerebellar neurological signs and deficits exist—and yet not exist? (3) How can dyslexia be present without "dyslexia"?*

The trick—"magical," of course—is to use Dr. Gold's neurological findings in dyslexia *after* his 1974 denials to solve the 100-year-old traditional riddles in dyslexia. And to do so, two additional neurological reports of Dr. Gold's are added here. These reports further substantiate a number of crucial points made throughout this book: (1) that hard and fast cerebellar neurological signs are the only ones found in dyslexics or learning disabled—despite Dr. Gold's denials; (2) that these cerebellar neurological signs continue to be found and reported by Dr. Gold—even after his 1974-75 private and public "scientific denials"; and (3) that Dr. Gold finds the very same cerebellar neurological signs in learning disabled or dyslexics with and without "dyslexia."

Until now, you had to take my word about the above concepts and that both forms of dyslexia (with and without "dyslexia") are cerebellar-related if not cerebellar-determined. Now we have *"hard and fast"* neurological data— "blindly" obtained by someone who didn't know what he was doing—to prove it all. And he's handed us this solution not only "blindly" but against a loud and clear denial of his reported content—a content that simply and easily solves the riddles created and enforced by the traditionalists. So listen and read carefully. All the proof and solutions my critics have been looking for have always been right before their very eyes—if only they weren't overcome by denial, perseveration or stubbornness, and related defense mechanisms.

The Hard Facts: Believe It Or Not

Dr. Arnold Gold is still finding and reporting cerebellar dysfunction and deficits in dyslexic children. Yet, to date I have found no other pediatric neurological reports to match Dr. Gold's in quality and thoroughness. And so I used them here to also serve as a *diagnostic model* and point of reference for all others attempting neurologically to understand and examine dyslexics.

To facilitate the objective solution of the riddles in dyslexia, I considered it essential to present the vital abstracts

of two of Dr. Gold's neurological cases with learning disabilities: one with a known current reading-score impairment, the other with past reading-score difficulties (didn't
read until the end of second grade—and then *spurted* [was
dyslexic with "dyslexia" and now is dyslexic without "dyslexia"]). See what you think, and judge *Dr. Gold and the traditionalist experts* against my views.

And upon viewing these reports note:

- the date of examination—since both cases were
  examined *after* Dr. Gold privately and publicly denied finding mild, moderate, or severe cerebellar
  deficits in dyslexia—regardless of whether or not
  the cases manifested *severe* reading-score impairments or "dyslexia," and

- the keenness with which Dr. Gold now recognizes
  the importance of multiple ear infections, vertigo
  and/or motion sickness and their possible relationship to cerebellar deficits, speech or language
  delays, and dyslexia (a factual and conceptual relationship I have been reporting since *1973*).

Patient # 1—A Dyslexic With "Dyslexia"

Lois Dalton[1]

Lois Dalton came to my office *after* seeing Dr. Arnold Gold.
He recognized that she had reading score and related academic symptoms. As a result, Lois was diagnosed by him
to have "static encephalopathy," despite the presence of
only cerebellar neurological signs and a past history of related motion sickness, multiple ear infections, as well as

[1]Only the patient's name, identifying data, and non-neurological words
were changed to preserve confidentiality. And important diagnostic
criteria and correlations were italicized—to enable easier understanding. Dr. Gold's "blind" neurological reports are contained in Appendix A.

an alleged "language difficulty . . . which mainly involved articulation and which all but disappeared by itself in 6 months." I ask the reader to keep the following questions in mind while reading the vital abstracts of Dr. Gold's outstanding neurological evaluation:

- Has not Dr. Gold in prior reports referred to articulation and slurring as cerebellar signs—rather than that related to a "language difficulty" with assumed cerebral or thinking-brain origins?

- Have not researchers repeatedly correlated speech disorders and delays similar to Lois' with repeated middle ear infections and fluid accumulations?[1]

- *Might Lois' spontaneous improvement in her language—really speech delay—within a short time (six months) be related to the clearing up of fluid in her middle ears?*

- *Might not all of Lois' symptoms—including her motion sickness since infancy—be simply explained by an inner-ear or cerebellar-vestibular dysfunction, without the need for the vague and frightening term, "static encephalopathy"?*

Dr. Gold's 1987 Neurological Evaluation

Lois was 7½ years old and in second grade when examined by Dr. Gold for academic difficulties. He assumed she had motion sickness since one month old—screaming whenever her carriage moved. Lois had sixteen ear infections between 1 to 2 years of age, associated with a significant speech delay. As a result, draining tubes were recommended and language therapy initiated for 1½ years. Although determined to be 2 years behind in language devel-

---

[1]My research as well as that of others (Silva et. al., 1982; Zinkus and colleagues, 1978) clearly shows that repeated ear infections in young children predisposes them to developmental speech and motor delays as well as behavior and learning disorders—dyslexia. Clearly, vertigo and motion sickness are also similarly determined by the resulting inner-ear dysfunction.

opment at 5 years, repeat testing 6 months later showed only a 6-month lag—involving mainly articulation. At the time, reading readiness was found deficient. Finally, in 1986, Lois was diagnosed to have "dyslexia" at Hofstra University.

An Abstract from Dr. Gold's Report

(5/22/87)—Academically, Dr. Gold noted *dysgraphia*, slowly performed calculations and a significant reading impairment. The latter was characterized by a first-grade level when reading a paragraph, word reversals ("*on*" for "*no*"), poor reading recall, and frequent word substitutions.

Her dysgraphia or poor graphomotor coordination was highlighted by: poorly formed and spaced letters and numbers, rotated and distorted Bender Gestalt patterns as well as indications of deficient visuomotor and spatial relationships. Also, Lois' figure drawing consisted of a stick figure with only three fingers on each hand. Lois' current language development was considered "fair" for both articulation and language content.[1]

Although hopping well, Lois had *difficulty with skipping*. Her motor examination was within normal limits. . . . Deep tendon reflexes were physiologic in the upper extremities but hyperactive in the lower ones. Babinski responses were flexor and pathological reflexes were absent. A complete sensory system exam revealed all modalities to be normal, including touch, position, vibration, and cortical sensation. Cranial nerve function was normal as were the visual fields to confrontation, and the fundoscopic exam was benign.

There was a cerebellar deficit with left finger-nose-finger dysmetria and past pointing, while rapid alternating movements were performed in a normal manner. There were however problems in fine finger movements, above all when both hands were utilized simultaneously, and this was associated with the previously described dysgraphia.

---

[1]Contrary to the theoretical fantasies of Vellutino and related traditionalists, language content may be "fair" or even above average in dyslexics with "dyslexia" —clearly refuting the conventionally accepted aphasic or linguistic origin of "dyslexia."

In summary, Lois revealed evidence of a prenatal static encephalopathy manifested by: auditory memory and suggestive
processing and perceptual difficulties, a visual perceptual dysfunction (impaired visual spatial and visuomotor problems), "*a
mild cerebellar deficit that primarily involves fine motor coordination, and an associated learning disability as evidenced by
dysgraphia, dyslexia with spelling difficulties and to a lesser extent, dyscalculia* . . .

At the time of the examination, Arnold P. Gold, M.D.
was professor of clinical neurology and professor of clinical
pediatrics at the Neurological Institute, Columbia Presbyterian Hospital.

Patient # 2—A Dyslexic Without "Dyslexia"

James Cone[1]

James Cone was 18 years old when initially seen by me in
1986 for diagnosis and treatment. He was having difficulty
in college keeping up with the pace and volume of required
reading due to eye-tracking difficulties. He still evidenced
writing (dysgraphia) and spelling difficulties noted by Dr.
Gold 10 years earlier, *more than 2 years after* Dr. Gold denied his cerebellar findings publicly and privately to all
who listened.

Of special interest in the report is the fact *that Dr.
Gold's final diagnosis is a "significant cerebellar deficit"—
rather than the usual minimal cerebral dysfunction or static
encephalopathy.* And the primary difference between this
report and the one preceding it is *that the patient compensated for his prior reading-score disorder when seen by Dr.
Gold and was thus mistakenly considered nondyslexic—despite the presence of dyslexic-related symptoms and a preliminary diagnosis of a "possible dyslexic syndrome."*

[1]The patient's name, identifying information, and non-neurological
data within Dr. Gold's report were changed to preserve confidentiality.

In other words, despite fixation, tracking, and reversal symptoms during reading as well as spelling and writing difficulties and cerebellar impairments identical to most "typical" dyslexics with severe reading problems, Dr. Gold appeared to deny an identity between dyslexics with and without severe reading-score impairments ("dyslexia"). As a result, this case clearly highlights a point I made in *A Solution to the Riddle—Dyslexia*: *In learning disability cases, Dr. Gold's final diagnosis appears completely dependent on whether or not he finds a significant reading-score disorder present—and independent of all other variables.*

Is this logical or sensible? Might there be significant degrees of "bias" here, to which no one until now has called attention? Does not Dr. Gold appear to equate *dyslexia* with *"dyslexia"*? Even worse, does he not also deny a cerebellar diagnosis in *"dyslexia"* but not in reading-score-compensated *dyslexia*?

Dr. Gold's 1976 Neurological Examination

James was 8 years 10 months old when examined by Dr. Gold for a "possible dyslexic syndrome." Important background history revealed delayed unassisted walking to 15-16 months, normal to precocious language development, poor coordination for walking and running—related to flat feet (pes planus), poor graphomotor skill as well as delay in learning to tie shoelaces, an average to good student despite poor spelling, "b-d reversals," and a need for "remedial reading programs."

An Abstract from Dr. Gold's Report

(2/28/76)—Jimmy evidenced minimal *word slurring*[1] . . . *Graphomotor skills were poor, relying on printed letters, which were poorly formed and spaced. His pencil grasp was slightly*

---

[1]Since Dr. Gold's final diagnosis in Jimmy's case is "a significant cerebellar deficit," it is apparent that Dr. Gold considers slurring and related articulation (motor) speech symptoms to be of a cerebellar vs. cerebral origin (see also Appendix A).

deficient. And all wrilting and drawing tasks required excess time and resulted in rapid fatigue. Bender Gestalt drawings reflected this poor graphomotor coordination, although there were no distortions or rotations.

Academically, Jimmy functioned within normal limits, other than the *graphomotor problem* and borderline spelling which appeared to be on a beginning third-grade level. Reading indicated good recall and was at least on grade level. Mathematics appeared superior.

Motor examination revealed normal muscle bulk, tone, and strength. Deep tendon reflexes were slightly hyperactive in the lower extremities and showed an unsustained ankle clonus bilaterally. These reflexes were physiological in the upper extremities. Pathological reflexes were absent and the Babinski responses were bilaterally flexive. Examination of sensation was normal for all modalities, including touch, position, vibration, and cortical sensation. Examination of the cranial nerves indicated exophoria in the left eye upon masking and convergence was poor. Visualization was benign on fundoscopic examination. Visual acuity was normal as were the visual fields to confrontation. *Oromotor coordination was mildly impaired with difficulty isolating the tongue from mandible on lateral tongue movements. There was a cerebellar deficit with finger-nose-finger dysmetria, past pointing and this was associated with significant deficiencies in catching, throwing, and kicking. There was an associated dysdiadochokinesis with poor performance in rapid alternating movements, as well as small finger-muscle problems with deficient performance in rapid succession movements.*

In summary, Jimmy presents with *a significant cerebellar deficit involving locomotion, eye-hand coordination, and small finger-muscle coordination skills. There is in addition, a slight extraocular muscle imbalance and a very mild impairment of oromotor coordination as well. The major deficit in function is that relative to small finger-muscle coordination which functionally is manifested by poor handwriting and the eye-hand coordination problems pose problems referable to athletic performance.*

At the time of examination, Arnold P. Gold, M.D. was professor of clinical neurology and professor of clinical pediatrics at the Neurological Institute, Columbia Presbyterian Hospital.

Considerations—In Retrospect

In retrospect, had Dr. Gold been able to read, understand, remember, and correctly verbalize what he clearly wrote and found—then together we could easily have solved the dyslexia riddles 20 years ago. And with Dr. Gold as a "club" member, the traditionalists' resistance to my CV-dyslexia research would probably have long ago disappeared rather than intensified.

In retrospect, it became readily apparent that in Dr. Gold's neurological reports his final diagnoses are different, depending almost entirely on whether he recognized the presence or absence of reading-score difficulties. In other words, Dr. Gold's final diagnosis in dyslexics: *(1) appears entirely dependent on whether he recognizes or is told that reading-score impairments are present, regardless of the presence of reading symptoms involving fixation, tracking and reversals, (2) appears completely independent of the presence of all other "typical" dyslexic symptoms (problems with writing, spelling, math, memory, speech, sense of direction and time, concentration and distractibility, balance and coordination, etc.), and (3) appears completely independent of his cerebellar and related neurological signs.*

Then why does he do a neurological examination on dyslexics or learning disabled, one might wonder, since he denies his own invariably present cerebellar findings, and since his final diagnosis appears determined solely by the recognized presence or absence of reading-score impairments.

For example, if a parent just told him, *"Lois has a reading-score disorder,"* then Dr. Gold seems to skip his neurological evaluation and just conclude "dyslexia secondary to minimal cerebral dysfunction or static encephalopathy." In response to the statement, *"James is a good reader now— but has writing and/or spelling and/or math problems and even visual fixation, tracking and reversal symptoms identical to Lois,"* then Dr. Gold's final diagnosis seems likely to be "a cerebellar deficit."

Hard to believe? Why should it be in the context of the previous chapters, each of which seems more *difficult if not impossible to believe than the last.*

Summary

As noted, Dr. Arnold Gold, professor of clinical pediatrics and professor of clinical neurology at Columbia-Presbyterian Hospital, *denied his own cerebellar findings* in dyslexia (1974-75)—despite the evidence presented in Chapter 4. And his colleague, Dr. Martha Denckla, (director of the developmental cognitive neurology department, Kennedy-Krieger Institute) and Dr. Larry Silver's "objective" colleague on dyslexia, helped to validate his denial before the Orton Society (1975).

Considering all this:

- Who would believe that Dr. Arnold Gold has the *chutzpa* to continue to report cerebellar findings in dyslexia—undaunted by his prior denials?

- Who would believe that he now emphasizes multiple ear infections and motion sickness in his history— symptoms and findings correlated with inner-ear (cerebellar-vestibular) dysfunction and thus predisposing individuals to dyslexia and related speech symptoms?

- Who would believe that Drs. Gold, Denckla, Masland, Silver, and the whole group of traditionalists denied and/or still deny the presence of cerebellar findings in dyslexia and related learning disabilities?

- Who would believe that *dyslexia* = *"dyslexia"*?

- *Who would believe that a cerebellar deficit is denied in "dyslexia" but not in dyslexics—considering both have identical cerebellar neurological signs?*

- *Who would believe the presence of a cerebral diagnosis in "dyslexia" but not in dyslexics—considering both groups have absolutely no evidence of cerebral neurological signs?*

Hopefully readers have been persuaded by what has thus far been presented and objectively supported. Otherwise the traditionalist "experts" will never solve the diagnostic/therapeutic riddles characterizing dyslexia. Otherwise countless millions of dyslexics will continue to suffer needlessly, without hope and medical treatment.

The Third
and
Last Critical Wave

CHAPTER 17

The Importance of Time, Timing, and Rhythm

After 30 years of clinical research and 20 years of biased "scientific" criticism such as that collected, analyzed, and reported throughout *A Scientific Watergate—Dyslexia,* my cerebellar-vestibular (inner-ear) and related temporal (timing) processing concepts of dyslexia were finally presented at a scientific meeting in 1992, co-sponsored by The New York Academy of Sciences. My cerebellar concepts in dyslexia were presented *without any reference* by the same "experts" and Rodin Academy organization *clearly and definitely* hearing and/or reading about these very same concepts in *1986, 1987, 1988, and 1989.*

Since my initial 1973 research paper, I have repeatedly defined dyslexia as a cerebellar-vestibular-determined spatial-temporal sensory-motor dysfunction in dynamic equilibrium with compensatory and even decompensatory mechanisms (see Chapter 3). Clearly, this definition was a far cry from the traditional concept of dyslexia being a reading disorder in which subjects *must* be at least 2 years below peers and/or potential in reading scores. As a result, my conceptualization of dyslexia was criticized roundly and referred to by dyslexia experts as "incomprehensible" and even "mystifying."

For those readers curious as to how I figured out that the cerebellar-vestibular or inner-ear circuits process (spatial-) temporal functions, the answers are quite simple:

- I listened carefully to the signs and symptoms of my dyslexic patients *with only CV dysfunction* and recognized that timing (and spacing or orientation and direction) errors often characterized their sensory-motor symptoms, and that misperception of speed and time were frequently present.

- I listened carefully to and observed the favorable responses of my dyslexic patients on CV- or inner-ear-enhancing medications and recognized characteristic improvements in all their many and varied (spatial-) temporal-related sensory-motor dysfunctioning symptoms.

To highlight these later points, I considered it helpful to present here the temporal or timing (and other) improvements reported by a social worker, William Simms (whose daughter, Jennifer, was presented in Chapter 7), and a dancer, Alba Caraballo. And as you recall the many dyslexic cases presented thus far, including those of Meg Fex (Chapter 1-A) and Joan Sparks (Chapter 10), think of both the symptoms and related therapeutic improvements dyslexics frequently experience with their *motor timing and rhythm.* Thus, for example, these important temporal-related observations include the following:

- timing difficulties with running, skipping, hopping, speaking (stuttering, stammering, etc.) as well as with sports and dancing,

- rhythmic difficulties with reading, writing, drawing, etc.—where the "flow" is dysrhythmic,

- difficulties in learning to sense and tell time as well as in judging speed,

- difficulty with certain rhythmic-related neurological tests (i.e., dysdiadochokinesis) diagnostic of cerebellar-vestibular dysfunction—such as those typically described but denied by Dr. Arnold Gold and to be highlighted further in Book II,[1]

- corresponding medication-triggered improvements in all the above—including increased or newly acquired dancing, musical or speech flow and/or time-related abilities.

In addition, data revealed by using my 3D Optical, Auditory, and Tactile Scanners have indicated:

- *that there is also a sensory-timing and related cognitive impairment amongst dyslexics with only cerebellar-vestibular dysfunctioning, and*

- *that these sensory and related cognitive timing impairments also frequently improve on CV- or inner-ear-enhancing medications.*

During testing, for example, dyslexics frequently experience the speed of moving visual, auditory, and tactile sequences as being much faster than they really are—and thus blur them out at speeds dramatically below normal.[2] In other words, it appears as if impaired cerebellar functioning results in a corresponding decrease in the inhibition of both the volume and rate of sensory-motor reception and transmission. Accordingly, there occurs the *illusion of enhanced speed*—even racing thoughts and "blurring." And CV-enhancing medications often triggered corresponding improvement in these temporal-related sensory-input functions as well as in processing capacity.

For a more thorough understanding of the many generalized and specific cerebellar-vestibular-determined and

---

[1]Dysdiadochokinesis represents impaired rhythm and symmetry in rotating extended arms towards and away from the midline.

[2]Note the dramatically reduced blurring-speeds observed and verified by Mrs. Chapman while watching her children tested with the 3D Optical Scanner. Stated another way, these inner-ear-impaired dyslexic children perceptually experienced the elephants racing much faster than they really were—faster than Mrs. Chapman and I perceived them (see Chapter 7).

related symptoms characterizing dyslexics, I encourage you
to read my many research papers and books and refer to
Chapter 13 here. But for those remaining skeptics requiring "proof"—objective of course—I refer you to my varied
scientific works in which I specifically discuss the role of
timing in dyslexics with only cerebellar-vestibular dysfunctioning, dating back to *1973*. And since the Orton and
Rodin societies' adherents were clearly aware of my "dangerous" books (*A Solution to the Riddle—Dyslexia* and *Smart
But Feeling Dumb*), I decided to present some of my temporal-related concepts from these works for review so that
you can objectively and independently judge what follows.

Timing—Extracts from
A Solution to the Riddle—Dyslexia (1980)

A Reconceptualization of Dysmetric Dyslexia

The clear recognition of specific and independent clinical, symptomatic and blurring-speed compensatory forces in CV dysfunction and dyslexia resulted in a modification and reconceptuali-
zation of the definition of dyslexia—a definition independent of
such overdetermined and nonspecific parameters as reading-
scores, IQ, etc. *Dyslexia, or DD, was thus redefined as a primary CV-induced dysmetric sensory-motor and spatial-temporal
sequencing and processing disorder in dynamic equilibrium with
compensatory forces*—resulting in a diverse spectrum of symptoms in varying states of decompensation, compensation, and
overcompensation. Thus, the dyslexic reading, writing, spelling,
arithmetic, grammatical, graphic, speech, memory, *temporal,* ori-
entational, and emotional symptoms may appear in any combination and in any degree of compensation and overcompensation. The author's definition and conceptualization of dyslexia,
as well as the traditionally accepted point of view, are illustrated
in Figure 7-5. The contrast will highlight the fallacious and incomplete assumptions characterizing the traditional descriptive

dyslexic concepts, as well as the author's attempt to capture both neurophysiologically and clinically the essence and totality of the dyslexic disorder and panorama (p. 178).

Speculations on the Role of the Cerebellum in Modulating Conscious and Nonconscious Perception

Prior to this research effort, conscious and nonconscious mental and perceptual events could not be explained neurophysiologically. Analysis of the blurring-speed and tracking data, however, has led to a new hypothesis of the cerebellar role in modulating conscious and nonconscious events, and the functioning of bilateral cerebral hemispheres or "2 brains"—perhaps enlarging Young's (1962) interesting speculations as to "Why do we have 2 brains?"

Utilizing the 3D Optical Scanner and blurring/recognition-speed methodology, blurring or nonrecognition was found to be a *cerebral cortical indicator* of maximum cerebellar tracking capacity. In other words, the dominant cerebral cortex is "blind," and thus cannot "see" and consciously "perceive" a *rapid input exceeding its conscious interpretive threshold.* However, reading score-compensated dyslexic individuals with significantly reduced blurring speeds were noted to utilize occasionally a special form of speed reading. These rapid-scanning dyslexics were found capable of absorbing and comprehending both fixated, conscious content and "blurred," "unseen," "background" or "non-conscious" content.

As a result of these observations, the author was forced to assume that DD individuals were able to derive the meaning of a paragraph, chapter, or book by a process of peripheral or background nonconscious perception. How else could one explain the overcompensated reading ability on the one hand and the decreased blurring speeds on the other? As a gifted dyslexic writer put it, "I've always been amazed by how much I know and how little I read. Reading was always so very difficult and frustrating for me; and yet as a child I scored in the 98th percentile for reading comprehension. I just don't know how I did it." She was amazed to learn that her blurring speeds were one-quarter normal and that she saw "absolutely nothing" when words were moving across a screen at one-half the average word blurring speed of a 5½-year-old child.

If, indeed, nonconscious perceptions occur and can be recovered by questioning and associations (as well as comprehension and reading tests), and if conscious or "nonblurred" cerebral perception depends upon the speed of sensory impulses received by the cortex, then the CNS mechanisms determining conscious and nonconscious perception may be conceptualized as follows:

1. Conscious and nonconscious perception depends on the sensory transmission speeds impinging on, or received by, the cerebral cortex.

2. *The cerebellum, through its processes of selective inhibition, disinhibition, and facilitation, modulates the input transmission speeds received by the cerebral cortex.*

3. *Through the process of selective disinhibition and facilitation, the cerebellum may either fail to slow down the ascending sensory input, or even speed it up,* so that the sensory input speeds reaching the perceptual cortex exceed its "interpretive threshold," and blurring or "nonrecognition" is perceived and reported.

4. *The cerebellum, by regulating transmission speeds,* dynamically influences conscious and nonconscious cerebral perception, as well as foreground/background perception.

5. *By virtue of controlling transmission speeds, the cerebellum is especially well suited to serve as a dynamic sensory-motor filter* capable of separating the sensory-motor input and output into foreground and background.

6. The cerebral hemispheres have developed as an extension of, and in relationship to, cerebellar function.[1] Instead of view-

---

[1]The cerebral and Ortonian theorists appear to have denied the role of the cerebellum in influencing and modulating cerebral dominance—normally and abnormally. (Refer also to research by Previc, 1991.)

ing the cerebral hemispheres as dominant and non-dominant for gnostic perception, both cerebral hemispheres may be considered dominant. One cerebral hemisphere is dominant for foreground perception and the other hemisphere is dominant for background perception. Might this hypothesis not serve to clarify Young's question, "Why do we have two brains?" Holistically speaking, both cerebral hemispheres are in dynamic equilibrium with each other, and the organism as a whole.

7. The cerebellum selects, modulates, and coordinates right and left "brains," and may play a significant role in determining and/or influencing cortical dominance, and even handedness.

8. If, indeed, the right and left "brains" are extensions and reflections of cerebellar function and sensory-motor "processing need," and if Snider and Stowell's findings (1958) of sensory mirrored "homunculi" projection areas in the cerebellum are correct, then one might speculate that: (a) there exist primitive right and left cerebellar "brains" for integrating and/or modulating the sensory-motor input, analogous to the right and left cerebral "brain"; and (b) the basic body-image sense is a reflection of the cerebellum's hypothesized role as the head ganglion of the total sensory-motor system.

9. These speculations imply that a form of "cerebellar dominance" may exist which, in turn, guides and shapes cortical dominance.

Should these hypotheses prove valid, a theoretical gap artificially separating psychoanalysis and neurophysiology will have been bridged; and one hopes that further crossings will eventually contribute a windfall scientific harvest to both fields (pp. 229-231).

Timing—Extracts From
Smart But Feeling Dumb (1984)

The inner-ear also acts as a timing mechanism, setting rhythms to motor tasks. A disturbance within this system may result in difficulty in learning to tell time and sensing time. Frequently, dyslexic children do not know *before* from *after* and can't sense whether a minute, and hour, or several hours have gone by. Accordingly, dyslexic individuals may become "compulsively" late or early. Speech timing may be off, resulting in slow or rapid talkers and even dysrhythmic talkers, or stutterers (p. 25).

Time

The inner-ear is a pacemaker imparting timing and rhythm to various motor skills. Accordingly a dysfunctioning inner-ear system may result in difficulty or delay in sensing time, as well as difficulty in learning to tell time.

Compensatory and overcompensatory processing may result in "gifted" timing mechanisms whereby dyslexics are able intuitively to measure time spans down to split seconds. Still, they may have difficulties reading an ordinary watch. The difficulties in reading time are manifold:

- Difficulty recalling number representation.
- Difficulty recalling hand representation, i.e., which hands tell minutes and hours.
- Directional disturbances such as clockwise and counter clockwise, before and after.
- Difficulty seeing numbers clearly, i.e., blurred vision.
- Eye tracking disturbances resulting in skipping and misreading the clock's numbers.

Although digital watches have been lifesavers for many dyslexics, they have presented difficulties for some. Thus 7:15 may easily be misread as 7:51 or any reversal combination thereof.

Speech

Speech disturbances of varying intensity and quality characterize a majority of dyslexics. While some speech difficulties are readily apparent, the vast majority are subtle and are elicited only upon careful questioning.

Many a future dyslexic will have been a late talker, while others will exhibit a variety of articulation or slurring speech errors requiring speech therapy.

Episodic stuttering was found to taint dyslexic samples periodically, suggesting that there is a relationship between stuttering, dyslexia, and inner-ear dysfunction. Later studies of mine clearly verified this relationship.

As stated earlier, *the inner-ear imparts timing and rhythm to motor tasks, speech included.* As a result of a disturbance in rhythmic activity, *speech functions may become dysrhythmic, resulting in starting, stopping, and sequential rhythmic errors.*

The concept that *rhythm is impaired in stuttering* is supported by an interesting observation: Stuttering frequently disappears when individuals sing. Some researchers even notice an improvement in stuttering when a metronome is placed next to the ear; the former acts as a rhythmic pacemaker. If rhythmic activity helps compensate for stuttering, then might we not further assume that a disturbance in rhythm underlies stuttering?

Starting and stopping speech activity in stuttering were found to be complicated by another factor already described—perseveration. In other words, a motor speech pattern becomes stuck and interferes with the normal speech flow. Not infrequently, stuttering may also be triggered by difficulty pronouncing or recalling a word or thought. The resulting hesitation will invariably affect speech rhythms, especially if preexisting disturbances are already present.

The most common and subtle disturbances found among dyslexics, often leading many to become shy and avoid unnecessary speaking, are *input and output speech lags.* In the presence of a drifting sound input, many dyslexics will hear the sound and not know its meaning until several seconds or even several minutes later. If the sound sequence coming into the brain drifts, it will take the thinking brain several minutes to compensate for the disturbance, and the patients will frequently ask "What?" This reflex response allows the patient time to compensate for this drifting input and eventually know what was said.

If the motor speech responses drift, or if there are impaired word memory or concentration mechanisms, then there will be a lag between the intention to say something and the actual motor speech response. Memory disturbances for word and thought recall may so complicate the spontaneous speech flow that many dyslexics develop "loose," rambling, and disjointed speaking styles, and are naturally viewed as scatterbrained. This dyslexic speech style must be clinically differentiated by a doctor from more serious neurological and psychological disturbances affecting the speech process, such as those that underlie the loose, rambling speech of psychotic patients or aphasic patients.

Directional disturbances frequently affect speech-processing and result in word and even thought reversals. For this reason dyslexics are prone to slips of the tongue, saying words out of sequence, or reversal of directions such as up and down.

Concentration and distractibility disturbances may further complicate all of the above speech disturbances and mistakenly give the impression of a hearing loss. Hearing tests are recommended in these circumstances.

The inability to inhibit or block out extraneous background noises or speech patterns while listening to someone nearby or in the foreground may result in severe confusion for some dyslexics. The background contaminates and scrambles the foreground sound sequence and results in an overall sound blurring. This type of situation is frequently present in crowds and restaurants and was found to result in crowd and restaurant phobias (pp. 124-126).

Spatial-Temporal Insights

Derived from Symptomatic Descriptions

Ron Tilly

Ron Tilly (48) was examined on May 4, 1993 for inner-ear-related dyslexic symptoms. And his spontaneous description of spatial (directional)-temporal impairments is typical of many patients with dyslexia. These simple clinical observations led me many years ago to redefine this disorder, accordingly, and to discuss these spatial-temporal and related mechanisms in my prior books and research papers. Ron states:

> Although I am a relatively high-functioning person (an attorney and musician), I have often felt as if certain parts of my brain do not function properly. Interestingly enough, the materials you sent to me seem to contain a checklist of many of my problem areas, which previously seemed unrelated to a single malfunction. Although the list which follows is lengthy, I have developed ways to compensate for many of the problems. What follows is a listing of my major symptoms, as requested in your letter.
>
> (1) *Poor sense of direction/trouble distinguishing right from left.* I have always had a problem with directional concepts, including right vs. left. I have a scar on my left pinky, and when I was younger I had to look at my hands prior to making a final decision.
>
> (2) *Poor coordination and rhythm/inability to learn certain motor skills.* As a child I had problems "judging the ball" which was very bad for development of a positive self-image. *I believe my reflexes are slow* (i.e., if somebody is falling, instead of jumping to help them, I process the information very *slowly* and think, "Look, she is falling. I should help." Often by the time I act it is *too late* to help, and I feel foolish.

It is very difficult for me to learn motor skills and sequential tasks from observation. Dancing has been very difficult for me. However, I play the piano very well and compose music. I have an extremely deep love for music. Even with the piano, although I have a good sense of harmonics and melody (it seems almost intuitive), *rhythm has always been my weak area.* This has made it difficult for me to join combos or participate in jam sessions. Although it would surprise people who have heard me play, *I never have any idea as to what tempo I might be playing a song in. Additionally, I have no understanding as to what various time signatures mean or how they translate into how a song should sound.* This is something so basic that it is understood by people who have no real sense of how to play an instrument.

The rhythmic deficit also affects my written expression, in that at times I'm unsure as to where the natural pause in a thought occurs which requires a comma.

Hopefully this brief clinical vignette will enable the reader to rapidly grasp concretely not only the directional (spatial or sequential ordering) symptoms described by Ron, but also his timing and speed-related reflex, thinking, musical, and writing difficulties.

Substantiating Letters

Although timing, or *"Temporal Information Processing in the Nervous System: Special Reference to Dyslexia and Dysphasia,"* was the topic selected for discussion (without reference) at the Rodin Society in September 1992, the reader must by now recognize *that there's much more to dyslexia than temporal processing, and that there's much more to temporal processing than the Rodin experts and their gifted dyslexic sponsor, Dr. Per Udden, have "newly discovered."*

However, before proceeding to William Simms' and Alba Caraballo's cases here and the next follow-up chapter, two substantiating letters may reassure remaining skeptics.[1] Their content clearly establishes: (1) that Dr. Per Udden, the founder of the Rodin dyslexia society, read *A Solution to the Riddle—Dyslexia* and *Smart But Feeling Dumb* in 1986 and recommended these works to the foundation's scientific committee (some of whom are even on the prestigious Nobel and Karolinska Institutes), and (2) that he appeared to agree with my cerebellar concepts—as did Nobel Laureate Sir John Eccles. Francis Lestienne also reported to the Rodin Society that the French-Russian cosmonauts began reading upside-down and backwards at zero gravity—an inner-ear-determined condition I call "space dyslexia."

Moreover, the second letter from Sir John Eccles to the scientific chairman of the Rodin Society in 1989 confirms his cerebellar-vestibular views on dyslexia—albeit modestly for someone who feels he lacks sufficient expertise in this area (personal correspondence, 1987). Unfortunately, he was not able to attend the scientific meetings in Europe (1989) at which I discussed my cerebellar-vestibular research on dyslexia and phobias, documented scientifically in a well known peer reviewed journal, *Perceptual and Motor Skills* (see references).

---

[1] If you're skeptical, you will never be disappointed—if you're right. And for parents with children who have improved on medication—it's great to be wrong. No one will ever criticize you for saying you're skeptical. It even has an intellectual—even egoistic—ring to it, depending on the user, of course. And for some interesting reason, very few people will challenge a "skeptic" to fully and scientifically explain and justify the basis of his or her skepticism.

Academia Rodinensis Pro Remediatione (The Rodin Remediation Academy)

Dear Gunther   Professor G. Baumgartner
                                Universitaetspital
                                Frauenklinikstrasse 26
                                8091 Zuerich

Harold Levinson: *A Solution to the Riddle—Dyslexia*, New York: Springer-Verlag 1980, was badly received by the dyslexia professionals. From these second hand reports of the antihistamine treatment, also I was very little impressed. Now I have read his book. He for sure has a point, that middle ear functions and thus also cerebellum, plays an important role in dyslexia. His last book *Smart But Feeling Dumb*, Warner Books Inc., 666 Fifth Avenue, New York, NY 10103, is well worth reading.

At the Cambridge and London meetings, *Eccles expressed his belief that the cerebellum is deeply involved, which view was strengthened by Francis Lestienne, who reported, that after some days of the French/Russian space mission, the cosmonauts could view anything in any direction, also read text upside down.*

                                Best regards,

Kerns, 10 July 1986   Per Udden
                                EXECUTIVE SECRETARY
                                HOFSTRASSE 1
                                CH-6064 KERNS
                                SWITZERLAND

Copy to: Eccles, Gaddes, Humm, Lestienne, Levinson, Przedpelska-Ober, von Rotz

Sir John Eccles' Letter

8, June 1989

Dear Professor Rudolf Groner,

I thank you for your letter of May 22nd with the invitation to the European Conference on Eye Movements in Pavia, Sept. 10-12th. Unfortunately I am already occupied at this time, so will not be able to come.

I met Dr. Levinson about 2 years ago in New York and we discussed dyslexia. I think that his cerebellar-vestibular fixation and tracking mechanisms could provide at least a partial explanation of dyslexia.

With my best wishes for your conference.

Yours sincerely,

Sir John Eccles

Improved Spatial-Temporal Functioning in Dyslexia—Two Brief Case Presentations

William Simms and Alba Caraballo are two dyslexics presented in order to demonstrate how their spatial-temporal functioning dramatically improved on inner-ear-enhancing medications. Their fascinating comments also illustrate how therapeutic responses such as these can highlight the many and varied spatial-temporal and related symptoms characterizing dyslexics and their disorder. Initially, the majority of these responses were completely unanticipated, since I considered dyslexia to be merely a severe reading disorder—as did (and do) all other "experts." Were it not for the meticulous study of these improvements and their corresponding symptoms, the true depth and scope of this CV- or inner-ear-determined disorder would never have materialized. Indeed, dyslexia would still be viewed as merely "dyslexia."

William Simms

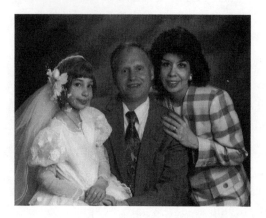

William is a 44-year-old social worker who reported his symptoms and improvements on antihistamines (March 1993) as follows:

Background

During grade school I was always considered a slow learner. There were always problems with writing, spelling, grammar, mathematics and speech—communication. However, my major problem was daydreaming: poor concentration, easily distracted, restlessness, impulsivity . . . And in sports I was bad—no matter how hard I would practice throwing a baseball or catching one, I almost always dropped the ball or missed the person I was throwing it to. The same problems were in dancing or music. *I just have no sense of rhythm.*

Recognizing the Problem

It has been my good fortune to have met, and to be treated by, Dr. Levinson. My introduction to his treatment and theories was either an accident or an act of grace. One Friday a friend had come over to our house. She looked tired and I asked if there was anything wrong. She started talking to me about her child who has dyslexia and the difficulties faced by the family. At the time she was unaware that both I and my then 7-year-old daughter were learning disabled. Later that day I went to the library to do research for a class paper. On entering the library I first went to the new books section. There was one book sticking out of the shelf and the title was *Total Concentration*, by Dr. H. Levinson.

At this time in my life I was having great difficulty at school. I was in a Master's Program in the School of Social Welfare at Stony Brook and doing poorly. *It seems that every time I would say something or try answering a question the words would come out incorrectly, people were upset at me and I couldn't figure out why.* The professor and my fellow students considered me insensitive. It was a total negative cycle (couldn't read the non-verbal facial and body language of others).[1] After reading Dr. L.'s book I called his office and made an appointment.

Favorable Responses

The first day that I took the medications that Dr. Levinson prescribed is still very vivid in my mind. Within 15 minutes my life changed. Colors were brighter. Lines looked different. This might seem odd, but for some reason when speaking to someone I was able to focus on their lips. It was the first time in my life that I was aware that the sound was coming out of a person's lips. Along with that came the awareness of hidden gestures in body language, and different patterns of speech.

The journey had begun. Each day new things would happen. My speech began to change. It was slower and I lost the slur in my voice. My eyes began to follow lines and shapes.

I was able to draw for the first time and so I couldn't put the pencil down. Balance and coordination improved dramatically. For the first time in my life I could throw a ball and hit a target. *But my favorite is the most recent de-*

---

[1]In many ways, William's speech—prior to treatment—resembled that attributed to President Bush (see Chapter 1-D).

velopment in the area of rhythm. My wife likes to dance, and she always had to lead. One day recently we went to a dance and she said, "Oh William, you are dancing in step with the music." For the first time in fifteen years I was really dancing. I have become more aware of music and melody, my piano playing also improved.[1]

Also, my powers of concentration are enormously enhanced and my distractibility is minimal—a decided improvement.[2]

Because of my treatment by Dr. Levinson, my life, and that of my family, is happier.

William's Figure Drawing

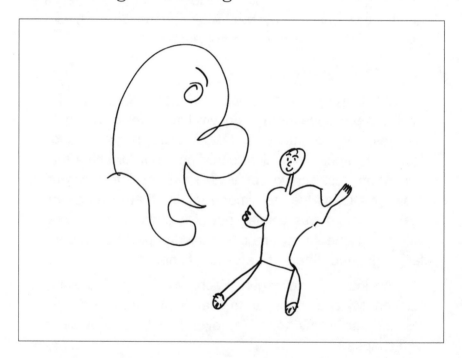

[1] Note these inner-ear-based improvements in *rhythm or timing*. And compare similar changes in my other patients—especially Joan Sparks (Chapter 10).

[2] The improvement in William's academic, speech, balance/coordination/rhythmic and concentration/distractibility or ADD symptoms when taking only an antimotion-sickness antihistamine clearly indicated that all four of these so-called "different" syndromes are most probably inner-ear-determined.

During neurophysiological testing, all dyslexics are required to draw figures as well as Bender Gestalt designs. Although many graphomotor skills among dyslexics are usually somewhat compensated by adulthood, some are not. Accordingly I thought it might be helpful to present William's figure drawing here.[1] Observe how his inner-ear-determined fine-motor incoordination manifests when attempting to draw fingers, arms, legs, etc. I'm sure you will now better understand his difficulties using a pen and pencil prior to treatment—and why he couldn't put them down after his improvements.

Alba Caraballo

Alba is a 32-year-old dancer. Her response to medication:

On antihistamine: Panic and Agoraphobia disappeared instantly—2 days after taking medication. Was a little tired at first—rested, and felt like a new person. More energetic now—working 7 days a week (easier than when compared to 2 days per week before medication).

I don't have this unknown anxiety any more—just realistic concerns. I'm able to work now on stage. Before, I was afraid of people and getting an anxiety attack in front of them. Gone! Now I go out alone and drive my car long distances. Before, I had to be driven—feared losing control of the car and hurting somebody. Also I had obsessive thoughts—that would hurt someone. Gone! Now these thoughts get corrected—even when they're there; they are fleeting and then they disappear. They don't stick.

I'm more personable and outgoing—and connect with people easier. Because I don't feel like a freak anymore.[2]

[1] It is crucial not to misinterpret these figure drawings psychologically—as many diagnosticians have been known to do. Although psychological conflicts and fantasies may be projected into drawings, these figures are significantly neurophysiologically determined.

[2] Contrary to Ortonian Priscilla Vail's "concern" and prediction that my therapy will trigger patients to feel like "freaks," Alba and countless others actually felt much better than before.

I feel normal—like I belong. Before, I'd turn new friends-to-be or people off. Feared they would reject me. I'm no longer afraid.

My reading is better. Words are not wiggling and jumping all around. And I can follow words and lines—without losing my place and going back and back over the same line. My eyes are not gluing on the word—and I could see no further. Now I can glide from word to word—and I can see 2-3 words at a time instead of only one—a short one.[1] Words are no longer *blurring.*

Concentration is much better. Can stay focused when doing needlepoint, reading or even during conversation—without getting distracted. No longer slurring when I talk. And I can use the word I want—instead of substituting. I can now remember and pronounce the word better. *No longer misspelling as much. My writing is sharper*—it flows more easily instead of a big blob of ink resulting where words should be!

Improved sense of space and timing. I'm a dancer. My movements are more concentrated—premeditated or in-tentional. They just don't come out of the blue. *I feel more sure-footed. Before I avoided sharing space with other girls—for fear of kicking or being kicked. That's gone. Now, I know where I stand. My sense of space or spacing is better. In all my years—if you were sitting in your chair and I was behind your desk—I'd feel our space was over-lapping—too close.*[2] Now I can be dancing on stage with others—sardined together—I feel my space is mine and theirs is theirs.

---

[1] The improved tunnel vision and its impairment prior to treatment occurs much more frequently than the preferred use of peripheral vision. By contrast, M.I.T. researchers Geiger and Lettvin reported the opposite: that peripheral vision is enhanced amongst dyslexics (*New England Journal of Medicine*, 1987).

[2] This difficulty with spatial perception was often found resulting in claustrophobia.

My sense of time has improved a great deal—in dancing and elsewhere. In general, I know what time it is when I go to sleep and get up. Not so confused—as before. I couldn't do it. I Just had no idea. 9-11 A.M. could have felt like 5-6 P.M. *I can now keep up with the music and rhythm.* Before I either went too fast or too slow.[1]

Although things are great—I was still skeptical that my agoraphobic cycle was just ending on its own. But then how come all the other improvements took place—that never happened before.

Do you think in time I'll get over my feeling *stupid*?

---

[1] Patients occasionally develop a negative therapeutic response to medications that were previously well tolerated and effective. Since Alba had reported one such experience following six months of drug therapy prescribed by another physician, it was anticipated that this negative response might reoccur with the antihistamine I gave her.

CHAPTER 18

Acceptance
Without Reference

Many years ago, I told a concerned and interested colleague: "Don't worry so much about
all the negative criticism I'm getting. The real
game will start once all the criticism stops. As
soon as my concepts begin to sink in and are
really politically and scientifically understood,
then these very same defensive critics will attempt to make my ideas their own."

On September 12-15, 1992, The Rodin Remediation
Academy, together with The New York Academy of Sciences, sponsored a conference entitled, "Temporal Information Processing in the Nervous System: Special Reference
to Dyslexia and Dysphasia." *For the first time, a conference
gathered speakers presenting hypotheses indicating that the
cerebellum and its timing mechanisms may be deficient in
learning and speech as well as other related sensory-motor
functions.*

Richard Ivry, Ph.D., of the University of California, Ber-
keley, presented a paper indicating cerebellar and cortical
involvement in the temporal processing of speech and non-
speech stimuli. And Peter Wolff, M.D., of Harvard Medical
School, presented research entitled, "Impaired motor tim-

ing control in developmental dyslexia," and suggested "impaired motor coordination may be one behavioral expression of a more general deficit of timing precision and temporal organization in perception and action of dyslexic individuals." (Although he did not mention the cerebellum, it could be inferred from his communication.) Most important, Rodolfo Llinas of the department of physiology and biophysics, New York University Medical Center, presented a paper with two titles. Although he spoke only about *"Cerebellar involvement in temporal sensory-motor processing,"* there was an additional title in the conference brochure: *"relevance for speech, reading and writing."*

Although Drs. Ivry and Wolff were as unaware of my research as I was of theirs, the circumstances were different with Drs. Udden and Llinas. No doubt in preparation for this meeting, Dr. Udden, the sponsor and benefactor of the Rodin Society, had invited Dr. Llinas and me to dinner (along with others) in 1989. He sat us next to one another and encouraged us to discuss our respective research endeavors which appeared to have much in common:

- My research highlighted the presence of a cerebellar-vestibular-determined spatial-temporal dysfunction in dyslexia and related symptoms.

- Dr. Llinas' neurophysiological research recognized that the cerebellum modulated timing in the central nervous system.

Since these independently determined findings sufficiently corroborated the validity of our respective concepts, a joint research endeavor was discussed. And to enlighten Dr. Llinas with my CV concepts on dyslexia, I personally delivered *all* my research papers and books to his offices at New York University Medical Center, since I was also on staff there at the time. As a result, it seemed strange: (1) that Dr. Llinas never acknowledged receiving the papers and books despite several follow-up calls and letters; (2) that there was no reference to my research in his presentation; (3) that Dr. Udden did not comment on the correlation between the two; (4) that not one of the Rodin experts receiving Dr. Per Udden's 1986 letter concerning my books, *A Solution to the Riddle—Dyslexia, Smart But Feeling Dumb,* as well as mention of Sir John Eccles' agreeing with my cerebellar-dyslexia views acknowledged this communication; and (5) that not one of the many Rodin experts who had access to my four research papers (published in Perceptual and Motor Skills) and/or heard my presentations during several 1989 meetings in Europe sponsored by this very organization attempted to link Dr. Llinas' research with mine.

The silence was deafening! As a result, I felt obliged to ask Dr. Llinas what he thought of my cerebellar research as well as the use of medications in relationship to the discussion we had in 1989 and his own data. His comment seemed somewhat oblique: "I've merely presented a hypothesis." Jokingly, I added, "Of course. Isn't a hypothesis an attempt to explain data in a logical and scientific way?" *In other words, he never answered my question anymore than he responded to the papers and books I sent him linking the cerebellum and its timing and spatial dysfunction to dyslexia and its many symptoms.* Although Llinas sidestepped my question and I "jokingly" responded, I *knew* then and there that *A Scientific Watergate—Dyslexia* would soon be initiated and completed.

Indeed, this book was the hypothesis I had in mind to scientifically explain this deafening silence and related "acceptance-without-reference." No doubt the Freudian significance underlying my "joke" was lost, since Llinas is a Nobel Prize contender in neurophysiology rather than Freudian psychology.

Since truth is often stranger than fiction, I wasn't surprised when a line from Goethe's *Faust* suddenly occurred to me: *"To make a world, strange people there must be."* Hopefully my past Freudian training and this resulting book will have enabled me to explain all the strange riddles characterizing dyslexia and its experts.

At the end of the conference, Dr. Per Udden stated that as a dyslexic he was among the *15 percent* of people who had some variation of a sensory-motor temporal dysfunction—receiving applause from the panel of experts on stage. Although I had previously decided not to comment any further, *I was inspired by Dr. Udden's having quoted both my statistics and my definition of dyslexia.* His quote—unreferenced, of course—contrasted sharply with that of the keynote speaker, Dr. Martha Denckla, who, I was told, still indicated that dyslexia was a pure reading disorder in which individuals have reading scores at least two years below peers or potential. On the basis of this non-realistic definition, only two percent of the general population are dyslexic—not 15 percent.

Accordingly, I got up, thanked Dr. Udden for quoting me (even though he left out the reference), and then attempted to answer difficulties with the prior and current definitions and research on dyslexia to date. My statement sounded something like this:

Twenty years have passed since I renamed dyslexia—Dysmetric Dyslexia and Dyspraxia (DDD). I did so to emphasize:

- its cerebellar-vestibular-determined spatial-temporal origin and its effect on balance, coordination, speech and basically all sensory-motor processes;

- that dyslexia was merely one of many syndromes derived from a cerebellar-vestibular dysfunction, i.e., ADD, anxiety disorders, dysgraphia, dyscalcula, dyspraxia, dysphasia, etc.;

- that the traditionally accepted reading-score-dependent definition of dyslexia (that one had to be at least two years below peers or potential) was based on highly selective or biased sampling and a fallacious analogy of dyslexia with alexia of cerebral cortical origin—the latter resulting in the complete inability to recognize the meaning of written symbols and thus leading only to severe reading impairments;

- that a patient-based or clinically-derived description of dyslexia and a related definition is needed before researchers can meaningfully investigate "microscopic" details in a "vacuum," as they have been doing;

- that my having defined dyslexia over twenty years ago as a cerebellar-vestibular-determined spatial-temporal dysfunction in dynamic equilibrium with compensatory vectors and other dysfunctioning forces offers the best way of looking at this syndrome to start with;

- that the detailed research of many must be consistent with the total clinical picture of this disorder, and the reverse;

- that it often appears as if many researchers publish findings and data about dyslexia inconsistent with, or impossible to reconcile with, the clinical reality of this syndrome; and

- that if researchers continue to function as they have in the past, it will take them another twenty years to get my concepts correct—since it took twenty years to almost get where I was in 1973.

With these last remarks, the conference officially ended. But hopefully, the effect of my summation did not. After all, criticism is a continuum and I will invariably need more content for a follow-up. No doubt, there will be quite a follow-up. The critics were verbally criticized. Will they listen or will they continue their attack, as did the Ortonians—albeit silently rather than loudly?

Prior to concluding, a word of interest. I was told by one of his colleagues that Dr. Udden was not taken seriously by the Orton Society and so formed his own. If indeed this is true, then: Did not Dr. Udden inadvertently create another Orton-like Society, albeit one with a new name and different, yet similar, experts? Dr. Denckla, as a keynote spokesperson for both societies, no doubt cemented this "identity." Might Dr. Udden have invited Dr. Denckla for political and economic as well as scientific expediency? And had he not counted on my giving her a hard time—for him? After all, he really believes in the cerebellar role in dyslexia as well as the related diagnostic value of eye-movement impairments. Were this not so, why else would he have an eye-tracking monitor designed for sale? And did he not "forget" to reference my dyslexia concepts in order to appease the traditionalist majority comprising his scientific advisory board and/or roaming "experts" who move with him from conference to conference?

I can only guess that my above reasoning is correct. Were it otherwise, then how might one explain or answer the following questions:

- Why else did Dr. Udden invite my wife and me to the speakers' dinner at The New York Academy of Sciences, when in fact I was not invited to be a speaker? And why did he personally call to invite me to all his other conferences? And even to have dinner with him and Dr. Llinas?

- Why did he express disappointment with my not participating *more actively,* or critically, from the audience before my final summation? I was only able to attend the last day—in time to hear *Dr. Llinas' presentation without reference.*

- And why did he consider using my 3D elephant testing parameters in his ocular tracking instrument?

- Why did he convey to me that Sir John Eccles, Nobel Laureate in cerebellar neurophysiology, espoused and supported my cerebellar research (1986, 1987, 1989), and that Francis Lestienne reported that the French-Russian cosmonauts started reading upside-down and backwards at zero gravity—an inner-ear condition I named "space dyslexia"?

- And why did he write to the other members of his society, conveying to them that my books, *A Solution to the Riddle—Dyslexia* and *Smart But Feeling Dumb*, were significant, despite their poor initial reception by the traditionalists?

Special Mention

Among those at the above-mentioned Rodin Society conference, I have chosen to highlight a few for review:

To *Dr. Denckla's* credit, one must say that she has attained many positions of respect. Currently she is director of the developmental cognitive neurology department at the Kennedy-Krieger Institute in Baltimore, Maryland. Indeed, she has attained these positions while believing and publicly stating: (1) that Dr. Arnold Gold's definite but "mild" and "moderate" cerebellar deficits are normal; (2) that dyslexics must be at least two years below peers and/or potential in reading-scores, regardless of the large number of dyslexics who have significantly compensated and eventually scored higher, including such famous dyslexics as Einstein, Edison, Da Vinci, Patton, and others; and (3) that dyslexia is a language disorder resulting from a defect or dysfunction within the language centers of the cerebral cortex—despite the absence of any proven language disorder and localizing cerebral neurological signs, and much cerebellar evidence to the contrary.

Although *Drs. Livingstone and Galaburda's* recent publication emphasizing a visual processing defect in dyslexia did, in fact, further refute the language theory of dyslexia which these researchers previously espoused, their visual concepts remained as incomplete in explaining and encompassing the vast majority of dyslexic symptoms as did the language theories. As repeatedly stated, my research in

1973 highlighted that visual processing in dyslexia was impaired, but that this impairment was secondary to a cerebellar-vestibular dysfunction. Despite my research and patented 3D Optical, Tactile, and Auditory Scanners indicating that there also exists auditory, tactile, and a total sensory dysmetria and dyspraxia in dyslexics manifesting most clearly during tasks requiring rapid processing, their studies and mine were never properly integrated.

In other words, how can a *visual magnocellular* theory explain *all* the auditory, proprioceptive, tactile, motion, compass, temporal, spatial, motor, balance, coordination, concentration, activity, mood, anxiety . . . symptoms experienced and reported by dyslexics? It can't—anymore than could the language theory it replaced. Yet this theory was proposed by traditionalist experts and thus accepted by other club members without question. Does not the "blind" proposal and acceptance of "tunnel theories" and data clearly prove my repeatedly voiced thesis that dyslexics know much more about dyslexia than their esteemed traditional experts—regardless of whether or not these experts have recently converted? And it also tends to confirm what I've said about the traditionalists sticking together—and even covering for each other.

Also Dr. Galaburda once again found and reported abnormal cells in the magnocellular layers of the brain which apparently modulates rapid visual processing. Indeed, when he thought dyslexia was due to an angular gyrus deficit within the thinking-speaking brain, he found abnormalities within the angular gyrus, and in only one case that was also epileptic. Since then, he's also found abnormalities all over the thinking brain of dyslexics. And he considered them all prenatal—occurring before birth and during early embryonic development.

And for unknown reasons, no one has asked Galaburda the following questions: *If visual as well as auditory, tactile and sensory-motor functions are impaired in dyslexia, are all corresponding cerebral brain centers modulating these functions also characterized by abnormal cell formations? And if so, how is it possible for so many bright and gifted dyslexics (Einstein, Edison, etc.) to have so many cellular abnormalities throughout their thinking brains?* In other words, were Galaburda and colleagues correct, there wouldn't be enough healthy brain cells in the thinking brain of dyslexics with which to function "normally"—let alone exceptionally. And were these prenatally (before birth) determined abnormal cellular formations truly required for dyslexic symptoms, how can one explain: (1) the triggering of dyslexic symptoms at any age following excessive spinning, zero gravity ("space dyslexia"), and a host of inner-ear impairments, e.g., ear and sinus infections, concussion states, whiplash injuries, etc; and (2) the reversal of dyslexic symptoms via inner-ear-enhancing medication and related therapies. One couldn't! Unless, of course, inner-ear disorders after birth also caused these "cellular" abnormalities and inner-ear-enhancing medications and helpful therapies dissolved them!

Consider an alternative hypothesis: *Might not these so-called "abnormal" cellular formations be accidental or coincidental findings (a view also shared by Sir John Eccles) and/or secondary rather than primary prenatal (occurring before birth) phenomena as maintained by Galaburda and his Harvard colleague Dr. Norman Geshwind?*

In addition, Geshwind and Behan postulated that *dyslexia occurs ten to one in left-handed males, that both are due to a hormonal imbalance triggering abnormal cellular formations within the brain during early embryonic development, and that dyslexia correlated significantly with such autoimmune disorders as allergies, migraines, etc.* By contrast, after having studied thousands of dyslexics, I found all of these statistics and theories impossible to realistically account for. They were and still are out of contact with the clinical and experimental reality of dyslexia. Yet so many researchers reference rather than re-think and integrate these articles with their own data and concepts. Perhaps they have insufficient data of their own and thus "parrot" the above—especially since the often-referenced authors are affiliated with prestigious institutions.

According to my research and that of Shaywitz and colleagues (1990) and Peter Wolff (personal correspondence, 1992), dyslexia is independent of handedness and gender. And if there is a higher incidence of autoimmune disorders such as allergies and migraines in dyslexia, as Geshwind and Harvard colleagues maintain, I reasoned that this phenomena might be largely of a *secondary origin*:

- Since dyslexics are predisposed to greater degrees of stress, might the latter secondarily trigger higher yields of autoimmune problems?

- Some allergic phenomena of the inner-ear may trigger dyslexia and/or intensify preexisting "mild" manifestation of dyslexic symptoms—thus influencing the recognized incidence. But it's doubtful that these origins can account for the significantly higher incidence and prenatal theories that Geshwind and colleagues claim. Allergies aside, I have not personally recognized any higher incidence of any severe autoimmune disorders such as they report.

And although dyslexics are often prone to *headaches* as they are to vertigo, nausea, abdominal complaints, motion sickness, etc., these psychosomatic symptoms are completely unrelated to autoimmune disorders. The inner-ear triggers these symptoms either directly or secondarily due to stress. And stress may also *secondarily* trigger migraines in those already predisposed to them. This reasoning is substantiated further by the fact that inner-ear-enhancing medications frequently reverse these psychosomatic symptoms by triggering compensatory inner-ear mechanisms—without directly affecting the autoimmune system.

If I am correct, then there is something very wrong with the research of researchers in the field of dyslexia. I can only assume that these experts never spent sufficient time talking to, listening to, analyzing or studying dyslexics over time. And at best, they appear to be experimenting and reporting on "test-tube" dyslexia—and "blindly" publishing "shots in the dark."

Have the traditionalist sanctioned clubs and theories blinded all within to external realities concerning dyslexics and dyslexia?

Although *Paula Tallal* came the closest to clinically recognizing a total sensory-motor involvement in dyslexia, she failed to clearly correlate the timing deficiencies with a cerebellar dysfunction, and she failed to reference my research indicating so—perhaps because she considers this defect to be of a primary thinking-linguistic cerebral origin. And perhaps because she was as previously unaware of these references as I was of hers.

Almost last but not least, and as previously noted, *Dr. Rodolfo Llinas* presented content within a paper indicating that the cerebellum modulates timing mechanisms. Despite his lecture's title relating this timing defect to reading, writing and speech mechanisms in dyslexia, Llinas avoided all explanations of these latter symptoms in his talk, such as those summarized in Chapters 13 and 17. And he avoided any mention of our prior discussion, *as if my cerebellar research never existed.* Had I not specifically mentioned before the audience that Llinas' neurophysiological research on cerebellar timing validated my research on the cerebellar-vestibular-determined spatial-temporal dysfunction in dyslexia and related disorders, the connection between the two would have remained silently hidden and disconnected throughout the conference.

Strange! Perhaps not—since I read nonverbal communications quite well. I can still feel my dismay at the shocking contrast between my incredible *enthusiasm* and Llinas' *surprising indifference* when I told him during our last supper in 1989 about my spending a day with Sir John Eccles two years before—and that Eccles shared my cerebellar-dyslexia views.

The contrast between us said it all—despite my wishing at the time it were otherwise. And so I went through the follow-up motions with Llinas until I knew for sure that my first gut feeling was correct. Needless to say, my instincts for reading dyslexia and related experts were razor sharp, considering all my "basic training."

Although *Dr. Per Udden*, a founder and financial supporter of the Rodin dyslexia organization, specifically invited me to attend this conference as a guest rather than as a speaker (His "experts" were no doubt still upset by my "controversial" cerebellar concepts which I presented to them in 1989.) and despite his having invited Dr. Llinas and me to dinner in 1989 so as to discuss our mutual research, he also remained ominously silent about my research throughout the conference. And although in 1989 he and Dr. Llinas were discussing a planned conference in which Dr. Llinas might get Barbara Bush to attend, they never mentioned any desire to target "timing" as a key conference parameter. Perhaps they hadn't yet decided. But then why would Llinas have been involved—since his research was on cerebellar timing and not dyslexia?

The After-Effect

As a result of this conference—especially the thunderous silence about my research—I was inspired to complete *A Scientific Watergate—Dyslexia*.

Postscript

An Independent Observation and Critique

Although by now even the most skeptical of readers might be willing to accept this continuously evolving "believe-it-

or-not" content without verification, I thought it essential to provide independent corroboration. Accordingly, I will present a letter about the Rodin conference by one of my dyslexic and ADHD patients, who happens to be a gifted violinist.

October 9, 1992

Dear Dr. Levinson:

I would like to share with you my experiences with the recent "Rodin sponsored" conference of the New York Academy of Science at the Vista Hotel (WTC, NYC 9/92).

The rude and obnoxious behavior exhibited toward me by a few of the attendees (and at least one of the speakers) was disheartening and shocking.

For example, the first day (Mon. 9/14) of my attendance, when taking some time off for a brief lunch, I had the unfortunate experience of having one of the attendees invite herself to sit with me (at lunch). Subsequent to her sitting down, she commenced a virtual non-stop litany of comments such as "You're not dyslexic, you're just a con-artist, a faker, an attention seeker who enjoys being pitied with her fake "learning disability status," etc., etc. She continued to make remarks with "hidden questions" and innuendos in them. Any feedback from me was interpreted by her in "Pseudo-Freudian" style. When I realized (quite rapidly) that she wanted obviously for me to "lose my cool," I then played back the part of a "Pseudo-Freudian" listener, while she "free-associated" these offensive remarks, obviously frustrated by my (silent) lack of verbal feedback. When the waiter brought my check and I left (my lunch unfinished due to her interruptive intrusion), she proceeded to follow me into a ladies room! The only thing that kept my "sanity" to stay the remainder of the two days were the very kind-hearted and gentle words of encouragement given to me by your friend Debby Levy. Thank God she was there for me when I really needed it, a "guardian angel" suddenly appearing in the nick of time.

The following day (Tuesday), the verbal abuse picked up in both frequency of occurrence and degree of rudeness! Many of my "critics" appeared to be hostile about my sharing my experiences (9/84 - present) going for treatment with you; their hostility in some instances was subtle but very apparent—in the climate/tone/body "nonverbal" language while others were directly critical/skeptical, in a "chilly," "icy" or arrogant manner (i.e., tone of voice). The "worst offender" was a psychologist Ph.D. "shrink" who tried to be a clone of the aforementioned lunch "guest" I had Monday (who incidentally was also a Ph.D. Psychologist "shrink").

Luckily, although Debby wasn't there Tuesday (or I didn't notice if she was), you attended. Thank God!!! I think that had you not attended, my temper would have gone off like a stick of TNT dynamite. That's how annoyed and angered I became, with comments that I speak poorly, that I cannot express myself articulately; comments questioning my intelligence, knowledge, intellect, academics (doctoral status, despite dyslexia), etc., etc.

Thank God for your "tirade" "tempest in a teacup" that you delivered to them at the end of the afternoon. It was so deserved and I felt proud that you "gave it back to them in spades." They really had it coming and deserved a "taste of their own medicine." Their narrow-mindedness, ignorance, refusal to listen, etc., was appalling. I have ADHD (Attention Deficit Hyperactivity Disorder) but they have a definite "Good Manners and Intellectual Deficit Disorder," a much worse and non-treatable (by medicine) problem! At least I have more common sense, empathy, compassion and you even told me that I was smarter than these "Pseudo-scientific intellectuals"! After you left, here and there I got "semi-apologies" from a few, but a definite "cold shoulder" or worse, from the majority of others.

If anything, the conference showed me how these prestigious scholars are at best "Pseudo-scientists," and at worst are 100+ years behind the times. In addition, their ethics sometimes were questionable, as in when the speaker cited your statistics, findings, etc. from your earlier works, and did not provide proper credit nor citation. "In my book," that goes beyond bad ethics, it's really not "plagiarism." At least they could thank you in a footnote or equivalent (or a bibliography, annotation, etc.). They call themselves scholars, but being a doctoral student myself, I know that such behavior is considered unacceptable in the Finance/Business/Accounting fields! Don't similar standards apply to Science and Medicine? I would think so! It also appalled me to see your colleagues act in such an "unfriendly" way to you at the conference. I detected subtle touches of sarcasm and hostility they tried to "cover up" (but they didn't succeed). Lastly, not one mention was made of how to help, i.e., inner-ear medicine. Imagine a diabetes conference without insulin mentioned!

P.S. Several people went over to me and took the Irlen lenses off my face without permission and made really inappropriate comments![1] Would they take braces off an orthodontic patient's mouth or a toupee from a chemo patient's head? Of course not! However, they thought it was perfectly in good taste to take the glasses off my face and try it on themselves, etc. "All in all," I was appalled to "bear witness" to this, especially in "Hi-Tech 1992"!

The two positive things about the conference were your "tempest in a teapot" and Debby Levy, two rays of sunshine among the black clouds!

Warmly, musically, your patient,

Ms. Marsha Lampert, MBA

---

[1] Irlen lenses, as previously discussed in Chapters 13 and 15, are tinted glasses used by inner-ear dysfunctioning dyslexics to filter-out specific light-wave frequencies. They were used by some of my other patients presented within this work.

Section III

Concluding Content

B<small>Y CHANCE</small> or inner design, this book "required" several concluding chapters. And only upon reflection did the reason become apparent: *Symmetry*. Thus, for example, these concluding chapters appeared to parallel corresponding pre- and formal vs. informal introductions. And *A New Beginning*, the last segment in the final chapter, presented the dramatic improvement of a dyslexic girl whose thank-you note symbolically opened *A Scientific Watergate—Dyslexia*.

And since "God" is discussed in these final chapters as a cosmic determinant influencing chance and inner design, I thought it important to define Him via the following poem taken from *A Solution to the Riddle—Dyslexia*.

> **G**od is cosmic and organismic mind,
>
> Mind is an electromagnetic computer field,
>
> Matter is energy transformed,
>
> Earth is a speck in the cosmos,
>
> Man is a cell in the dust,
>
> Science is an electron in search of its orbit,
>
> Theory is one of many orbits,
>
> Fact is fiction in perspective,
>
> The end is just a new beginning . . .

CHAPTER 19

Beyond Criticism?—
No Way!

Before concluding this work, I want to assure my readers that this clinician *is not beyond criticism.* As mentioned throughout my prior research, I have repeatedly been mistaken and have attempted to correct the errors made wherever and whenever found. And these errors were invariably discovered: (1) when data did not materialize as expected or when statistical exceptions to the rule appeared and had to be explained, (2) when critics were correct—and I was able to listen to them, and (3) when I was able to listen to my own criticism and make appropriate corrections.

Thus far I've attempted to present the obvious bias and clearly negative motives characterizing my critics. But as you can see from this book and research, no one is perfect. So realistically one must be able to separate out the *pluses* and *minuses* in all scientists and their research if the scientific endeavor is to maintain momentum.

The constructive critics and criticism enabled me to advance. And as I've repeatedly said within this text and emphasized within my dedication: the negative critics and criticism, although initially slowing me down, eventually highlighted the bias, confusion and hidden motives of

dyslexia researchers who unwittingly wasted their otherwise bright and God-given talents and learning merely to
create and cement the dyslexia riddles in place for the last
hundred years. Moreover, the analysis and resolution of
this negative criticism as well as the reactive adrenaline-re-
lated energies unleashed within me eventually catalyzed
the completion of *A Solution to the Riddle—Dyslexia* and *A
Scientific Watergate—Dyslexia*, as well as the other scientific works in between.

Although this book has thus far concentrated almost
exclusively on the darker side of my critics and the motives
underlying their criticism, much of what they had to say
was superficially valid. Thus, for example, I've repeatedly
been accused of not performing "double blind" medication
studies to objectively determine if the reported favorable responses—not cures—are really real or just wish fulfilling
sugar coated fantasies.[1] And I have also been correctly accused of not doing this or that. Needless to say, some of
the endless list of "nit-picking" is valid and justifiable.

But just step back and review the quality of my negative critics' statements and thus their underlying intent:

- Why wasn't I given credit for what I did do rather
  than just criticized away for what I didn't?[2]

- Didn't these critics understand that the prime function of a sole, unfunded medical practitioner is to

---

[1] In "double-blind" medication studies, neither the patient nor evaluating physicians know whether "real" medications or "placebos"—sugar
pills— were used. However, as you have noted, the "blind" cerebellar
studies, even when performed, were denied by the very same critics
demanding "blind" medication studies. Also, most of the medication-
triggered results were initially unanticipated—and so "double blind."
And many small unpublished "double blind" drug studies were conducted—and usually patient responses such as that described by Joan
Sparks in Chapter 10 signalled the use of an active drug vs. placebo.

[2] There is sufficient research in my books for hundreds of scientific papers—were my interests directed at quantity vs. quality. Research papers
can only present one variable at a time for presentation. My interests

help and heal suffering patients and not to fool around and experiment with their pain while testing them "to death"—for personal egoistic and even academic needs?

- Why hadn't these critics realized that *one single practitioner and "hobby researcher"* such as myself could never have discovered *The Solution* rather than merely *A Solution to the Riddle—Dyslexia*, stated right up front in the preface of the above-mentioned medical text?

- Didn't my critics realize that only "scientific malingerers" or psychopaths could have delivered "perfect" and "complete" scientific copy or data, completely free of the untold, unknown and unexpected variables that underlie and overdetermine all disorders—dyslexia included; and thus free of criticism, albeit equally free of reality and realistic considerations?

- Why was I attacked for admitting to my limitations and correcting my mistakes?

- Isn't this a "normal" scientific process—or is it? I thought it was until I realized it wasn't! Just observe the *mercurial* nature of my critics and their theories—*changing opportunistically with the political tides and never a moment to acknowledge—or reference—the change.* (See Chapter 15, What's in a Color? and others as well.)

- Hadn't my critics understood that most of what I reported and discovered was initially unanticipated

were aimed at investigating and pursuing all the many and varied parameters needed for *A Solution to the Riddle—Dyslexia*. There were thousands, and I was driven to link them all together so they made sense. As this book and my others indicate, I feel assured that my primary aims were accomplished.

Obviously, I published many scientific papers as well, but I could have published many hundreds more. I could not do both. So I documented my findings in books where I had sufficient time and space for explanations—a luxury not present in scientific papers.

and thus, in fact, was found in error and/or by correcting errors?

- Didn't they realize that I never pretended, nor was I trained, to be a highfalutin researcher working with equally trained staffs, statisticians, lab technicians, etc.?

- Wasn't it obvious to them that I had my hands more than full by merely sketching the CV-dyslexic findings so that those better equipped might work out the details—however needed? Obviously! For I repeatedly acknowledged these considerations—as I do now.

- *Why did my critics—with all their available research and funding resources—never attempt to perform the research they thought was necessary? Were they unable or unwilling? And if unwilling—did they fear finding I was right rather than wrong? In other words, was their criticism positively or negatively intended—even when valid?*

- And if this criticism—even when correct—was well intended, why was it never applied and directed to club members—especially when what was reported was not only incomplete but way out in left field?

But these negative critics could not accept reality as it is or was: neither mine, nor that of dyslexics and dyslexia, *nor even their own—especially their own.*

Perhaps in retrospect, that's why it took a psychiatrist to figure out what other scientists, perhaps trained and positioned with the latest and costliest tools and labs at their disposal, could not. Might they have been too sophisticated and thus over-trained for the job at hand? Might they have been unwittingly looking for "elephants," not only in the wrong place but with an electron microscope instead of binoculars? Worst of all, were they fearful of finding data supporting CV rather than their 100-year-old erroneous cerebral-linguistic (aphasic-alexic) dyslexia conceptualizations? *Were they not captives of their own denial?*

As previously noted, sometimes simplicity is the best scientific gift and tool of all. And often defensive complexity, especially of a condescending kind, is a detriment to the extent that it masks and offensively rejects the simple findings of simple-minded clinicians like myself without an academic axe to grind or prove, and having only an interest in understanding and treating people in need. In retrospect, my greatest ability was recognizing my limitations and not being afraid of admitting what I didn't know and asking repeated questions of patients, their parents, other experts, and repeatedly analyzing the resulting content.

I asked questions until I was either given clear understandable answers or clues with which to ask more and better questions. And eventually, clarity and simplicity replaced the traditionally maintained and defended mystery and riddles characterizing dyslexia and its research efforts for almost 100 years.

In this regard, I must once again take issue with one of my most enthusiastic Ortonian critics, Priscilla Vail. As you might recall, she *warned* parents as well as adult dyslexics who can read and even read very well—and professionals without sufficient expertise—about being taken in by *clarity.* And to emphasize this scientific absurdity, she resorts to the following quote: *"It is dangerous to apply simplistic formulas to complicated human questions. As Alfred North Whitehead said, 'There is danger in clarity—the danger of overlooking the subtleties of the truth.'"* (See Chapter 6: The Orton Society Sanction.)

And so for those of you familiar with my prior books, I feel it worthwhile asking: Are my "formulas" in *A Solution to the Riddle—Dyslexia* and *Smart But Feeling Dumb* either too complex to be understood or simplistic? Are they not

merely realistic? And is realistic scientific simplicity a danger—or a vital necessity? Have not the traditional experts—Drs. Gold, Silver, Denckla, Vellutino, etc.—taken
simple truths and made them "complex" and taken complex concepts and oversimplified them into inaccurate and
erroneous versions, e.g., *dyslexia* = *alexia* and *dyslexia* =
"dyslexia."

As a medical clinician and researcher and former mathematics student, I have invariably felt and stated that: Errors are unavoidable when pursuing unknowns in a scientific vacuum. And if errors are to be made, it's best to err
in the direction of clarity than defensive and even offensive
pseudocomplexity and scientific naivety. And in retrospect,
it was the traditionalists bias that rendered simple and
clear insights "dangerous" and thus difficult to understand.

To emphasize and redramatize the above-stated point, I
have instinctively followed a basic and intuitive dictum:
*You don't really understand something sufficiently until you
can simply and successfully explain it to a child.* And to
prove this dictum, I wrote two "therapeutic novels" for children which clearly and simply explain most symptoms
characterizing dyslexics, and most methods of therapy for
dyslexia—and why and how they work. As a result, I an-
ticipate that the dyslexic children and readers of *The Upside-Down Kids* and *Turning Around—The Upside-Down
Kids* may know more about their disorder and how to treat
it than *all* my critics—collectively. *By comparison, I know of
no traditionalist work that appears able to explain more
than "dyslexia" in dyslexia.*

And although my Ortonian and related traditionalist
critics have claimed that my medical text, *A Solution to the
Riddle—Dyslexia,* is too complex to be understood, they
have also cautioned their readers about its *clarity.* Are
these Ortonians not acting as allegedly "overconcerned ex-

perts" to their dyslexic patients? To protect them? *Or are they attempting to protect them from clear insight—insight which will render dyslexics free of those "experts" egoistically and financially thriving from their untreated suffering—and thus dependency.* Were this not so, would these "overconcerned critics" be so fearful of "100% cures?"

Accordingly, let me provide the reader with a *simple, clear* scientific rule of thumb I learned during my dyslexia research efforts: Everything real and helpful in dyslexia came from the mouths of dyslexics and their loved ones. And as *A Scientific Watergate—Dyslexia* will repeatedly attest to: Experts provided only fantasy, fiction—and far worse. As previously noted for purposes of corroboration, Nobel Laureate in physics Richard Feynman once stated, "Experts don't know more than the average person."

CHAPTER 20

Personal Reflections— Freely Associated

Is it by chance or design that I should have initiated dictating this book on (sundown) Rosh Hashanah, a holiday celebrating the beginning of the Hebrew New Year. Having recognized the date, I decided to attempt its completion, at least conceptually, ten days later, on Yom Kippur—the day of atonement.[1]

Obviously, both dates were highly significant. Indeed, they were symbols of my New Year's commitment to complete rapidly this work and its intended cleansing and healing process—so vital if millions are to receive the benefits of the research characterizing *A Solution to the Riddle—Dyslexia*.

Around and Around It Goes

Internal harmony was needed to *order* and deal with the external scientific chaos. Isn't it strange that the resolve to go ahead with this book, and especially my initially having begun writing it, should correspond with another circular completion: the desire to return again to my religious roots. The first time I thought of writing *A Scientific Watergate—Dyslexia* was twenty years ago, approximately the last time I attended a religious service.

[1]These dates follow the Rodin Dyslexia Society conference, September, 1992.

In retrospect, I had to wait twenty years to mature and understand enough so as to feel integrated with the reality of both religious and scientific systems—sufficiently so to attempt a scientific exploration and exposé of ignorance, bias, and scientific denial. I had to pass the test of time—a lifelong endeavor that many are not fortunate enough to survive. In other words, *I had to emotionally resolve and inwardly accept* A Scientific Watergate—Dyslexia *before I could write it.*

What's In A Name?

Why then did I call this book *A Scientific Watergate?* Because Watergate simultaneously represented or symbolized diametrically opposing processes: both political and personal imperfection vs. attempts at cleansing the system. There was much pain and disappointment during and after the political Watergate process. But in the end, many lessons were learned. The system grew stronger in several ways: it had survived the ordeal, but it almost did not. It warned others to be more careful, respect the law, respect the system. It also taught us not to again endanger these vital processes for personal gains. *Hopefully, scientists will benefit by this Watergate-like exposure as did the politicians from theirs.*

Looking back, I realized, as the reader must also by now, that *there appeared to be entirely too much politics in science.* And as expected, the politician-experts rose to the top and attempted to stay in "scientific office," no matter what. Needless to say, some were dangerous to science and deadly to the countless millions of patients needing science for hope and help.

Accordingly, this book, via exposing this deadly self-serving process, attempts to skim the surface so that the majority of dedicated scientists hidden beneath can breathe fresh air and attain their intended God-given goals. *For scientists to truly achieve, they must surely have a large measure of religious give vs. egoistic "pseudoacademic" take so as to propel them forward and help overcome life's interminable chaos.*

Surviving

This book is in many respects an autobiography of a stumbling, fumbling student attempting to become a scientist. More than that, it is the story of someone devoting his life to a medical cause— *trying to help people.* Trying to save millions undue suffering. And what it took to get there. And how I almost didn't. And how many others failed, who perhaps weren't psychoanalytically and religiously trained or equipped to handle the inevitable Watergate-like and related chaos that man is heir to —and invariably acts out. And as stated in my dedication, my wife's love and loyalty as well as her sacrifice played no small role in my survival as a clinical researcher. *And the love for our children projected itself onto the children of others. And so there was nothing short of death that would block my determination to succeed, to help them.*

This book is as much a survivor's manual for dyslexic patients and their loving parents as it is for budding physicians and scientists, and those determined colleagues attempting to maintain the faith, despite "Satan's chaos and temptations." In retrospect, these free-associations and the analysis of Satan-like projected content of the traditionalist experts within *A Scientific Watergate—Dyslexia* attempts to warn others: Let all know what is out there. What is real. And how to side-step the mine fields to succeed so as to carry out God's true scientific purposes—to help mankind no matter what detours and suffering we undergo between our aims and their completion. *And as I only recognized in hindsight, the worst mine field of all is premature acceptance and adulation of an idea or person, often forcing one into early emotional and scientific retirement: egoism.*

The Catalyst of Criticism

In many ways, the continued storm and stream of criticism has forced me to continue to grow, to overcome, to rethink, to re-explore, to re-explain . . . In retrospect, I really owe most of my accomplishments to my relentless critics, for they forced me to resolve for myself, and by myself, what they were incapable of resolving within themselves. In the final outcome, my prior training allowed me to resolve and thus overcome sufficient bias and denial mechanisms within myself so as: (1) to recognize that dyslexia, LD, and a host of phobias and mood disturbances were of a physiological, rather than of an emotional, origin; (2) to understand the true meaning and significance of the defensive and offensive criticism attempting to derail me from my destination; (3) to realize that science and religion had more in common than my esteemed teachers snobbishly thought and even mistakenly taught: that science was based on fact and religion on belief; and as all who read this content will realize, *there is significantly more belief vs. fact in science than most realize.*

The Right Way

In retrospect, it was the initial antagonism I felt towards the defensive critics and "betrayers of truth" that most certainly fueled my fire to succeed—to overcome whatever necessary. This line of thought led me to recall a story I told a colleague about myself as a very young boy. I laughed while telling it for the very first time, surprised how little I have changed over the years.

My family was the only Jewish one on the block. It was just prior to the United States entering World War II. We were located in a house on 41st Street, centered between 8th and 9th Avenues, Brooklyn, New York. Every day, I walked to 8th Avenue to attend grade school, located on 44th Street between 6th and 7th Avenues. And I had to fight God-knows how many Italians to get where I was going. But every day I went to school, no matter what. I doubt that my parents knew what I encountered en route. I never told them. Eventually, we all became very good friends—and still are. (Were we—and are we still—fighting for such basic instincts as "turf" and control?)

In telling this story, I realized that I could have avoided the daily fights, if only I had walked to 9th Avenue, walking to school a very, very slightly longer way around. That area was Jewish.

The thought of being forced to go a longer way, to surrender, never entered my mind. Maybe I was just stupid? Who knows what I would have done had the thought occurred to me. Then again, I feel the same way now. The thought of backing off, or going another perhaps safer route with my research, never occurred to me throughout my medical and research career. And here I am, still alive and kicking. And still fighting my way to learn something new every single day—although I did eventually learn how to bypass my determined critics. But in retrospect I wondered:

- Was there some purpose or meaning—symbolic— to recalling and repeating this story here? And if so, what? Might the difficulties I encountered in getting to and through school have been a predetermined "proving ground" or basic training for what was to follow: *A Scientific Watergate—Dyslexia*? Was my destination already "fixed" by cosmic and related unconscious forces a long time ago? And was history to repeat itself?

- Did not the above "proving ground" as well as the universality of "bias" suggest that the latter may be derived from rather basic biological instincts? Might species-specific *herding* and *fighting* for turf—dating back to the territoriality of our animalistic origins— currently result in *exclusion* and other modern-day bias phenomena, even among scientists? Do not "turfing" and "herding" (societies, clubs, etc.) and the resulting bias characterize the traditionalist critics and critical content within *A Scientific Water-gate—Dyslexia?*

Proving the CV Hypothesis

Who would have guessed that ultimately an analysis of the critical content within *A Scientific Watergate—Dyslexia* was needed to prove my thesis and life's work relating to dyslexia and its cerebellar-vestibular (CV) or inner-ear origin? Was all this due to chance alone? Or were God's dice loaded?

In other words, dyslexia and the critical resistance forces attempting to mask its scientific solution were somehow linked together and thus required a common or unified answer. The same is true with neurotic disorders in which the defensive or resistance perimeters must be continuously peeled—like an onion—until reaching the hidden core. And thus I realized that to ultimately solve the hidden riddles underlying dyslexia, the defensive and offensive criticism and critics or scientific superstars had to be dealt with, understood, and thereby explained away. And since so many "*stars*" have seen fit to document the scientific horizons with their critical comments concerning my work, it seemed only reasonable to significantly reference and analyze them in this work on dyslexia, regardless of their "God-like" or eminent professional positions and connections.

Although I only periodically responded to critics in writing—and certainly some confrontations were necessary and unavoidable—I deliberately side-stepped time-wasting and disorienting confrontations whenever possible. And also I did not want to appear defensive or confrontational. Yet that is the way repeated rebuttals would look. And their effect would have negated my life-long ambition—to turn people on to concepts I believe to be valid and helpful to millions. Yet I periodically was driven to respond in force attempting to remind critics that criticism is a double-edged sword; and despite their "club-sanctioned" immunity and resulting impunity, that they might one day be called to task for their bias, ignorance and self-serving denial (e.g., *A Scientific Watergate— Dyslexia*).

The Science of Criticism

Fortunately, I knew how best to handle criticism from my psychiatric background: collect it, study it, collate it, and then analyze it for common denominators and determinants. In this work, I've done just that—mirroring the way I've studied and detailed the dyslexia and CV-related content. Although some critical comments were witnessed by me and many others, too, the vast bulk of data has been presented from printed material to ensure the reader of its factual and reliable nature. And I willed myself to analyze the critical content as if it were coming from a neurotic patient. Mind you, neurotic and even psychotic patients often voiced objective criticism as well. Accordingly, it is extremely important to attempt the separation of positive and negative (non-objective) criticism.

Often, this separation is no easy matter. And it takes more than intellect alone to do so. Internal emotional steadiness and security, a feeling of oneness with God and His scientific wisdom—without "illusions of grandeur"— are the most important ingredients and qualities. Without being able to separate and clearly analyze positive and negative criticism, one cannot grow. One cannot properly help others—whether we be called psychoanalysts, researchers, clinicians, physicians, parents, ministers, rabbis, priests, etc.

Having been repeatedly and extensively exposed to criticism, I can almost hear some new versions: This book is a vendetta! This is merely an attempt to get even! No doubt these motives were and are still present, despite the last twenty years of reflection: Few can forget important and painful past and present experiences. Only a liar will deny important and inevitable emotional reactions to both positive and negative criticism. Only the aimless and mindless would waste precious time and engage only in the above.

The resulting analysis of criticism here served several important functions: (1) It added perspective, background, color and meaning to what otherwise might have been viewed as mere black vs. white, flat, two-dimensional sketches. (2) It allowed the critics to benefit from the analysis—should they be able. (3) It put other critics on notice, that they may one day be called to task for what they say and do—and thus should take time and care to ensure the objectivity of their content.

Hopefully, this book will end the immunity that traditional critics, such as those presented here, have always had! Hopefully, this book will create greater degrees of scientific tolerance and acceptance of "controversial" or new ideas—ideas coming from "non-club members"—thus ending the traditionalists' impunity as well as their immunity! Hopefully?

Maintaining the Status Quo

For every Watergate-like exposure, there are millions of similar events that are covered up. After looking at the scientific functioning or "dysfunctioning" in dyslexia over a 20-30 year period, it appears truly amazing how any meaningful discovery ever took place. *The waste and fallout is tremendous! And although scientific motives may play some role in scientists and scientific organizations, this role appears far too small to produce the yields it should.* And if my study of dyslexia and the underlying bias and neurotic forces governing its related science and scientists are correct, then we now have an answer explaining why breakthroughs in science either take forever, or are covered over, despite the presence of brilliant minds and billions of dollars. In retrospect, I was forced to ask myself: *Is there an unconscious force attempting to prevent discoveries and thus change? Does not God and Man or Science have to contend with Satan and his attempts to reverse and at best maintain the status quo?*

Why I Left the System

All too often, what we do is governed more by intuition than conscious logic. And intuition is, in turn, determined by unconscious drives and motives, most of which I came to significantly understand during many years of psycho-analysis. Having recognized a high degree of illogic and distortion motivating many researchers in dyslexia, I instinctively felt that the forces I was dealing with: (1) would never allow me to breathe fresh air from within, until I was strong enough to handle it; and (2) would never give me the room and freedom I needed to survive as a scientist, completely free of dues and obligations to those sponsoring me.

I felt I needed time and distance, as did my research, otherwise contamination and defeat would occur. Although my "cerebellar spatial-temporal" ideas were simple, too many "bigshots" were firing "nuclear weapons" at them, and at me as well. This suspicion led me to go my own way in order to independently explore whatever avenues might open up.

This journey was truly an eye-opener. I came across gifted clinicians, researchers and therapists who appeared to function "autistically"! And the most frightening part of the whole experience was that these "autistic giants" often gathered the greatest number of followers. Accordingly, I was forced to wonder whether they were all serving one master: The status quo? Satan? Or was God napping?

Are We All Threatened by Dyslexia?

There was something puzzling about my research. Why didn't one plus one equal two for the majority in control? Couldn't they add? I already knew they couldn't read. Had they been able to read, then their criticism would have been significantly different. Not so way-out. Not so distorted.

Were they all dyslexic, I wondered? Might most of us have some dyslexia or inner-ear dysfunctioning in us—albeit to different compensatory extremes? Have we been attempting to deny this in ourselves by: (1) defining us *out* of the disorder via ridiculous quantitative definitions requiring dyslexics to be at least two or more years behind their peers or potential in reading-scores, etc.; and (2) attacking all others like myself whose research is aimed, willy nilly, at defining us *in*?

Must We Deny Our Evolutionary Links

The more I reasoned, the more questions arose: Might the experts' simultaneous needs (1) to worship the "thinking-speaking" brain, while (2) denying the crucial role of the cerebellum in sensory-motor, perceptual, cognitive and even language functioning—serve one and the same purpose? Might these seemingly different needs serve to egoistically separate man and his special thinking-speaking brain from his evolutionary origins and beastly ancestors— the latter having only a cerebellum to "think" and communicate with rather than a cerebral cortex—man's pride and joy? Might the neurophysiologic force governing our unconscious drives, instincts, feelings and thoughts be also hidden within the cerebellum and/or its control?

Were all this so, it would certainly help explain the bizarre nature of the critics and criticism I've met along the way—especially their denial. Then add to it all of the other neurotic and infantile tendencies that motivate people— scientists and clinicians included—and we have the basis to explain all that I've encountered: *Reality!*

A Method to the Madness

The study of dyslexia and its various psychological and neurological theories over the last thirty years *forced me to recognize and overcome* a host of nonsensical conceptualizations often espoused by the most esteemed experts around. Hopefully, you've gotten to know them as I did, unbelievable as it may be.

Being psychiatrically and religiously trained, I was also forced to reckon with another question: *Is there any method to the scientific madness I've encountered in dyslexia research—and researchers?* And as usual, associations occurred to me: *barriers, frustration, overcoming.* And suddenly I had an answer—right or wrong—but an answer nevertheless: *For science and scientists to progress beyond the existing status quo, they must be challenged and forced to do so.* And so the resistance of my critics forced me to function at my maximum in order to survive and succeed while opening up new ways to bypass their "brick wall." Had not Darwin described similar survival-of-the-fittest mechanisms to account for evolution's advance?

Bypassing the Experts

Although my analytic techniques were sufficient to see through the transparent disguises of the traditional dyslexia experts, I still had to find a way of bringing my scientific message to those dyslexics in need. No, I couldn't shout, rant and rave. I had to wait, and wait, and wait some more, until twenty years elapsed. I had to mature. I had to bypass the status-quo experts. I had to get directly to those with the problem, those that needed insight and help. So I enlisted the help of the media. I wrote books that patients and/or parents—even children—would be able to read and understand. I carried the problem directly to those in need who would be forced to understand and thus accelerate a change.

This dyslexic "bypass" no doubt upset my critics even more. Did they really expect me to continue knocking my head against their brick wall? Obviously! That was the way it should have been done according to the rules set by the traditionalists. After all, was that not the reason the wall was built and maintained? And isn't preserving the status quo—at all costs—not the job of traditionalists?

Bypassing got me to those with the problem first, so I could help them. And eventually they would help me promote my concepts by spreading them to others. That seemed to me to be the simplest way around the traditional wall. I knew I could not do it all alone. I needed lots of help. And there was little within the scientific community on which I could rely to sustain this effort. For as you've seen, "the club" and its political strength reigned supreme from within. And the majority of others were forced to follow ("herding") by virtue of a common underlying bond—the instinctive need to preserve the status quo, at all costs.

I also felt that over time and with *new* and *less-biased* scientists in the field, the resistance would lessen significantly—eventually. Hopefully? But inwardly I always knew that only an analysis of the critical content and intent presented within this book will catapult the development of this new breed of clinicians and researchers, free to feel and think for themselves, free to benefit from modern research concepts such as those of Leiner, Leiner and Dow (1991). Free to take a step beyond their "easy" status quo.

The Changing Shape of the Critics

Having studied the critical resistance and egos of the traditionalists over the last twenty years, I felt that their blocking tactics would merely change over time, before really allowing breakthroughs. For that was the nature of the status-quo beast. And because I had carefully observed the mercurial nature of my critics and the way they suddenly switch theories—without reference, depending on the direction of the political tides—I told a concerned and interested colleague many years ago that the real game will start once all the criticism stops and the defensive critics attempt to make my ideas their very own. And as you've read, the game has begun.

Looking back, denial and defensive egoism were found responsible for both the political and scientific (rejection vs. acceptance) Watergates. And although the political Watergate was clearly illegal, the scientific Watergate was merely immoral. But which was worse? Which did the most damage and caused the greatest suffering?

CHAPTER 21

Looking Back— Where I Came From

Although exposing and thereby resolving ignorance, bias, and self-serving denial among those experts controlling dyslexia research (via their "pseudo-scientific monopoly") would more than have justified *A Scientific Watergate— Dyslexia*, I instinctively felt more was needed—more was possible. Indeed, the feeling that *more was possible* has always driven me forward in medicine, fueled by the inner fire needed to overcome the suffering of countless millions.

This fire did not just start twenty years ago when "The First Big Denial(s)" (Chapters 3, 4 and 5) initially darkened my naive medical horizons. This fire started years and years before, when I saw my family practitioner coming to my house with his medical bag trying to help relieve my suffering as a child.

And he didn't have a limousine drive him. And he didn't wear fancy clothes and shoes. And he didn't try to impress our family with his sophistication. And his office wasn't really "slick"—just ordinary chairs for the sick and an old examining table. And it wasn't in a fancy Park Avenue, New York City area. In fact, his office was on the Lower East Side of Manhattan—an area which housed a significant majority of the Jewish peasants that just barely escaped the Czar's crucifixion or persecution and the endless wars and cruel starvation ravaging Europe. And they escaped with nothing to show for it except the skin on their bones and an inner drive and flame to survive and enable their children to have a better life than they did.

And *my doctor*—Dr. Rose—came to help me in Brooklyn whenever I was sick. And he came by train, over an hour's ride from his shabby office in a shabby old house in a shabby old area of New York City that looked like what it was to everyone—that is, everyone except those escaping from the pre-concentration camps known as Jewish ghettos. And to these refugees from *hell*, their shabby streets really seemed lined with *gold and silver* (no pun intended). And their slums and tenements were magnificent Fifth Avenue brownstones when compared to the peasant huts, starvation, and pogroms they were used to.

And to a little boy—frequently ill with overconcerned and pretraumatized parents witness to a prior hell and scourges without any medical treatment available—Dr. Rose was God, albeit not a fancy-looking one. But we saw right through his shabby facade. And what *we saw inspired us to sacrifice* so that one day I could follow in Dr. Rose's footsteps:

- Almost 60 years have passed since I first met Dr. Rose, shortly after I was born.

- Almost 60 years have passed since my father first began working as a "seltzer and soda man"—carrying 20-60 pound boxes up 2, 3, 4 . . . flights of stairs to immigrants and others wanting beverages.

- Almost 50 years have passed since I began helping my father in this gruelling task, without once ever hearing him complain of his long hours and exhausting work.

- Almost 40 years have passed since my own academic and medical work-load was too much and too time-consuming to help him—and so my younger brother jumped in.

This was my background. Those were my inspirations. And my aspirations were simple: *To be like Dr. Rose. To be a doctor and help sick and suffering people.*

Clear? Simple? I would certainly think so. But I'm sure my critics will once again project their own thoughts onto me and thus look at the darker side: What about getting rich and famous?

Considering my background, I became rich and famous when I entered and completed medical school.[1] And I was flying high as an intern and resident: *helping sick and suffering people—mostly indigent—on death's firing line at Cook County Hospital (Chicago, IL) and later Kings County Hospital (Brooklyn, NY).*

---

[1]In contrast to the above-mentioned positive feelings, I have always felt that the medical school training process during the first two years completely overloaded bright and gifted students with memorization rather than clinically-based and mathematical-like conceptual solution-tasks. As a result, this process:

- contributed significantly to the inability of graduates and later "experts" to think and reason and thus re-evaluate new, "controversial" or untaught realities for themselves,
- contributed to a mental process whereby many bright students gaveup their time-wasting reasoning capabilities so as to better function—and thus pass—on tests designed for parrots and so continued to function as intelligent-sounding autistic-like "traditional experts,"
- contributed to a syndrome I discovered amongst colleagues called "*medical-school phobias*" whereby gifted physicians remain traumatized—like dyslexics—by their prior overloading education experiences, even thirty years later.

In retrospect, I believe my past mathematical and psychoanalytical training—emphasizing understanding and reasoning vs. memory—saved me from becoming just another "traditional expert"—like the rest. But it took me years after my medical school "memory bashing" to bounce back to my old mathematical-self. Fortunately, I made it, driven by an inner force to always understand and thus be better able to help those in need. Unfortunately, too many did not make it and so continue to function as mere parrots—repeating or perseverating memorized phrases in a logical vacuum.

My parents' dream came true. And so did mine. And everything after that was clear sailing until I was confronted with the events constituting *A Scientific Watergate—Dyslexia*, events overcome by my identification with Dr. Rose's image and his true medical aims—helping the sick and suffering. Little did I know then that Dr. Rose's "slum practice" was really gold and silver—compared to the Gold and Silver I later came across. Little did I know then what determination and endurance it took for him to become a doctor so many years ago—the endurance and determination defining Dr. Rose. Little did I know then that I would have to pay the same price to carry out my dream, Dr. Rose's dream, the dreams of my parents and, no doubt, the dream and tradition of our ancestors going back God-knows how many years—a dream defined by *love, sacrifice, endurance, charity, knowledge, science and medicine—religion aside. And of course, survival.*

And as I write this "ending" to *A Scientific Watergate— Dyslexia*, or is it really *a new beginning*, my father lies dying in Maimonides Hospital in Brooklyn—the very place I was born in. Is this chance? Or is there real significance to Einstein's incredible remark that "God does not play dice with the universe"? In other words, is there really a God-like cosmic force guiding us from without as there is one— the unconscious—guiding us from within? *Was I born and being driven to complete* A Scientific Watergate—Dyslexia *before my father's death as a symbol: a symbol representing my gift to God and/or my father for His gift to me?*

In any event, I suddenly needed time and a digression before continuing. Emotions were getting too hot and heavy. And I must have required a change or mental pause. And so to defuse, I (my unconscious) suddenly recalled a thought that once popped into my head one student day as a psychiatric resident: *Moses and Jesus aside, Einstein and Freud must surely have been God's children.*

Was this above thought not related to cosmic and un-conscious determinism? And since it was not random, did this thought not prove the existence of this determinism? To get back to my dying father and seeing the suffering in the intensive care unit and the many Dr. Roses caring for him. And suddenly these flashbacks. And suddenly these insights. And suddenly diversions or resistance to my con-tinuing. And once again—clearly and simply—I saw my predetermined purpose in life: *To help relieve suffering. To restore hope—and replace despair. To complete* A Scientific Watergate—Dyslexia.

No doubt I was initially detoured, by some greater force, from Dr. Rose's medicine to psychiatry. And then once again driven back to medicine after gaining the psychiatric and Freudian psychoanalytic insights needed to under-stand and help mental and emotional suffering—as well as the critical resistance or blocking forces which only God knew would follow.

Although driven to complete this cycle or circle, the ends didn't quite meet when I finished my basic training. And so I came out different—better equipped to handle the task before me. A task revealed to me on Rosh Hashana—and conceptually completed on Yom Kippur—a task I called *A Scientific Watergate—Dyslexia.*

In many ways, my "learning curve" or "cycle" was not too different from that characterizing evolution's. And suddenly my mind felt a need to redefine and re-explain the concepts: phylogeny, ontogeny, survival-of-the-fit-test, etc.[1]

---

[1]*Phylogeny* represents the "developmental stages" in evolution from our animalistic origins to our present form. *Ontogeny* represents the rapid repetition of these evolutionary developmental stages in the em-bryo—and even continuing out of the embryo during early childhood and perhaps even young adulthood. And so *ontogeny recapitulates phylogeny* or the history of evolution's stages—perhaps even account-ing for the cycles and circles responsible for *history repeating itself!*

In many ways, the obstacles forever blocking needed insights and perhaps even premature dissemination of the steadily evolving CV or inner-ear concepts led me to recognize:

- that the resistance barriers to success as well as the survival-triggers forcing those who can to overcome are akin and no doubt related to the survival-of-the-fittest mechanisms characterizing the progress-curves, -circles and -cycles over evolutionary time spans,

- that my slow, tedious, bumbling, fumbling and stumbling progress over the last 20-30 years merely followed evolution's learning curves—often characterized by detours, set-backs, side-tracking, and even regression,

- that the cycles and circles or repetitive patterns I kept recognizing were merely echoes of ontogeny recapitulating phylogeny—or history repeating itself.

Oops, I've no doubt done it again. I've no doubt added unnecessary confusion and seeming complexity to what was, until now, a rather simple discussion of the motives and drives leading me to where I am now and the completion of this work. But as always, unexpected complexity occurs and thereby forces those who can to understand and overcome and those who can't to forever deny or block it out and thus hide in the past—as do "traditionalists."

In other words, evolutionary mechanisms appear to have an "ambivalent" life of their own—forever pushing the existing status quo another notch forward while at the same time often appearing to slow down or derail this very same progress. Needless to say, this latter resistance—symbolized by the traditionalists—attempts to maintain the status quo at all costs. In retrospect, might not the resistance—the traditionalists—serve evolution's purposes also by slowing down the speed of progress so that it might be properly assimilated and integrated into the "total game plan"—whatever that is and whoever guides it—God? Do not these seemingly opposing mechanisms—progress vs. resistance—serve one master as well as shape the resulting zig-zagging and detours characterizing the progress of evolution's eventual advance. But in the final analysis, we either eventually advance or slide backwards. And it is truly impossible over an extended time span to stay put— exactly in one spot.[1]

This is no doubt what history or looking back is all about—teaching us that if we do not learn from past mistakes we will either be forever repeating them and thus forced to follow *the same truly circular paths and patterns* guiding our scientific ancestors or worse:

- Suddenly I understood my need to discuss ontogeny and phylogeny.

- Suddenly I realized that the ontogeny/phylogeny cycle is forever operative—over short and long evolutionary time spans both in and out of the womb.

- Suddenly I understood the reason for my footnote concerning "memory bashing" in medical school and thereafter, forcing bright and gifted students into "parroting"—repeating what they are taught without either time or inclination to rethink and reconceptualize yesterday's "facts" with today's realities, forcing them to parrot history over and over again— endlessly, forcing them to think and reason like traditional dyslexia "experts."

- Suddenly I understood that—"mutants" or exceptions aside—the traditional majority are forced by instinctive mechanisms to forever repeat the slow, tedious and often regressive patterns of their predecessors, regardless of whether or not these patterns are *currently most* adaptive or "logical."

[1]That's the spot maintained by the dyslexia traditionalists for the last century—until my rather recent "push."

- Suddenly I realized what scientific "herding," "turf-ing," and exclusion or bias are all about and why traditionalists invariably attract the majority to their "ancient" and even illogical views—excluding all "controversial others" who disagree and thereby threaten status quo instincts.

- Suddenly I saw myself as a "mutant," an exception to what appears to be the underlying traditional sci-entific rule which attempts to maintain the status quo or existing equilibrium at all costs—regardless of manifest "scientific claims" to the contrary.

- Suddenly I understood my prior "free associations" leading me to discuss genes, predetermined drives, "God-like" or cosmic and unconsciously-rooted forces as well as cycles and circles, etc.

- Suddenly I understood associations indicating that my family was the only Jewish one on the block—a break in "herding."

Hopefully, my freely associated reflections and looking back as well as attempts at analyzing them have been as helpful to you all as they were to me. Hopefully, you better understand that the inner mechanisms slowing down my own progress during the past 20-30 years were similar to those of the traditionalists. Hopefully, you will recognize that a mere twenty year "evolutionary time-span" was needed for this genetic variant within me to break loose and spread via *A Scientific Watergate—Dyslexia* so that the cerebellar-vestibular concepts might dominate the scien-tific dyslexic scene in the evolutionary or "God-driven" in-terests of survival—help for countless millions. Hopefully, you will see that Acceptance Without Reference (Chapter 18) highlighted this new evolutionary change, albeit a few of the "new breed of experts" claimed to be "the fittest" and the "first." Hopefully, you will recognize and understand that my father's imminent death served both as an obstacle and a stimulus—refueling the fire and energy needed to finally catapult me over the last hurdle or resistance barrier.

And in retrospect or looking back, I better understand my need to explain:

- that we were all dyslexic in the past—until another mutant began to read, write, spell and calculate,

- that compensatory mechanisms and genes developed over an evolutionary time span in those fittest to survive so that the majority currently define themselves as "*nondyslexic*," or perhaps even "*dyslexic without 'dyslexia'*,"

- that our momentary and permanent lapses into dyslexia—scientific and otherwise—are mere ontogenetic signals of this past stage in phylogeny (and thus history repeating itself), and

- that ontogenetic development continues after birth, explaining the normal dyslexic symptoms in young children and even "developmental delays" until compensatory mechanisms dominate—then called "spurting" if compensation is dramatic; or stated another way, are not these latter "embryonic" or ontogenetic stages merely reflections of how dyslexic man eventually spurted or compensated and so became increasingly nondyslexic over an evolutionary time span?

And upon further reflection, I also realized how important it was to highlight and stress the diagnostic/therapeutic value of basic *clinical research* in solving the many and varied riddles characterizing dyslexia. This simple and clear *patient-based and -grounded* methodology (listening to and observing symptoms and attempting their *qualitative* and quantitative analysis)—often snobbishly referred to as "subjective"—confirmed Sir William Osler's century-old dictum that history is more than 90% of diagnostic insight—since it led to all my diagnostic/therapeutic breakthroughs.

This "subjective" method also helped explain the century-old theoretically-based confusion and denial of the traditionalists as well as their completely ineffective but "objective" hands-off and distant attempts at *quantitatively testing* dyslexics to death using a variety of highfalutin investigatory and statistical tools. But their tools were mistakenly aimed at the normal and compensatory cerebral cortex or the thinking-linguistic centers of the brain. So the results they obtained were often out of sync with scientific dyslexia realities, and/or unwittingly forced to fit preexisting and erroneous convictions. And the vast majority of refuting data had to be denied—including my CV-determined diagnostic/therapeutic results as well as dyslexic samples greater than 25,000 patients. No small feat of denial—even for a monopoly.

Suddenly, my inner need to express all these often rambling and complex thoughts made sense—although it didn't initially. Mind you, I knew from past experience that there was a logic and pattern to the unconscious forces driving me and leading me to think what I did, but it took 20-30 years to understand them better—in perspective. In other words, my prior unedited thoughts were "dyslexic"—resembling President Bush's alleged speech patterns as previously presented. And it took a rather short 20-30 year "evolutionary time span" to render my "dyslexic" thoughts and data nondyslexic. Once again: *Is not history repeating itself in the present? Or, is not ontogeny recapitulating phylogeny?*

By contrast, if my preexisting concepts were "dyslexic," then, by analogy, those of my critics appeared "alexic" or "aphasic." And in the final analysis, I realized that "God" hadn't been asleep, as I had often previously thought. Obviously I was—as are the traditionalists.

Summary

In retrospect, I feel this work is God's—not mine. *He* (cosmic and unconscious determinism) gave me the genes to survive as He gave them to my ancestors. And He programmed or willed them to complete the works I was born and raised and sacrificed for.

And with this work, *A Scientific Watergate—Dyslexia,* I feel God's will—gift—within me will survive and have its predetermined effect: *to carry mankind another step forward with help and hope. And as stated earlier: This work is my gift to Him and His children for His gift to me and my children; and to my dying father—who will forever live via this research and its potential help to countless millions.*

As we all know, the purpose of looking back is to see more and better—clearer—when we once again refocus and look ahead. And so for those of you readers who deserve much more than just reading about and analyzing criticism, I repeatedly attempted to inspire you—as I was inspired—with dyslexic patients, young and old, whose suffering was relieved, albeit not cured. A far contrast to the self-serving diagnostic/therapeutic void offered suffering dyslexics by the traditionalist critics for the past 100 years.

And in retrospect, I hoped that my image of Dr. Rose—a currently extinct form of family doctor—*would inspire and ground all those medical researchers in ivory towers who have lost touch with both the feelings and pain of the suffering millions as well as the instinctive drives motivating us as healers and researchers to help them—at all costs. Not theirs—ours!*

Hopefully, looking back and exposing life's resistance barriers will catalyze scientists and thus science to *spurt* forward. Hopefully, mankind will benefit currently rather than in evolutionary generations to come. Hopefully, *A Sci-*

entific Watergate—Dyslexia will rapidly *add* a new stage in phylogeny and thus ontogeny. Hopefully, we will, in the near future, be repeating the history of man's progress vs. his traditionally acceptable *status quo*.

CHAPTER 22

The End is Just a New Beginning

A

The End—Book I . . .

To Isidore, my father: who saw and approved this manuscript and its aims, but who will never read again.

To my dyslexic critics: who saw and read only themselves instead of their patients, and thereby unwittingly inspired and catalyzed *A Scientific Watergate—Dyslexia.*

To the countless dyslexic millions whose hope and help I was raised and sacrificed for, and who will forever after "spurt" and thus see daylight instead of gloom and darkness.

To science and scientists—freed and thus catalyzed to perform God's predetermined wonders and "miracles."

To God's evolutionary process—and a new advanced "compensatory" generation of *dyslexics without "dyslexia"* and even man without dyslexics.

To A New Beginning—Book II.

B

A New Beginning

As the reader might have guessed by now, this book "avoids" ending. Rather, I avoided ending it. And upon reflection, a number of associations occurred to me: *there's so much more to say*—hence the reason for Book II. *There are so many more dyslexics I'd like to present to you, something appears missing, a further need for symmetry; the end is just a new beginning.*

And upon analysis, I recognized that all these associations zeroed in on the fact that I had omitted something of importance and was thus stalling. Suddenly I recalled using Elizabeth Woof's *thank-you card* to open up this book— a card she sent me without even her parents' knowledge. And on second thought I realized that Elizabeth's appreciation and delight at her favorable responses to medication were symbolic of *the very essence—hope and help*—catalyzing both the initiation and completion of this work and all my other efforts to date.

Suddenly I understood my stalling and Freudian slip of mind—the omission of Elizabeth's favorable responses until this book's completion—or almost completion. My subconsciously-driven intuition was once again telling me something very important. And fortunately I was trained to listen. The message was clear: *The end is just a new beginning.* Since I began this work with Elizabeth, it should symmetrically end (or rather *begin anew*) with the hope and help inspiring and motivating Elizabeth's *thank-you.*

Suddenly the "blurred" message I was consciously getting became even clearer. I had to end this work with my own thanks to the thousands of dyslexic patients and their loved ones who refused to surrender to the diagnostic/

therapeutic void of the traditionalists. To those who made this research possible. May Elizabeth's favorable responses as well as those of all others within this work symbolize a comparable new beginning for millions and millions of other dyslexics freed from the ignorance and denial characterizing the traditionalist dyslexia monopoly.

Elizabeth Woof

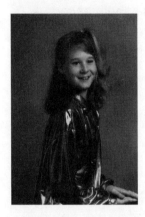

After three months of treatment, Mrs. Woof wrote the following progress note (10/25/92):

> The change in Elizabeth has been remarkable. She has changed from a stubborn, difficult child to a happy, cooperative one.
>
> I have enclosed her report card. It's remarkable. She has never gotten such good grades. Her assignments are done on time, and the right assignments are completed (she used to get instructions mixed up). Notice her reading level is 4 (was 2!).
>
> Just as important as is her progress at school, her progress at home is great. She wakes up alert in the morning, ready for the day. It used to be a battle to get her on the school bus every morning. She follows instructions at home, and her room is neat! (Mostly—she's not perfect yet—but it's a great improvement.) Much less fighting with her brother.

She was always complaining of some physical problem. That's all disappeared. Last year she was in the lowest reading group, at the very bottom, and was described
by her teacher as "inattentive with a poor attitude." At conferences this year, she is at the top of the middle group
and is described by her teacher as "bright and a delight."
Thank you does not begin to express our appreciation to you.

On weekends, when no medication is given, we can
see some regression of symptoms. So Elizabeth asked us
to continue the treatment seven days a week—so she can
enjoy the weekends. And we can better enjoy her.[1]

---

[1]This consideration and others as well eventually led me to *reverse* the
traditional practice of stopping medications on weekends and holidays. Medication is now given seven days per week to patients unless
there are reasons to do otherwise. Indeed, this reversal is one of many
characterizing my research. It highlights the "dyslexia-like" clinical-
theoretical errors characterizing prior traditional conceptualizations.

Elizabeth's Report Card

Student's Name Elizabeth Woof

EXPLANATION OF MARKS

A – Exceptional
B – Above Average
C – Average
D – Below Average
U – Unsatisfactory

S – Satisfactory
N – Needs Improvement

LEVELS
(as determined by teacher assessment)

Reading

Grade 1:
  R – Readiness
  PP – Preprimer
  P – Primer

Grade 2
Grade 3
Grade 4
Grade 5

Mathematics
Grades 1 – 5

SUBJECTS	1	2	3	4	5	6	Year	TEACHER COMMENTS (DATE)
READING	A							
Reading Level	4							
LANGUAGE	A							
SPELLING	B							
HANDWRITING	S							
MATHEMATICS	A							
Mathematics Level	5							
SOCIAL STUDIES	A							
SCIENCE	B							
HEALTH and SAFETY	A							
ART	S							
MUSIC	S							
PHYSICAL EDUCATION	S							

✱ Indicates that the curriculum in this subject has been modified to meet the student's individual needs.

BEHAVIOR

GRADING SCALE: A/B/C/D/U

TEACHER	1	2	3	4	5	6	Year	COMMENTS (DATE)
Fellers	A							
Fisher	A							
McMurray	A							
Lee	A							

WORK HABITS

GRADING SCALE: S/N

TEACHER	1	2	3	4	5	6	Year	COMMENTS (DATE)
Lee	S							

RECORD OF ATTENDANCE

	1	2	3	4	5	6	Year	COMMENTS (DATE)
Days Present	30							
Days Absent	0							
Days Tardy	0							

Additional Comments: Elizabeth is making great progress! 10/12

GRADING SCALE
A - 93 - 100
B - 85 - 92
C - 77 - 84
D - 70 - 76
U - 0 - 69

Appendices

(Appendices B and C as well as a complete list of references will be included in Book II.)

Appendix A

Dr. Gold's and Carter's Verbatim "Blind" Cerebellar Data in 22 Dyslexic Children[1]

In order to confirm the author's CV neurologic findings in dyslexia, twenty-two CV-impaired dyslexic children were randomly selected and referred to Drs. Arnold Gold and Sidney Carter for "blind" neurologic examinations, and the neurologic data quantitatively and qualitatively analyzed.

The specific aim of this appendix is to present the reader with the "raw," "blind" cerebellar dyslexic data base, so that the background from which the author derived his foreground quantitative and qualitative insights may be "seen," and thus independently corroborated.

Inasmuch as the quantitative analysis of all the "blind" cerebellar dyslexic findings has already been presented in Chapter 4, the task at hand is "merely" to present abstracted verbatim quotations of the cerebellar (and vestibular) findings characterizing twenty-one of the twenty-two "blindly" examined dyslexic cases.

Chapters 4 and 16 included qualitative abstracts for demonstration purposes. This data was taken from Appendix B—*A Solution to the Riddle—Dyslexia*, pp. 327-337. Also Appendix C of the above text includes six complete and typical "blind" neurological reports as well as their analyses—despite the criticism by Ortonian-related experts that this "dangerous" book provides no evidence for its cer-

---

[1]Although the names were changed to initials in order to preserve confidentiality, all other quoted content is exact. The use of "cerebellar deficit" and directly associated neurological signs by Dr. Gold have been italicized for emphasis. These very same signs are also found in Dr. Carter's cases, although he only mentions the cerebellar diagnosis in one.

ebellar-vestibular (CV) basis. After reviewing this content, judge the critics and criticism for yourselves. And I hope you better understand why this book is dangerous. And who amongst my critics feel the danger.

Learning-Disability Cases
Examined by Dr. Arnold P. Gold

K.G. is a 7-year-old boy: "There was a slight slurring of words which may be due to the delayed eruption of the upper incisor teeth . . . He held a pencil in a deficient fashion with the index and middle finger over the pencil and very close to the point. This was associated with slight deficiency in graphomotor skills with mildly impaired formation of letters and numbers. His reproduction of the Bender Gestalt patterns reflected this mild graphomotor difficulty . . . Station revealed a bilateral pes planus with a tendency to toe outwards . . . Motor examination revealed a mild decrease in muscle tone with slight hyper-extensibility of joints involving the intrinsic muscles of the fingers . . . *Cerebellar examination showed normal finger-to-nose function with reasonably good catching, throwing, and kicking. There was, however, a mild impairment of rapid alternating movements such as with alternating pronation and supination. However, small finger muscle coordination such as rapid succession movements involving the intrinsic muscles of the fingers was moderately impaired and associated with mirror movements . . .*

"In summary on neurologic examination this seven and a half year old youngster *showed evidence of a mild degree of muscular hypotonia with hyperextensibility of joints, and this was associated with a mild to moderate impairment of small hand muscle coordination.*

"The family history is of significance in that the father who obtained an equivalency high school diploma had a significant learning disability and when tested, Mr. G., who is of normal intellect, was only able to spell at a third or fourth grade level and his reading was below a fifth grade level with multiple omissions and substitutions. In addition to the learning disability there was a significant speech problem with stuttering which in large part, is related to the frustration that Mr. G. encountered with his academic performance."

D.W. is an 11-year, 11-month-old boy: "He held a pencil in a rigid and awkward fashion in the right hand and the graphomotor coordination was immature for age and letters were poorly printed. Copies of the Bender Gestalt patterns were likewise deficient with mild distortions and these reproductions were complicated by irregular lines and poor angulations . . . *There was no cerebellar deficit other than that involving graphomotor function.* The child encountered no difficulty with throwing, catching, and kicking and on formal cerebellar examination there was no abnormality in finger-nose-finger or the performance of rapid alternating and rapid succession movements."

M.C. is a 6-year-old boy: "Coordination is poor above all for visuomotor and small hand-muscle coordination skills. He did not button clothes until six years of age. He was unable to tie his shoelaces until recently . . . Speech patterns were deficient in that the child spoke with a slight to moderate slurring of words and this was associated with salivary accumulation . . . Prehension was markedly deficient in that he held a pencil in a very awkward fashion with four fingers . . . This was associated with deficient graphomotor skills with very poor formation and spacing of letters . . . The reproduction of the Bender Gestalt patterns were likewise deficient and in part was related to the poor graphomotor skills but in addition there were distortions and immature reproductions which suggested the presence of an associated perceptual problem with visual spatial difficulties . . . The gait patterns were characterized by a tendency to toe inwards above all on the right, but was otherwise unremarkable for the regular heel, toe, and tandem walking. *Hopping was slightly deficient . . . There was a significant cerebellar deficit with finger-nose-finger dysmetria above all on the left and this was associated with poor catching, throwing, and kicking. Of greater significance was moderate to marked impairment of alternating rapid succession movements as well as the presence of mirror movements.* Cranial nerve examination revealed the previously described speech patterns and this was associated with an immature oropharyngeal coordination with an inability to isolate tongue from mandible on lateral tongue movements.

"The mother had a significant learning disability. Mrs. C. is left-handed and as previously stated has marked right-left confusion . . . There is only one sibling, J., age 8½ years, who is poorly coordinated and has difficulty with spelling, but apparently is an extremely bright boy and has not encountered any significant academic problems.

"In summary, on neurologic examination this 6-year, 9-month-old child showed evidence of a static encephalopathy of prenatal origin and in view of the prominent history it is highly probable that this is of genetic etiology. This is manifested by a hyperkinetic behavioral syndrome, deficient coordination, poor speech patterns, impaired visual perception and a learning disability as delineated above."

R.V. is an 8-year-old girl: "She was late in both buttoning her clothes and tying her shoelaces . . . Graphomotor coordination is poor for age and grade placement. A pencil was held rigidly in the left hand and there was a slightly deficient formation and spacing of letters. Reproductions of the Bender Gestalt revealed immature appearing copies that were slightly distorted with irregular lines and poor angulations . . . Small hand muscle coordination was below that expected for age and there was deficient performance of rapid succession movements, above all on the left.

"In summary, *on neurologic examination R. . . . showed on examination a mild but definite impairment of cerebellar function which primarily involved small muscle coordination.*"

A.K. is an 11-year-old boy: "His copies of the Bender Gestalt were slightly immature with irregular lines and poor angulations. He held a pencil in an awkward and rigid fashion in the right hand and his graphomotor coordination was significantly below that expected for age. He wrote with printed letters that were poorly formed and spaced . . . Gait patterns were normal with a slight tendency to toe outwards on the left . . . *There was a mild cerebellar deficit which primarily involved fine muscle coordination in the hand with poor succession movements.* Cranial nerve examination was unremarkable other than an intermittent and mild convergent strabismus of the left eye. There was excessive salivary accumulation and the child could not dissociate tongue and mandible on lateral tongue movements . . . There is also impairment of small muscle function involving the oral pharynx and extraocular muscles.

"The family history is of interest in that there are three older siblings; the older two boys had a mild reading and a spelling problem, but presently are doing quite well."

A.H. is a 12-year-old boy: "He spoke with a slight slurring of words . . . His graphomotor coordination was grossly deficient in that there was poor formation of letters and numbers that were poorly written and spaced. The reproductions of the Bender Gestalt patterns were immature for age with irregular lines but there were no true distortions or rotations . . . *Cerebellar function was normal other than a slight impairment of small finger function with awkwardness in the performance of rapid succession movements.* Cranial nerve examination other than the minimal speech deficit was unremarkable . . . In addition, there was a very mild expressive language problem associated with deficient small muscle coordination.

"This disorder is usually secondary to a static encephalopathy of genetic origin and it is highly probable that this is related to the father's disability."

S.T. is a 7-year-old boy: "He spoke with a slight but definite slurring of words and this was associated with salivary accumulation . . . Copies of the Bender Gestalt were immature in appearance but at no time was there distortion or rotation. These reproductions had irregular lines and poor angulations. Graphomotor coordination was poor with printed letters that were poorly formed and spaced . . . *There was a cerebellar deficit and this was manifested by slightly awkward gait for regular, heel and toe walking. Hopping was poorly performed and there was evidence of tandem ataxia. In addition to problems with locomotion there was a significant extremity deficit and this was manifested by a minimal finger-nose-finger dysmetria and a moderate to marked impairment of rapid alternating and rapid succession movements. Catching and throwing were poorly performed. It is of interest to note that this youngster's deficit in cerebellar function was most marked in small muscle function.*

"It is my impression that this youngster with a hyperkinetic behavioral syndrome shows *evidence of organic dysfunction of the central nervous system that primarily involves cerebellar function.* I do not believe that there is evidence of true dyslexia but the child does have a mild learning disability."

W.H. is a 9-year-old boy: "The acquisition of developmental milestones revealed a significant delay in motor function and a mild delay in the acquisition of speech patterns . . . Coordination is stated to be poor for all functions except for walking and buttoning . . . His speech patterns were poor and this was associated with slurring of words and slight stuttering . . . Copies of Bender Gestalt patterns were immature for age and in addition were slightly rotated to the right with irregular lines and poor angulations . . . Graphomotor coordination showed that the child held a pencil in an awkward and rigid fashion in the left hand and there was significant deficit in both the formation and spacing of printed letters . . . Reading was characterized by poor cadence . . . Station was characterized by a mild pes planus with a slight scoliosis of the thoracic vertebra to the left. *His gait patterns were awkward for regular, heel and toe walking. Tandem gait was deficient and hopping was poorly performed, especially on the left foot . . . There was a significant cerebellar deficit manifested by a moderate impairment of finger-nose-finger function as well as a significant deficit in the performance of rapid alternating and rapid succession movements.* He threw only with distal musculature such as observed in females and was very deficient in catching, throwing and kicking . . . This child with a delay in the acquisition of all developmental milestones showed at the present time *deficient* motor, *cerebellar,* and expressive language problems as well as the mild but definite learning disability."

S.D.R. is a 9-year-old boy: "Coordination was stated to be poor for handwriting and catching. He first buttoned his clothes at 5-6 years of age and first tied his shoelaces at 7 years of age . . . Past history and review of symptoms revealed that the child has an impairment of the extra-ocular muscle function for which corrective glasses have been prescribed. There have been many episodes of recurrent pharyngitis and otitis with febrile reactions which rose as high as 105 to 106 degrees . . . His copies of Bender Gestalt were of poor quality. These reproductions were mildly distorted with irregular lines and poor angulation. *Graphomotor coordination was deficient* with poor formation of both letters and numbers . . . *There was a deficient cerebellar deficit that was manifested by a mild finger-nose-finger dysmetria and a moderate impairment of rapid alternating movements. Catching, throwing and kicking were poorly performed.* Cranial nerve examination revealed a prominent alternating convergent strabismus which was most apparent in the right eye. There was a prominent difficulty in the youngster fixing for any prolonged period of time. The eyeglasses tended to correct this problem.

"It is my impression that this youngster with a relative micro-cephaly shows unequivocal evidence of organic dysfunction in the central nervous system that is often referred to as 'minimal cerebral dysfunction or minimal brain damage.' The evidence to support this impression of neurologic dysfunction is the perceptual problems with visuo-spatial muscle function, above all in the hands, as well as an extraocular muscle imbalance.

"The family history is of interest in that the mother was a slow learner and presently has a marked alternating convergent strabismus. The father had likewise encountered significant problems with academic function.

"Concerning etiologic factors it is possible that this is of genetic etiology and may well be related to the parents who also had significant learning problems."

D.S. is a 7-year-old boy: "His copies of the Bender Gestalt tests were markedly abnormal with gross distortions, rotations, irregular lines, and poor angulations. These were highly diagnostic of a marked perceptual problem with visuo-spatial difficulties . . . Graphomotor coordination was likewise deficient with poor formation and spacing of both letters and numbers. The gait was regular for normal, heel and toe walking. *There was evidence of slight tandem ataxia . . . There was a significant cerebellar deficit with poor performance of finger-nose-finger function as well as deficient function in the performance of rapid succession movements, especially that which involved small muscle groups. Catching, throwing and kicking were poorly performed.*

"It is my impression that this youngster shows evidence of abnormal neurological function which is commonly referred to as 'minimal cerebral dysfunction.' This is manifested in this youngster by a failure to establish dominance with right-left confusion, the marked perceptual deficit, *a mild to moderate cerebellar deficit that was most marked in fine muscle function and finger dexterity.* The entire clinical picture is then associated with a marked learning disability that not only involves reading but other spheres of academic function. Etiologic factors appear to be obscure but it is highly possible that there is a genetic basis in view of a paternal uncle who is left handed and has an associated learning disability."

C.O. is a 7-year-old girl: "The child has frequent falls but upon questioning it is more probable that this is secondary to her mild coordination problem with hyperkinesis, rather than any inner ear disease. C. was recently evaluated at Lenox Hill Hospital and apparently vestibular function studies as well as an audiogram was performed and this showed some questionable findings . . . The child's speech patterns were slightly deficient in that on occasion she showed evidence of poor articulation of words with slurring . . . Her prehension was slightly deficient in that she held a pencil with the index finger over the pencil and very close to the point. This was associated with poor graphomotor skills and her letters were deficiently formed and poorly spaced. She could produce most numbers but had difficulty with the number 9 which was subsequently written in a mirror reversal . . . Reproductions of the Bender Gestalt patterns were grossly deficient with distortions, rotations, and immature copies. These were indicative of a deficient visual memory and impaired visual perception as well as poor visuomotor and visual spatial relationships . . . Gait was complicated by a slight tendency to toe inwards with mild pes planus . . . *There was slight deficiency in hopping on the left lower extremity . . . There was a cerebellar deficit with a slight finger-nose-finger dysmetria associated with poor catching, throwing and kicking and this was associated with a moderate dysdiadochokinesis and poor performance of rapid succession movements.* It is of note that despite the impairment of coordination in small finger muscle function, the child had no difficulty in snapping her fingers.

"Mrs. O. . . . shows evidence of a mild learning disability. . . It is apparent, likewise, when evaluating Mr. O. that he shows evidence of a significant residual learning problem."

N.C. is an 8-year-old boy: "Coordination is stated to be good for walking, running, catching and throwing. In contrast, he has problems with small muscle coordination which involves handwriting, buttoning, and shoelace tying. Even at the present time N. is unable to tie his own shoelaces . . . Prehension consisted of a tripod positioning of the pencil but his graphomotor skills were poor with deficient formation and spacing of both letters and numbers. Reproductions of the Bender Gestalt patterns were likewise impaired with distortions, irregular lines and poor angulations; in part this was due to the deficient small hand muscle coordination. It is of note that reading is N.'s most proficient subject in that he is reading at grade level and both immediate and intermediate recall was good. Spelling was poor and at the second grade level while number concepts were poor and limited to finger counting. He was unable to tell time. The child's fund of knowledge and general intellect appeared to be normal for stated chronological age. Former neurologic examination revealed bilateral pes planus with the knees in genu recurvatum . . . His gait was on a slightly widened base but otherwise unremarkable for regular, heel, toe, and tandem walking. Hopping was well performed on either foot. Motor examination showed a generalized *decrease in muscle tone, and this hypotonia was associated with slight hyperextensibility of joints . . . There was a mild cerebellar deficit and this primarily involves small finger muscle function such as in the performance of rapid succession movements and this became more impaired when both hands were utilized simultaneously.* Cranial nerve examination revealed an alternating divergent strabismus and the child was unable to maintain fixation for any period of time. This was further complicated by photophobia which in part may be due to his present upper respiratory infection.

"In summary . . . N. is an 8-year, 5-month-old child who showed evidence of a neurologic deficit that was manifested by muscular hypotonia, impaired small hand muscle coordination, an extraocular muscle imbalance, and a learning disability as delineated above. These findings would be consistent with what is commonly referred to as 'minimal cerebral dysfunction or minimal brain damage.'"

M.M. is an 8-year-old girl: "Behaviorally there is evidence of a prominent hyperkinetic behavioral syndrome which is most prominent in the home setting . . . Past history and review of systems revealed that at 2 years of age the child had a one minute seizure in which she woke up in the morning screaming and this was associated with eye rolling and head shaking . . . In addition she was clumsy and would frequently fall . . . At the completion of my evaluation the mother related that the child was seen at New York Hospital for an ENT evaluation which was normal as well as obtaining normal audiogram but apparently the calorics were abnormal. I would be most appreciative if you could supply me further data concerning this vestibular function study. M. was also seen by Dr. K. in neurological evaluation who stated that the child showed no evidence of neurologic deficit . . . Physical examination revealed . . . child tended to speak from the right side of her mouth with a tendency to tilt her head to the left . . . A pencil was held in a rigid fashion with hyperextension of the index finger. Graphomotor coordination was poor in that the child wrote with printed letters that were deficiently formed and spaced. Reproductions of the Bender Gestalt patterns were moderately deficient with immature reproductions that were distorted and rotated associated with irregular lines and poor angulations; these reproductions were characteristic of a perceptual problem with visuo-spatial difficulties. Auditory memory and auditory perception were likewise deficient . . . *Gait patterns were slightly awkward with a tendency to toe inwards on the left . . . There was a significant cerebellar deficit that was manifested by a slight left finger-nose-finger dysmetria, a moderate impairment of rapid alternating movements with dysdiadochokinesis and a moderate to marked impairment of small finger muscle coordination with deficient performance of rapid succession movements, above all involving both hands. Catching, throwing and kicking were all poorly performed.* Cranial nerve examination revealed a very slight slurring of words and this was associated with a mild impairment in oropharyngeal coordination with an inability to isolate tongue from mandible.

"In summary, on neurologic examination this 8-year, 8-month-old child showed evidence of a static encephalopathy of prenatal or perinatal origin that is commonly referred to as 'minimal cerebral dysfunction or minimal brain damage.' The evidence to support this clinical impression is the impaired auditory and visual perception, the deficient coordination which was most prominent for small finger muscle function, the learning disability as delineated above, and historically a hyperkinetic behavioral syndrome."

P.R. is an 8-year, 11-month old girl: "At 2½ years of age P. fell from a swing and this resulted in a laceration of the right scalp . . . at 3½ years of age, the child began to present with recurrent eye pain which is often triggered by exposure to bright light or sunlight . . . Approximately 2 years ago during the course of a routine school physical examination hearing was noted to be deficient on the left side . . . Subsequent audiological evaluation revealed a nerve deafness on the left . . . Reproductions of the Bender Gestalt patterns were mildly deviant from the norm but there were no distortions or rotations. The copies had irregular lines and poor angulations. Graphomotor coordination was deficient with poor formation and spacing of letters and numbers . . . Gait patterns showed a tendency to toe outwards with mild pes planus . . . *There was a very mild cerebellar deficit with slight finger-nose-finger dysmetria and a mild small finger muscle coordination such as in the performance of rapid succession movements.*"

C.S. is a 9-year-old girl: "At 4½ years of age she was seen at the Brooklyn College Speech and Hearing Center where no therapy and a diagnostic impression of a 'late talker' was made. Coordination is stated to be poor, above all for fine muscle function as manifested by difficulty in tying shoelaces and poor graphomotor coordination. School performance revealed that the youngster is presently in the third grade and is a B student for all subjects other than reading where she has obtained a C grade . . . Past history and review of systems revealed that the youngster has been seen by an optometrist who states that there is poor eye coordination . . . Copies of the Bender Gestalt were below that expected for age and were highly suggestive of a perceptual problem with visuo-spatial difficulties. Number concepts were adequate for age while spelling and reading were slightly below average. None of the subjects showed gross deficiencies, certainly there was no evidence of a true dyslexic syndrome . . . . Station was characterized by a lumber lordosis and the *gait was slightly awkward for regular, heel, toe, and tandem walking . . . There was a mild cerebellar deficit with finger-nose-finger dysmetria, above all on the left, poor performance of rapid succession movements and deficient catching, throwing and kicking.* Cranial nerve examination was normal other than poor disassociation of tongue and mandible on lateral tongue movements . . . This youngster with a history of hyperkinetic behavioral syndrome shows a mild to moderate perceptual problem as well as *a mild cerebellar deficit.* These findings would be consistent with a diagnosis of minimal cerebral dysfunction or minimal brain damage.

"The family history is of interest in that Mrs. S. was slow in school and 'had to work to obtain grades.' She is a slow reader and this has continued until the present time. Coordination is poor and she did not participate in physical activities as a child."

M.D. is an 11-year-old boy: "Academically the child has had problems since kindergarten . . . and was nervous and hyperactive. Station was complicated by a slight bilateral pes planus but his gait was otherwise unremarkable for regular, heel, toe, and tandem walking . . . Sensory examination was normal for all modalities including touch, position, vibration, and cortical sensations. *There was a significant cerebellar deficit with a moderate finger-nose-finger dysmetria above all on the left and this was associated with poor catching as well as dysdiadochokinesis and above all a prominent impairment of small finger muscle coordination such as with rapid successive movements and this was associated with mirror movements* . . . In summary, on neurologic examination M. shows evidence of a brain damaged syndrome that is characterized by a prominent perceptual problem with visual spatial and visuomotor difficulties, deficient auditory memory, *poor cerebellar function,* and an associated learning disability."

A Chronological Study of a Case of Benign Paroxysmal Vertigo

P.S. was a 6-year-old youngster when he was first seen by Dr. Arnold Gold. January 1968: "This six-year, ten-month-old youngster was evaluated with the chief complaint of 'severe' headaches. He was previously diagnosed by Dr. S. and Dr. B. as a vascular migraine secondary to food allergy . . . The acquisition of developmental milestones revealed that handedness has not been established in that he writes and eats with the right hand and throws and catches with the left. Gait was delayed until 17 months of age . . . Coordination reveals a child with excellent catching and throwing ability and who does well with fine muscle coordination. At the present time he is an excellent student in first grade . . . The family history revealed that the father had two vertiginous episodes secondary to a middle ear infection . . . Approximately two years ago the child began with vertigo episodes . . . All episodes occur at night with the child suddenly gagging, spitting up phlegm and holding his eye (the parents state the right eye; the child the left). There is very little pain but he describes true vertigo with the child spinning around the room and this is associated with a markedly ataxic gait. During the entire episode there is marked photophobia and the child is neither able to lie down or stand but prefers to assume a sitting position. When the episode has terminated there is no residual complaint . . . Physical examination revealed a bright, verbal youngster who was obviously superior in intellect for his stated chronological age . . . Spelling and number concepts were superior . . . The gait was characterized by the head tilting to the right and the head was maintained stiffly in this position. There was a tendency towards pes planus and genu recurvatum when standing; when walking, there was a tendency to toe-in on the left. Motor examination revealed a generalized decrease in muscle tone . . . There was no evidence of a cerebellar deficit.

"Impression: Episodic vertigo—rule out vestibular dysfunction versus vascular anomalies involving the cerebellum or brain stem."

March 1968: "P. was admitted to the Babies Hospital from January 31st to February 13th, 1968 . . . An electroencephalogram was performed and this was an abnormal record due to well defined bilateral synchronous paroxysmal discharges present both in the alert and drowsy states . . . An audiogram was performed and this was normal. Vestibular function studies with calorics and rotational tests were normal. These normal studies would rule out a vestibular etiology for the vertiginous spells . . . Despite the atypical nature of the spells, the possibility of a convulsive disorder must be considered especially in view of the abnormal electroencephalogram. For this reason, the child was placed on Dilantin in the dosage of 100mg. twice daily.

January 1972: "I had the opportunity to re-evaluate P. on Jan. 14, 1972 . . . the child was last evaluated by me during a hospitalization at the Babies Hospital . . . in Jan. 1968. At that time he was discharged on Dilantin . . . the medication was decreased and ultimately discontinued after a period of six months. P. was essentially asymptomatic until Jan. 10, 1972, when at 4:00 a.m. the child awoke screaming 'help me' or 'I'm dizzy.' This time he was holding his right eye, was unable to open his eyes and complained of a headache. The child could not lie down or stand but ultimately could only sit. After a period of three to four hours the symptoms improved and by 12:00 noon P. was asymptomatic . . . *Neurologic examination revealed a slight slurring of words . . . His reproductions of the Bender Gestalt patterns were of poor quality and in large part this was due to a slight impairment in graphomotor skills. These reproductions had irregular lines and poor angulations.* Academic function was at grade level.[1]

Gait patterns were normal for regular, heel and toe walking but tandem gait was poorly performed . . . Cranial nerve examination showed a mild bilateral eyelid ptosis . . . P.'s neurologic evaluation was essentially unchanged from my initial evaluation of the child. At this time, I could not delineate any evidence of head tilt which was previously noted. The episodic 'dizziness' is most unusual for which I did not have an adequate explanation. The possibility of inner ear disease or a vascular etiology must be considered. Despite the abnormal electroencephalogram noted four years ago I would seriously question whether this is a convulsive disorder."

February 1972: "An electroencephalogram was obtained on P. on Jan. 25, 1972 . . . this tracing was only mildly abnormal and was significantly improved when compared to the prior electrical tracing of 1968."

September 1972: "From September 10th until September 13, 1972, P. has presented with daily episodes and as previously noted, these would always awaken him from his sleep. Although they are characterized as being right eye pain, in reality this is a sensation of subjective vertigo which is localized primarily to the right eye, but can also be found on the left side as well, and this is associated with headache. During the episode the child is unable to lie supine or stand and can only

---

[1]This child was referred to the author in 1974 for evaluation of his learning disabilities. And upon neurophysiological evaluation was found to have all the signs and symptoms characterizing DDD—including a significant reading disorder. An ENG performed at Lenox Hill Hospital revealed "direction fixed, positional nystagmus, reduced vestibular response—right, during bilateral bithermal caloric stimulation." In other words, the ENG showed evidence of an inner-ear dysfunction. Also, this child's graphomotor incoordination is consistent with Dr. Gold's diagnosis of a "cerebellar deficit."

walk with his head flexed forward. It is of note that the previously prescribed Dilantin was discontinued over three years ago. Antivert (meclizine), one half of a tablet three times a day was prescribed on September 12th, and as noted no further episodes were experienced after September 13, 1972."

"Gait patterns were normal for regular, heel and toe walking, but *there continued to be a mild impairment of tandem gait patterns* . . . It is apparent that this is not a migraine headache but the *entire clinical picture would be most consistent with either a benign paroxysmal vertigo or intermittent vestibular neuronitis.*"

November 1972: "Ancillary studies were obtained on P. . . . the electroencephalogram . . . noted . . . this was mildly and nonspecifically abnormal which in itself would not be indicative of a convulsive disorder. I am also enclosing a copy of correspondence from Dr. M. S., as well as the results of the vestibular function studies and audiological evaluation. I do believe that his comments are self explanatory and certainly the *findings would be consistent with benign paroxysmal vertigo.* For this reason it is suggested that if spells should occur Antivert should be prescribed on a PRN [when needed] basis."

October 1972 (Correspondence from Dr. M. S.): "As you will see, the *two vestibular labrynths are symmetrical with cold water but asymmetrical with hot water. This finding is consistent with the diagnosis of benign paroxysmal vertigo.* His hearing test remains completely normal.

Learning-Disability Cases
Examined by Dr. Sidney Carter

S.W. is a 9-year-old boy "who demonstrated trouble in hopping on either foot, impaired succession movements in both upper extremities."

G.A. is an 8-year-old boy: "Coordination is somewhat impaired. He is still having difficulty learning to ride a two wheeler, and he has trouble tying his shoelaces . . . There was some speech impairment. He had difficulty hopping on either foot."

S.L. is an 8-year-old boy: "His attention span is short, and he has difficulty in coordination with his small muscles. For example: at age eight, he cannot tie his shoelaces and has trouble with small puzzles . . . His clumsiness was evident in his hopping, but the remainder of the examination was unremarkable."

K.E. is an 11-year-old boy: "I had occasion to see K. . . . because of a history of having difficulty in school despite what is considered to be a very high IQ . . . I would emphasize a few minor facts in the history: specifically, K. has always been clumsy but despite that, is good at sports. He had right-left confusion as a smaller child, but this corrected itself . . .

"The positive findings were very minimal. *There was a very slight unsteadiness on finger-to-nose testing, particularly on the left and he had a very minimal impairment of succession movements—at the left more than the right. Quite honestly, I was not particularly impressed with his degree of cerebellar dysfunction. The remainder of his neurological examination was entirely normal.* His drawings were well done.

"It was my impression [based on history] that this boy could be classified as having minimal brain dysfunction, manifested in his case by behavioral difficulties and clumsiness and awkwardness."

D.L. is a six-year-old girl: "I saw little D. because of the complaints from the parents indicating that the child was said to have impaired visual perceptual function and to have right-left confusion . . . At four years of age an optometrist suggested that she might be having visual perceptual difficulties . . . Some right-left confusion was noted when she was in kindergarten, but this is of no real significance.

"The family and past histories are of significance in that the father is a physician and the mother is an ex-speech therapist . . . The examination proper was entirely within normal limits. It was my impression that this was a normal child."

Summary

In many ways, Dr. Gold's and Carter's "blind" cerebellar-dyslexia or LD data is the most important content within this work.[1] As a result, its print size and spacing are larger than they were in *A Solution to the Riddle—Dyslexia* (Appendix B) so as to facilitate its readability.

Ironically, this very same "blindly" reported data and its analysis not only solved the neurophysiological and medical diagnostic/therapeutic riddles characterizing dyslexia, LD, ADD or ADHD, etc., it also solved the psychological riddles preventing eminent scientists from advancing their research efforts for the past 100 years. In other words, the neurophysiological and psychological analysis of this content as well as its denial by all leading traditionalists provided the inspiration and insights characterizing *A Scientific Watergate—Dyslexia*. As a result, this crucial content provides a fitting ending to this book and a new beginning for other unbiased scientific works to follow.

---

[1] Upon rereading Dr. Gold's excellent neurological abstracts, you will find clear evidence that he considers impaired muscle tone, balance, and gross and fine motor coordination (graphomotor, ocular, oral or tongue, etc.) to be diagnostic of a cerebellar deficit. As a result, Dr. Carter's evidence of dyscoordination and clumsiness in his LD cases is consistent with that of Dr. Gold's. Most important, all cases are characterized by a complete absence of localizing cerebral neurological signs—despite the often-noted diagnosis of minimal cerebral dysfunction or brain damage.

In retrospect, it is readily apparent that Drs. Gold and Carter: (1) equate dyslexia with "dyslexia," and (2) via a circular logic, use balance/coordination or cerebellar signs to diagnose minimal cerebral dysfunction.

Bibliography

Bibliography

Adrian, E. D. 1943. Afferent areas in the cerebellum connected with the limbs. *Brain*, 66, 289-315.

Allington, Richard. 1981. Dyslexia has little to do with reading: A riddler's solution. *The Review of Education* 7 (2): 153-158.

Ayres, A. J. 1972. *Sensory integration and learning disorders.* Los Angeles: Western Psychological Services, 1972.

Barany, R. 1916. Some new methods for functional testing of the vestibular apparatus and cerebellum. In *Nobel Lectures, Physiology and Medicine, 1901-1921.* Amsterdam: Elsevier, 1967, 500-511.

Blythe, P., and McGlown, D. J. 1979. *An organic basis for neuroses and educational difficulties.* Chester, Eng.: Insight Publ., 1979.

Boniver, R. 1974. Influence du Piracetam sur le fonctionnement du systeme vestibulaire. *Acta Oto-Rhino-Laryngologica Belgica* 28: 293-299.

Brain, R. 1955. *Diseases of the nervous system.* London: Oxford University Press, 1955.

Broad, W., and Wade, N. 1982. *Betrayers of the Truth: Fraud and Deceit in the Halls of Science.* New York: Simon & Schuster, 1982.

Brody, J., 1974. Two doctors offer dyslexia theory: Faulty link is suspected between brain and ear. *New York Times*, April 29, 1974: 20.

Carter, S. and Gold, A. 1972. The syndrome of minimal cerebral dysfunction. In Barnett, M. H. and Einhorn, A. (eds.) *Pediatrics.* New York: Appleton-Century-Crofts, 1972.

Critchley, M. 1969. *The Dyslexic Child.* Springfield, IL: Thomas, 1969.

Delacato, C. H. 1959. *Treatment and Prevention of Reading Problems: (Neuro-psychological Approach).* Springfield, IL.: Thomas, 1959.

Denckla, M. B. 1991. Brain behavior insights through imaging. Paper presented at the Learning Disabilities Association National Conference, Chicago, IL, February 25, 1991.

_____. 1992. A neurologist's overview. Presented at The New York Academy of Sciences and The Rodin Remediation Academy, The XX Rodin Remediation Conference: Temporal Information Processing in the Nervous System: Special Reference to Dyslexia and Dysphasia, New York, NY, September 12-15. 1992.

De Quiros, J. B., and Schrager, O. L. 1979. *Neuropsychological-fundamentals in Learning Disabilities*. Novato, CA: Academic Therapy, 1979.

_____. 1976. Diagnosis of vestibular disorders in the learning disabled. *Journal of Learning Disabilities* 9: 39-58.

Dow, R. S., and Moruzzi, G. 1958. *The Physiology and Pathology of the Cerebellum*. Minneapolis, MN: University of Minnesota Press, 1958.

The Dyslexia Dilemma. *Harper's Bazaar*, November 1988: 212, 243.

Dyslexia: Does this unusual childhood syndrome begin as an ear infection? *Infectious Diseases* 4(7) July 1974: 15.

Eccles, J. C. 1973. The cerebellum as a computer: Patterns in space and time. *Journal of Physiology*. 229: 1-32.

_____. 1986. Learning in the motor system. *Progress in Brain Research* 64: 3-17.

Eccles, J. C., Ito, M., and Szentagothai, J. 1967. *The Cerebellum as a Neuronal Machine*. New York: Springer-Verlag, 1967.

Ente, Gerald, M.D. 1982. Ask the Doctor, Nassau County, NY Chapter of the Association for Children with Learning Disabilities *Newsletter* 1: 1 (Dec. 1982 - Jan. 1983): 4.

Fagan, J., Kaplan, B., Raymond, J., and Edington, E. S. 1988. The failure of antimotion-sickness medication to improve reading in developmental dyslexia: results of a randomized trial. *Journal of Developmental and Behavioral Pediatrics*. 96: 359-366.

Fawcett, A. J., and Nicolson, R. I. 1992 Automatisation deficits in balance for dyslexic children. *Perceptual and Motor Skills* 75: 507-529.

Fernandes, C. M., and Samuel, J. 1985. The use of Piracetam in vertigo. *South African Medical Journal* 68: 806-808.

Frank, J., and Levinson, H. N. 1973. Dysmetric dyslexia and dyspraxia: hypothesis and study. *Journal of American Academy of Child Psychiatry* 12: 690-701.

_____. 1975-1976. Dysmetric dyslexia and dyspraxia: synopsis of a continuing research project. *Academic Therapy* 11: 133-143.

_____. 1976. Compensatory mechanisms in cerebellar-vestibular dysfunction, dysmetric dyslexia and dyspraxia. *Academic Therapy* 12: 5-27.

_____. 1976-1977. Seasickness mechanisms and medications in dysmetric dyslexia and dyspraxia. *Academic Therapy* 12: 133-149.

_____. 1977. Antimotion-sickness medications in dysmetric dyslexia and dyspraxia. *Academic Therapy* 12: 411-425.

Furman, J. 1992. The Speech Thing. *The New Republic*, August 17 1992: 14-15.

Galaburda, A. M. 1992. Neuropathological evidence for elective affliction of the magnocellular visual subsystem. Presented at The New York Academy of Sciences and The Rodin Remediation Academy, The XX Rodin Remediation Conference: Temporal Information Processing in the Nervous System: Special Reference to Dyslexia and Dysphasia, New York, NY, September 12-15. 1992.

Galaburda, A., and Kemper, T. 1979. Cytoarchitectonic abnormalities in developmental dyslexia: a case study. *Annals of Neurology* 6: 94-100.

Galaburda, A., Sherman, G. F., Rosen, G.D., Aboitiz, F. and Geschwind, N. 1985. Developmental dyslexia: four consecutive patients with cortical anomalies. *Annals of Neurology* 18: 222-223.

Geiger, G., and Lettvin, J. Y. 1987. Peripheral vision in persons with dyslexia. *New England Journal of Medicine* 316: 1238-1243.

Geschwind, N. 1986. Dyslexia, cerebral dominance, autoimmunity, and sex hormones. In G. Pavlidis and D. Fisher (Eds.), *Dyslexia, Its Neuropsychology and Treatment*. New York: Wiley, 1986: 51-63.

_____. 1982. Why Orton was right. *Annals of Dyslexia* 32: 13-30.

Geschwind, N., and Behan, P. 1982. Left-handedness: association with immune disease, migraine, and developmental learning disorder. *Proceedings of the National Academy of Sciences of the USA*, 1982: 5097-5100.

Halliwell, J. W., and Sloan, H. A. 1972. The effects of a supplemental perceptual training program on reading achievement. *Exceptional Children* 38: 613-619.

Helfgott, E., Rudel, R. G., and Kairam, R. 1986. The effect of Piracetam on short- and long-term verbal retrieval in dyslexic boys. *International Journal of Psychophysiology* 4: 53-61.

Huston, A. M. 1987. *Common Sense About Dyslexia.* Lanham, MD: Madison Books, 1987.

Ito, M. 1984. *The Cerebellum and Neural Control.* New York: Raven Press, 1984.

Ivry, R. 1992. Cortical and cerebellar involvement in processing temporal information. Presented at The New York Academy of Sciences and The Rodin Remediation Academy, The XX Rodin Remediation Conference: Temporal Information Processing in the Nervous System: Special Reference to Dyslexia and Dysphasia, New York, NY, September 12-15, 1992.

Jordan, D. R. 1992. *Attention Deficit Disorder: ADHD and ADD Syndromes.* second edition. Austin, Texas: Pro-Ed, 1992, 5.

Kerr, J. 1897. School hygiene in its mental, moral, and physical aspects. *Journal of the Royal Statistical Society* 60: 613-680.

Koestler, A. 1968. *The Ghost in the Machine.* New York: Macmillan, 1968, 164.

Kohen-Raz, R. 1986. *Learning Disabilities and Postural Control.* London: Freund, 1986.

Kohl, R. L., Calkins, D. S., and Mandell, A. J. 1986. Arousal and stability: the effects of five new sympathomimetic drugs suggest a new principle for the prevention of space motion sickness. *Aviation, Space, and Environmental Medicine* 57: 137-143.

Kolata, G. 1992. Study reports dyslexia is not unalterable, as experts have been assuming. *New York Times*, January 16, 1992, A18.

_____ . 1990. Studies dispute view of dyslexia, finding girls as afflicted as boys. *New York Times*, August 22, 1990, A1, B6.

Leiner, H. C., Leiner, A., and Dow, R. S. 1986. Does the cerebellum contribute to mental skills? *Behavioral Neuroscience* 100: 443-454.

_____ . 1991. The human cerebro-cerebellar system: Its computing, cognitive, and language skills. *Behavioral Brain Research* 44: 113-128.

Lenzi, P., and Milanesi, I. 1969. Étude clinique d'un nouvel antivertigineux: la 2-pyrrolidone acetamide. *Clinica Otorinolaringologa dell'Universita de Milano* 24: 513-521.

Levinson, H. N. 1980. *A Solution to the Riddle—Dyslexia.* New York: Springer-Verlag, 1980.

_____ . 1989. Comment on Richard Allington's review of *A Solution to the Riddle—Dyslexia,* (*The Review of Education* 7[2]: 153-158), *The Review of Education* 7[2]: 235-244.

_____ . 1984. *Smart But Feeling Dumb.* New York: Warner, 1984. Revised Edition, 1994.

Levinson, H. N. with Steven Carter. 1986. *Phobia Free.* New York: Evans, 1986.

_____ . 1990. *Total Concentration.* New York: Evans, 1990.

Levinson, H. N. with Addie Sanders. 1991. *The Upside-Down Kids.* New York: Evans, 1991.

_____ . 1992. *Turning Around—The Upside-Down Kids* New York: Evans, 1992.

_____ . The cerebellar-vestibular basis of learning disabilities in children, adolescents and adults: hypothesis and study. *Perceptual and Motor Skills* 67: 983-1006.

_____ . 1989. Abnormal optokinetic and perceptual span parameters in cerebellar-vestibular dysfunction and learning disabilities or dyslexia. *Perceptual and Motor Skills* 68: 35-54.

_____ . 1989. Abnormal optokinetic and perceptual span parameters in cerebellar-vestibular dysfunction and related anxiety disorders. *Perceptual and Motor Skills* 68: 471-484.

_____ . 1989. A cerebellar-vestibular explanation for fears/phobias. *Perceptual and Motor Skills* 68: 67-84.

————. 1989. The cerebellar-vestibular predisposition to anxiety disorders. *Perceptual and Motor Skills* 68: 323-338.

————. 1990. The diagnostic value of cerebellar-vestibular tests in detecting learning disabilities, dyslexia, and attention deficit disorder. *Perceptual and Motor Skills* 71: 67-82.

————. The use and efficacy of the antimotion-sickness medications in the treatment of learning disabilities or dyslexia. (Submitted for publication)

————. 1991. Dramatic favorable responses of children with learning disabilities or dyslexia and attention deficit disorder to antimotion-sickness medications: four case reports. *Perceptual and Motor Skills* 73: 723-738.

Livingstone, M. 1992. Parallel processing of form, color, motion, and depth: anatomy, physiology, art and illusion. Presented at The New York Academy of Sciences and The Rodin Remediation Academy, The XX Rodin Remediation Conference: Temporal Information Processing in the Nervous System: Special Reference to Dyslexia and Dysphasia, New York, NY, September 12-15. 1992.

Livingstone, M. S., Rosen, G. D., Drislane, F. W., and Galaburda, A. M. 1991. Physiological and anatomical evidence for a magnocellular defect in developmental dyslexia. *Proceedings of the National Academy of Sciences of the USA* 88: 7943-7947.

Llinas, R. R. 1992. Cerebellar involvement in temporal sensory-motor processing: relevance for speech, reading and writing. Presented at The New York Academy of Sciences and The Rodin Remediation Academy, The XX Rodin Remediation Conference: Temporal Information Processing in the Nervous System: Special Reference to Dyslexia and Dysphasia, New York, NY, September 12-15. 1992.

Llinas, R. 1975. The cortex of the cerebellum. *Scientific American.* 232: 56-71.

Masland, R. L. 1985. Review of *Smart But Feeling Dumb.* Reprinted from the New York Branch of the *Orton Dyslexia Society Newsletter.* 8 (3) February 1985.

Masland, R. L., and Upsrich, C. 1985. Review of *A Solution to the Riddle—Dyslexia. Bulletin of the Orton Society.* February 1985, 8(3): 256-261.

Morgan, W. P. 1896. A case of congenital word blindness. *British Medical Journal* 2: 1378.

Murphy, J. M. 1981. Review of *A Solution to the Riddle—Dyslexia*, Understanding dyslexia: a story of scientific detection. *International Schools Journal* 1: 83-91.

Oosterveld, W. J. 1980. The efficacy of piracetam in vertigo. *Arzneimedizinische-Forschung* 30: 1947-1949.

Orton, S. P. 1937. *Reading, Writing and Speech Problems in Children*. New York: W. W. Norton, 1937.

———. 1942. Discussion of a Paper by Dr. J. G. Lynn, *Archives of Neurology and Psychiatry* 47: 1064.

Polatajko, H. J. 1985. A critical look at vestibular dysfunction in learning-disabled children. *Developmental Medicine and Child Neurology*. 27: 283-292.

Previc, F. H. 1991. A general theory concerning the prenatal origins of cerebral lateralization in humans. *Psychological Review* 98: 299-334.

Raymond, J. E., Ogden, N. A., Fagan, J. E., and Kaplan, B. J. 1988. Fixational instability and saccadic eye movements. *American Journal of Optometry and Physiological Optics* 65: 174-181.

Sekitani, T., McCabe, B. F., and Ryu, J. H. 1971. Drug effects on the medial vestibular nucleus. *Archives of Otolaryngology* 93: 581-589.

Shaywitz, S. E., Shaywitz, B. A., Fletcher, J. M., and Escobar, M.D. 1990. Prevalence of reading ability in boys and girls: results of the Connecticut longitudinal study, *Journal of the American Medical Association* 264: 998-1002.

Shaywitz, S. E., Escobar, M. A., Shaywitz, B. A., Fletcher, J. M., and Makuch, R. 1992. Evidence that dyslexia may represent the lower tail of a normal distribution of reading ability. *New England Journal of Medicine* 326 (3): 145-150.

Silva, P., Kirkland, C., Simpson, A., Stewart, I., and Williams, S. 1982. Some developmental and behavioral problems associated with bilateral otitis media with effusion. *Journal of Learning Disabilities* 15: 417-421.

Silver, L. B. 1984. *The Misunderstood Child: A Guide for Parents of Learning Disabled Children*. New York: Tab Books, 1984; second edition, 1991.

Silver, L. B. 1987. The "magic cure": A review of the current controversial approaches for treating learning disabilities. *Journal of Learning Disabilities* 20: 498-505.

Snider, R. 1958. The Cerebellum. *Scientific American* 174: 84-90.

Snider, R. S., and Stowell, A. 1944. Receiving areas of the tactile, auditory and visual systems in the cerebellum. *Journal of Neurophysiology* 7: 331-357.

Tallal, P. 1992. Neural basis of temporal perceptual motor processing: implications for speech and reading. Presented at The New York Academy of Sciences and The Rodin Remediation Academy, The XX Rodin Remediation Conference: Temporal Information Processing in the Nervous System: Special Reference to Dyslexia and Dysphasia, New York, NY, September 12-15. 1992.

Vail, P. 1982. Review of *A Solution to the Riddle—Dyslexia, Independent School*, February 19, 1982.

Wilsher, C. R., Bennet, D., Chase, C., Connors, K., DiIanni, M., Feagans, L., Hanvik, L. J., Helfgott, E., Koplewica, H., Overby, P., Reader, M. J., Rudel, R. G., and Tallal, P. 1987. Piracetam and dyslexia: effects on reading tests. *Journal of Clinical Psychopharmacology* 7: 230-235.

Wiss, T. 1989. Vestibular dysfunction in learning disabilities: Differences in definitions lead to different conclusions, *Journal of Learning Disabilities* 22 (2): 100-101.

Wolff, P. H. 1992. Impaired motor timing control in developmental dyslexia. Presented at The New York Academy of Sciences and The Rodin Remediation Academy, The XX Rodin Remediation Conference: Temporal Information Processing in the Nervous System: Special Reference to Dyslexia and Dysphasia, New York, NY, September 12-15. 1992.

Wood, C. D., Cramer, B., and Graybiel, A. 1988. Antimotion-sickness drug efficacy. *Otolaryngology, Head and Neck Surgery* 89: 1041-1044.

Wood, C. D., and Graybiel, A. 1970. A theory of motion sickness based on pharmachological reactions. *Clinical Pharmacology and Therapeutics* 11: 621-624.

Zinkus, P., Gottlieb, M. I., and Shapiro, M. 1978. Developmental and psychoeducational sequelae of chronic otitis media. *American Journal of the Disabled Child* 132: 1100-1104.

Index

Index

Emphasizing Major Themes

IF any of those who doubt your program would like to test me or hear from me, I would be happy to do so. I refer here to other "professionals" in the many fields who regard dyslexia as their province. Perhaps, as I experience such vast differences of perception when not taking the medication as opposed to when I do take it, I may be of some interest to them. It occurs to me, however, that they would rather study someone whose symptoms coincide with their theories and treatment.

Nonetheless, I continue to marvel at the improvement Christopher continues to enjoy. Many, many thanks.

—Joan Sparks [Chapter 10, p. 228]

(OPPOSITE)
VISUAL DISTORTION IN DYSLEXIA.
DESIGNED BY LISA ORANGE.

If any of those who doubt your programs would like to test
other "professionals" in the many fields who regard dyslexia
perception when not taking the medication as opposed to who

Sincerely,

Joan Sparks

province. Perhaps, as I exper

Nonetheless, I continue to

and treatment.

Nonetheless, I continue to marve

Joan Sparks

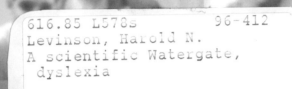

DATE DUE

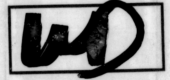

**This item is Due on
or before Date shown.**